Osteoarthritis: Biological Aspects

Osteoarthritis: Biological Aspects

Edited by **Sharlton Pierce**

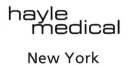

New York

Published by Hayle Medical,
30 West, 37th Street, Suite 612,
New York, NY 10018, USA
www.haylemedical.com

Osteoarthritis: Biological Aspects
Edited by Sharlton Pierce

© 2015 Hayle Medical

International Standard Book Number: 978-1-63241-309-3 (Hardback)

Contents

Preface

Osteoarthritis is described as an abnormality of joints, but the severity does not certainly produce pain. The book elucidates the nature of the most common form of arthritis in humans. The sections focus on metabolic and cellular aspects of Osteoarthritis. If osteoarthritis is certain, it is extremely important to facilitate its diagnosis, prevention, indications and options for treatment. Development in comprehending this disease has taken place with recognition that it is not simply a degenerative joint disease. Causative factors, like ligamentous abnormalities, malalignment, overuse, and biomechanical and metabolic factors have been identified as responsible for intervention. The diagnosis of this disease is based on recognition of overdevelopment of bone at joint margins.

This book is a comprehensive compilation of works of different researchers from varied parts of the world. It includes valuable experiences of the researchers with the sole objective of providing the readers (learners) with a proper knowledge of the concerned field. This book will be beneficial in evoking inspiration and enhancing the knowledge of the interested readers.

In the end, I would like to extend my heartiest thanks to the authors who worked with great determination on their chapters. I also appreciate the publisher's support in the course of the book. I would also like to deeply acknowledge my family who stood by me as a source of inspiration during the project.

Editor

Part 1

Metabolic

Proteases and Cartilage Degradation in Osteoarthritis

Judith Farley, Valeria M. Dejica and John S. Mort

Genetics Unit, Shriners Hospital for Children and Department of Surgery,
McGill University
Canada

1. Introduction

Osteoarthritis, the most common joint disease, affecting millions people world-wide, involves the degradation of the articular cartilage which provides frictionless contact between the bones in a joint during movement. To a first approximation, this tissue is composed of two components, a collagen framework and entrapped proteoglycans. The framework consists of type II collagen fibrils built on a type XI collagen core, and decorated with type IX collagen molecules and small proteoglycans. These composite fibrils give the tissue its integrity, tensile strength and ability to retain large proteoglycan aggregates. The extremely large size of the proteoglycan aggregates and their high negative charge endows them with an immense hydration capacity, giving cartilage the ability to absorb compressive loading by the slow displacement of bound water. Partial destruction or loss of the proteoglycans is the first step in the deterioration of cartilage as seen in arthritis. Subsequently, irreversible loss of collagen occurs leading to permanent cartilage degeneration. While glycosylhydrolases and free radicals could also participate, it is believed that proteolytic enzymes are the main agents responsible for the degradation of cartilage components in osteoarthritis. Currently two classes of proteases are thought to be the major mediators of collagen and proteoglycan cleavage. Collagen degradation was thought to be majorly due to the action of MMP (matrix metalloproteinase) collagenases while members of both MMP and ADAMTS (a disintegrin and metalloproteinase with thrombospondin motifs) families are important mediators of the degradation of proteoglycans which due to their extended core protein conformation are susceptible to the action of many proteases (Mort and Billington, 2001). Recently however, there is increasing evidence for the role of the cysteine protease cathepsin K in collagen degradation in articular cartilage (Konttinen et al., 2002).

The cleavage of cartilage proteins often occurs at specific sites on these molecules depending on the particular protease mediating the event. This results in the generation of characteristic N- and C-terminal epitopes that can be used for the production of antibodies specific for these cleavage products (anti-neoepitope antibodies) (Mort et al., 2003). A series of such antibodies has been produced and their specificities validated. These allow evaluation of the roles of different proteases in the degradation of collagen and proteoglycans in mouse models of osteoarthritis and in human and equine osteoarthritic cartilage using immunohistochemical methods and immunoassays.

2. Matrix metalloproteinases

Matrix metalloproteinases (MMPs) are a family of functionally and structurally related zinc endopeptidases that cleave proteins of the extracellular matrix, including collagens, elastin, matrix glycoproteins and proteoglycans (Martel-Pelletier et al., 2001) and are considered to be responsible for much of the degeneration of articular cartilage.

Most MMPs are composed of three distinct domains: an amino-terminal propeptide involved in the maintenance of enzyme latency; a catalytic domain that binds zinc and calcium ions and a hemopexin-like domain that is located at the carboxy terminal zone of the protease and that plays a role in substrate binding (Nagase, 1997). All MMPs are synthesized as preproenzymes and most of them are either secreted from the cell or bound to the plasma membrane in an inactive or proenzyme state. Several proteolytic cleavages are required to activate them and are critical steps leading to extracellular matrix breakdown (Nagase, 1997). Most of the MMPs are optimally active at neutral pH (Martel-Pelletier et al., 2001).

The human genome codes for 24 MMPs which can be classified depending on which components of the cartilage matrix they degrade (Birkedal-Hansen et al., 1993; Lee and Murphy, 2004). The MMPs that are the most important in cartilage extracellular matrix degradation are the collagenases (MMP-1, -8 and -13), the stromelysins (MMP-3, -10 and -11) the gelatinases (MMP-2 and –9), matrilysin (MMP-7) and the membrane type MMPs, in particular MMP-14 which can also act as a collagenase (Nagase and Woessner, 1999).

2.1 Collagenases

Matrix metalloproteinases with collagenolytic abilities are termed collagenases. These proteases mediate the initial cleavage of the collagen triple helix, occurring at three quarters of the distance from the amino-terminal end of each chain, forming collagen fragments of three-quarter and one-quarter length (Harris and Krane, 1974) (Fig.1). This site is susceptible to cleavage due to a reduced proline and hydroxyproline content which results in lowering of the stability of the triple helix. The collagenases are able to unwind this region of the triple helix and cleave all three collagen strands (Chung et al., 2004). This initial cleavage allows other MMPs to further degrade these unwound collagen molecules (Burrage et al., 2006). There are 3 collagenases: collagenase-1 or interstitial collagenase (MMP-1); collagenase-2 or neutrophil collagenase (MMP-8); and collagenase-3 (MMP-13). In addition, MMP-2 and MMP-14 also have the ability to cleave triple helical collagen.

2.1.1 Collagenase-1 (MMP-1)

Collagenase-1, which is primarily produced by synoviocytes (Wassilew et al., 2010), has been found in increased concentration in synovial fluid of patients suffering from joint injuries and osteoarthritis (Tchetverikov et al., 2005). It can also degrade aggrecan and different types of collagen: type I, II, III, VII, X, IX and denatured type II (Martel-Pelletier et al., 2001; Poole et al., 2001). This collagenase preferentially degrades type III collagen and its expression is mainly found in the superficial zone of articular cartilage in well-established osteoarthritis (Freemont et al., 1997). Even though its affinity towards type II collagen is lower than for collagenase-3, it is found in higher concentration in osteoarthritic joints (Vincenti and Brinckerhoff, 2001). *In vitro* studies showed that human chondrocytes can produce significantly more collagenase-1 than collagenase-3 following stimulation with proinflammatory cytokines, namely TNF-α and IL-1 (Yoshida et al., 2005).

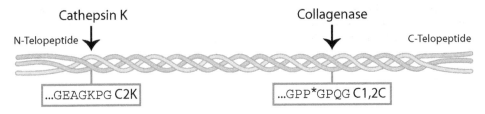

Fig. 1. Cleavage sites on type II collagen.
The type II collagen triple helix and non-helical telopeptides are indicated schematically. In reality there are many more turns in the triple helix. The ¾ / ¼ cleavage site for collagenases and the cleavage site for cathepsin K towards the N-terminus (Kafienah et al., 1998) are indicated along with the peptide sequences used to produce anti-neoepitope antibodies for the cleavage products. Asterisk indicates modification of proline to hydroxyproline.

2.1.2 Collagenase-2 (MMP-8)

Collagenase-2, which is mainly the product of neutrophils, degrades type I collagen with high specificity, but also cleaves collagen type II, III, VIII, X, aggrecan and link protein (Poole, 2001). It has been shown that collagenase-2 protein and mRNA are also produced by normal human chondrocytes (Cole et al., 1996), though recent data show that mRNA expression is very minor in normal and osteoarthritic chondrocytes (Stremme et al., 2003). Collagenase-2 is able to cleave the aggrecan molecule at the aggrecanase-site, between Glu^{373}-Ala^{374}, but cleaves preferentially between Asn^{341}-Phe^{342}, the MMP-site (Fosang et al., 1994) (Fig. 2).

2.1.3 Collagenase-3 (MMP-13)

Collagenase-3 was first cloned from human breast carcinoma in 1994 (Freije et al., 1994). It is predominantly a product of chondrocytes (Reboul et al., 1996) and has been shown to be expressed in human osteoarthritic cartilage (Mitchell et al., 1996), subchondral bone and hyperplasic synovial membrane in an osteoarthritis mouse model (Salminen et al., 2002). This collagenase is mostly expressed by chondrocytes surrounding osteoarthritic lesions (Shlopov et al., 1997) and can be found in superficial (Wu et al., 2002) and deep layers of osteoarthritic cartilage (Freemont et al., 1999; Moldovan et al., 1997). Matrix metalloproteinase-13 expression is strongly induced by interleukin-1 (IL-1), an important proinflammatory cytokine encountered in osteoarthritis (Gebauer et al., 2005; Vincenti and Brinckerhoff, 2001). Collagenase-3 degrades type II collagen preferentially, but also cleaves collagens type I, III, VII and X, aggrecan and gelatins (Poole et al., 2001). *In vitro* studies have shown that MMP-13 can cleave type II collagen about 5 times faster than type I collagen and about 6 times faster than type III collagen (Knäuper et al., 1996). Because type II collagen is its preferred substrate and because it can cleave type II collagen a least 5 to10 times faster than collagenase-1, collagenase-3 is considered to be one of the most important MMPs in osteoarthritis (Mitchell et al., 1996). It is also the collagenase with the most efficient gelatinolytic activity (Knäuper et al., 1996).

Many different *in vivo* studies have shown the importance of MMP-13 in osteoarthritis. Administration of specific MMP-13 inhibitors to animal models of osteoarthritis has shown a significant reduction in the severity of the pathology (Baragi et al., 2009; Johnson et al., 2007; Settle et al., 2010). Its importance in osteoarthritis was demonstrated, in a transgenic mouse line expressing constitutively active human MMP-13 in hyaline cartilage where excessive MMP-13 expression resulted in articular cartilage degradation and joint pathology similar to osteoarthritis (Neuhold et al., 2001). Recently, MMP-13 knockout mice have been developed and surgical induction of osteoarthritis by destabilisation of the medial meniscus in these animals demonstrated that structural cartilage damage is dependent on MMP-13 activity (Little et al., 2009).

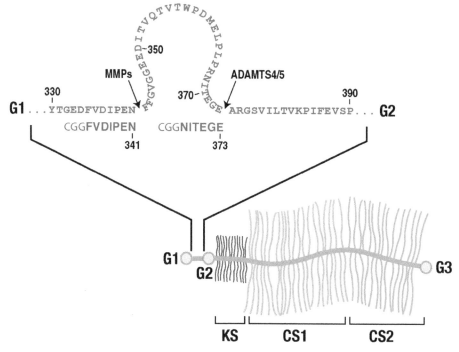

Fig. 2. Peptides used to generate anti-neoepitope antibodies to metalloproteinase cleavage products of aggrecan in the interglobular domain.
The domain structure of the aggrecan molecule is illustrated. The core protein (green) consists of two globular domains (G1 and G2) separated by an interglobular domain. A region rich in keratan sulfate (KS) follows along with two extended chondroitin sulfate rich regions (CS1 and CS2) which are substituted with glycosaminoglycan chains (blue). The CS1 region consists of a series of tandem repeats which can vary in number (Doege et al., 1997). The interglobular domain is susceptible to proteolytic attach. The sites of cleavage by MMPs and aggrecanases are indicated along with the sequences of peptides used to prepare anti-neoepitope antibodies which recognize the new C-termini of the G1-containing fragments that remain in the tissue following cleavage.

2.2 Gelatinases
Gelatinases are proteases that can further degrade denatured collagen, once the triple helix has been cleaved by collagenases. There are two gelatinases: gelatinase-A also termed 72 kDa or MMP-2 and gelatinase-B also termed 92 kDa or MMP-9.

2.2.1 Gelatinase-A (MMP-2)

Gelatinase-A degrades FACIT (fibril-associated collagens with interrupted triple helices) (Gordon and Hahn, 2010) collagens such as type IV collagen in the basement membrane and is a very efficient gelatinase degrading denatured fibrillar collagens and aggrecan (Poole, 2001). Gelatinase-A is mostly important in the completion of collagen degradation after specific cleavage of the triple helical region of fibrillar collagen molecules by collagenases (Nagase, 1997). This enzyme also cleaves the aggrecan molecule at the Asn^{341}-Phe^{342} site close to the G1 domain (Fosang et al., 1992) (Fig.2) and is mostly expressed in late stage osteoarthritis (Aigner et al., 2001).

It has been shown that in the horse, several joint cells, like chondrocytes and synovial fibroblasts, can produce gelatinase-A *in vitro* (Clegg et al., 1997a) and that the enzyme activity is increased in synovial fluid of joints of animals suffering from osteoarthritis (Clegg et al., 1997b). The activity of gelatinase-A was found to be increased in synovial fluid and synoviocytes of dogs with osteoarthritis, but was also detected in healthy joints (Volk et al., 2003). Recently, it has be shown that gelatinase-A deficiency in humans causes a disorder characterized by osteolysis and arthritis termed multicentric osteolysis with arthropathy, a disease that can be reproduced in gelatinase-A knockout mice (Mosig et al., 2007). Even if this enzyme seems to be implicated in the pathogenesis of osteoarthritis, it also plays a direct role in skeletal development.

2.2.2 Gelatinase-B (MMP-9)

Gelatinase-B has similar activities to MMP-2 but it can also act as an elastase. Though involved in collagen destruction, its collagenase action is at a very much lower level than that of gelatinase-A (Soder et al., 2006). Gelatinase-B can also cleave the aggrecan molecule at the same site as gelatinase-A, the Asn^{341}-Phe^{342} site (Fosang et al., 1992) (Fig. 2). This enzyme has been found in synovial fluid of humans (Koolwijk et al., 1995) and horses (Clegg et al., 1997b) with osteoarthritis, and its activity is increased in synovial fluid and synoviocytes of dogs (Volk et al., 2003) suffering from the same disease. Equine chondrocytes are also able of producing gelatinase-B *in vitro* (Clegg et al., 1997a).

2.3 Stromelysins

There are three stromelysins: stromelysin-1 or MMP-3, stromelysin-2 or MMP-10 and stromelysin-3 or MMP-11.

2.3.1 Stromelysin-1 (MMP-3)

Stromelysin-1 can degrade aggrecan, denatured collagens and interhelical collagen domains, as well as aggrecan and link protein. Importantly, stomelysin-1 can cleave the aggrecan molecule at the MMP site, at the Asn^{341}-Phe^{342} bond, to liberate the G1 domain from the remainder of the molecule (Flannery et al., 1992) (Fig.2). It has been shown that stromelysin-1 can activate the pro forms of collagenases and that this activation is a key step in cartilage degradation (Suzuki et al., 1990). In osteoarthritic cartilage, stromelysin-1 is localized in chondrocytes of the superficial and transition zone (Okada et al., 1992) and its strongest mRNA expression is found in early degenerative articular cartilage (Bau et al., 2002). In a rabbit model of surgically induced osteoarthritis, stromelysin-1 was found to be upregulated in the synovium initially, and in chondrocytes in the later phases of the disease (Mehraban et al., 1998), indicating that both cell types can produce stromelysin-1. It has been shown that in humans, the plasma level of stromelysin-1 was a significant predictor of joint space narrowing in knee osteoarthritis

(Lohmander et al., 2005). The concentration of this enzyme in human joint fluid can distinguish disease joints form healthy joints (Lohmander et al., 1993a). Another indication of the action of stromelysin-1 in the development of osteoarthritis is the significant decrease in severity of joint pathology in 2-year-old MMP-3 knockout mice (Blaney Davidson et al., 2007)

2.3.2 Stromelysins-2 and -3 (MMP-10 and MMP-11)

Stromelysin-2 has similar activities to MMP-3. This stromelysin can also activate procollagenases, and has been identified recently in synovial fluid and tissues from osteoarthritis patients, demonstrating the importance of this protease in articular cartilage degradation processes (Barksby et al., 2006).

Stromelysin-3 has been more implicated in general proteolysis, and shown to be up-regulated in osteoarthritic chondrocytes (Aigner et al., 2001). Unlike other MMPs, stromelysin-3 is activated intracellularly by the serine protease, furin, which processes many other proteins into their mature/active forms. MMP-11 is then secreted from cells in its active form (Pei and Weiss, 1995).

2.4 Other MMPs

Matrilysin (MMP-7), the smallest of the MMPs, lacking a hemopexin domain, is a protease that degrades aggrecan, gelatin, type IV collagen and link protein. Matrilysin cleaves the aggrecan molecule at the MMP-site (Fosang et al., 1992) and is mainly expressed in the superficial and transitional zones of osteoarthritic chondrocytes (Ohta et al., 1998). Matrilysin is the MMP with the highest specific activity against many extracellular matrix components (Murphy et al., 1991) and can also activate the zymogens of MMP-1 and MMP-9 (Imai et al., 1997).

There are six membrane-type matrix metalloproteinases (MT-MMPs) (Nagase and Woessner, 1999). Only MT1-MMP and MT3-MMP have been implicated in osteoarthritis (Burrage et al., 2006). The most important is MT1-MMP (MMP-14), expressed in human articular cartilage (Büttner et al., 1997) and synovial membrane. It degrades aggrecan, but also collagen type I, II, III and gelatin. It has been shown that MT1-MMP is highly expressed in osteoarthritic cartilage and could be responsible for the activation of progelatinase A in the extracellular matrix (Imai et al., 1995).

3. Aggrecanases

Aggrecanases are members of the 'A Disintegrin And Metalloproteinase with Thrombospondin motifs' (ADAMTS) family of proteins. Synthesized as inactive pre-proenzymes, the ADAMTSs have a catalytic domain containing a zinc binding motif with 3 histidine residues, HEXXHXXGX-XH, and a critical methionine residue located in a 'Met-turn' downstream of the third zinc-binding histidine (Kuno et al., 1997). The propeptide is removed by the action of the proprotein convertase proteases furin (Koo et al., 2007) or PACE-4 (Malfait et al., 2008). Currently there are 19 ADAMTS genes known in humans, numbered ADAMTS-1 to ADAMTS-20, the same gene product being described as ADAMTS-5 and ADAMTS-11 (Porter et al., 2005).

The degradation of aggrecan leads to articular cartilage softening and loss of fixed charges (Maroudas, 1976). Two major cleavage sites of the aggrecan molecule are situated in the IGD region of the core protein, allowing aggrecan molecules lacking the G1 domain to freely exit the cartilage matrix and so to no longer contribute to cartilage function (Sandy et al., 1991). The first cleavage site at the Asn^{341}-Phe^{342} bond, creating the neoepitope VDIPEN, was found to be generated by MMPs (Flannery et al., 1992; Fosang et al., 1991; Fosang et al., 1992). The second site at the Glu^{373}-Ala^{374} bond, creating the NITEGE neoepitope, was found to result from aggrecan cleavage by enzymes that were called aggrecanases (Sandy et al., 1991). There are 4 other aggrecanase cleavage sites situated in the GAG rich region (CS2) of aggrecan molecules between the globular domains G2 and G3 (Glu^{1545}-Gly^{1546}, Glu^{1714}-Gly^{1715}, Glu^{1819}-Ala^{1820}, and Glu^{1919}-Leu^{1920}, human sequences) (Tortorella et al., 2000) and a fifth cleavage site closer to the G3 domain that has been identified recently in bovine cartilage (Durigova et al., 2008). It was shown that aggrecan cleavage at the aggrecanase sites is responsible for cartilage degradation, *in vitro*, (Malfait et al., 2002; Tortorella et al., 2001) and, *in vivo*, ((Janusz et al., 2004), and that aggrecan neoepitopes generated by aggrecanases are found in synovial fluids of patients suffering from osteoarthritis (Lohmander et al., 1993b; Sandy et al., 1992). Moreover, it was also shown that contrary to MMP-inhibitors, aggrecanase inhibitors can block aggrecan degradation in human osteoarthritic cartilage (Malfait et al., 2002), demonstrating the importance of aggrecanases in cartilage matrix destruction.

The ongoing search for activities responsible for cartilage matrix degradation indicates that the ADAMTS family members are the most important aggrecanases. Of all of the ADAMTS enzymes, the phylogenetically closely related ADAMTS-1, -4, -5, -8, -9, -15 and -20 (Collins-Racie et al., 2004) are considered to be potential aggrecanases. All of the ADAMTS messenger RNAs except ADAMTS-7 were found to be present normal and/or osteoarthritic cartilage from hip or knee joints (Collins-Racie et al., 2004; Kevorkian et al., 2004; Naito et al., 2007). They have been shown to be able to cleave the aggrecan molecule at the Glu^{373}-Ala^{374} bond, except for ADAMTS-20 for which this cleavage site has not been tested to date (Collins-Racie et al., 2004; Rodríguez-Manzaneque et al., 2002; Somerville et al., 2003; Tortorella et al., 2000; Tortorella et al., 2002). The only 3 ADAMTSs that have been shown to be able to cleave aggrecan at the 4 aggrecanase sites located in the GAG rich region are ADAMTS-1, -4 and -5 (Rodríguez-Manzaneque et al., 2002; Tortorella et al., 2002), making them potent aggrecanases.

3.1 Aggrecanase-1 (ADAMTS-4)

Aggrecanase-1 has been well studied and evidence for its importance in aggrecan catabolism in cartilage is becoming stronger. ADAMTS-4 protein has been shown to be co-localized with aggrecan degradation products *in vitro* and *in vivo* (Naito et al., 2007). Selective inhibition of ADAMTS-4 and ADAMTS-5 has been shown to block the degradation of type II collagen by its protective effect on aggrecan molecules (Pratta et al., 2003). However, even if ADAMTS-4 has been shown to be able to cleave the aggrecan molecule *in vitro* (Tortorella et al., 2001), studies carried out with ADAMTS-4 knockout mice failed to show a protection against aggrecan loss after destabilizing knee surgery (Glasson et al., 2005). A similar study by Stanton et al. showed that, *in vitro*, ADAMTS-4 expression is not induced by IL-1α in mice suggesting that ADAMTS-4 may not be an important aggrecanase in osteoarthritis in mice (Stanton et al., 2005). However, in human osteoarthritis, ADAMTS-4 seems to play an important role in aggrecan degradation. In fact, this aggrecanase is induced in human cartilage, *in vitro*, by proinflammatory cytokines (Song et al., 2007), and is increased in osteoarthritic cartilage (Naito et al., 2007; Roach et al., 2005).

3.2 Aggrecanase-2 (ADAMTS-5)

ADAMTS-5 has also been well studied and its importance in aggrecan catabolism in cartilage has been shown. As mentioned for ADAMTS-4, selective inhibition of ADAMTS-

4 and ADAMTS-5 has been shown to have a protective effect on aggrecan molecules (Pratta et al., 2003). Studies carried out with ADAMTS-5 knockout and ADAMTS-4/-5 double knockout mice showed that these animals are more resistant to cartilage degradation after destabilizing knee surgery (Glasson et al., 2005; Majumdar et al., 2007; Stanton et al., 2005). In vitro, ADAMTS-5 expression is induced by IL-1α in mice, demonstrating its importance in osteoarthritis in that species (Stanton et al., 2005). ADAMTS-5 is also important in osteoarthritis in humans, its expression is high in human osteoarthritic cartilage and it is responsible for aggrecan degradation in normal and diseased cartilage (Bau et al., 2002; Plaas et al., 2007; Song et al., 2007). However, in the human, putative damaging polymorphisms in the ADAMTS-5 gene did not show any modification in susceptibility to osteoarthritis (Rodriguez-Lopez et al., 2008). The search for the most important aggrecanase in human osteoarthritis is still going strong (Fosang and Rogerson, 2010).

3.3 ADAMTS-1
ADAMTS-1 mRNA and protein are present in normal and OA cartilage (Kevorkian et al., 2004). This enzyme can cleave aggrecan at the Glu^{373}-Ala^{374} bond and at 4 additional aggrecanase sites between G2 and G3 (Rodríguez-Manzaneque et al., 2002). Concerning the expression of ADAMTS-1 in inflammatory conditions, ADAMTS-1 expression in articular chondrocytes is downregulated in vitro by human recombinant interleukin-1β (IL-1β) (Wachsmuth et al., 2004). An ADAMTS-1-KO mouse (Mittaz et al., 2004) showed that overall, ADAMTS-1 does not seem to be a key enzyme in normal and diseased cartilage, or in bone development and growth (Little et al., 2005).

4. Cathepsins

While the triple helical regions of the fibrillar collagens such as types I and II are resistant to the action of most proteases except the MMP collagenases (Nagase and Fushimi, 2008) which make an initial cleavage at the three quarter point, the cysteine protease, cathepsin K, is also able to degrade triple helical collagens (Garnero et al., 1998). Rather, this protease appears to erode the collagen fibrils from their termini, gradually reducing the chains to peptides with concomitant unwinding of the triple helix. Unlike the MMPs, cathepsins are single domain proteases which do not rely on additional modules to bind to their extracellular matrix substrates (Turk et al., 2001). However, the collagenolytic activity of cathepsin K is dependent on the presence of chondroitin 4-sulfate CS (Li et al., 2000) a major component of the aggrecan molecule which forms well-defined complexes with the enzyme (Cherney et al., 2011). While it was originally assumed that cathepsin K is unique to the osteoclast (and this cell does indeed contain huge amounts of the protease), many other cell types are now known to produce the enzyme (Anway et al., 2004; Sukhova et al., 1998). Its increasing abundance in chondrocytes close to the articular surface (Konttinen et al., 2002) suggests that its action may contribute to cartilage fibrillation seen with aging and joint disease.

5. Anti-neoepitope antibodies

The anti-cleavage site (anti-neoepitope) antibody approach has proven very productive as a means of detecting specific cleavage products in the extracellular matrix, thus demonstrating the action of one or a particular group of proteases (Mort et al., 2003; Mort and Buttle, 1999). In addition, since these cleavage products can accumulate in body fluids – synovial fluid, blood or urine – their quantitation can represent a measure of disease activity.

Our work has centered on aggrecan fragments generated by the action of MMPs and aggrecanases (ADAMTS family members, particularly ADAMTS-4 and -5) (Hughes et al., 1995; Sztrolovics et al., 2002) (Fig. 2) and on collagen cleavage epitopes generated by the action of collagenases (Billinghurst et al., 1997; Lee et al., 2009; Song et al., 1999) as well as the degradation of collagen in cartilage by cathepsin K (Dejica et al., 2008; Vinardell et al., 2009) (Fig. 1).

6. Immunohistochemical demonstration of protease action in cartilage

Anti-neoepitope antibodies can be used to demonstrate the effects of increased MMP activities in articular cartilage. This is illustrated in sections of joints of mice lacking the endogenous MMP inhibitor, tissue inhibitor of metalloproteinases-3 (TIMP-3). *Timp3-/-* mice are phenotypically normal, although old animals show some lung pathology (Leco et al., 2001) (Fig.3). However, detailed examination of the articular cartilage of adult animals demonstrates a decrease in glycosaminoglycan content (weaker Safranin O staining) and damage to the articular surface. Compared to wild type animals, there is a dramatic increase in the staining of the articular cartilage with an anti-VDIPEN antibody (Lee et al., 1998) which recognizes the G1 domain of aggrecan that remain located in the tissue following cleavage by MMPs. Although the aggrecanase cleavage site in mouse aggrecan generates the G1 terminating in the sequence …NVTEGE rather than …NITEGE, the antibody raised to the human epitope is fully functional with the mouse epitope and can be used to investigate the role of aggrecanases in cartilage degeneration in animal models of arthritis (van Lent et al., 2008).

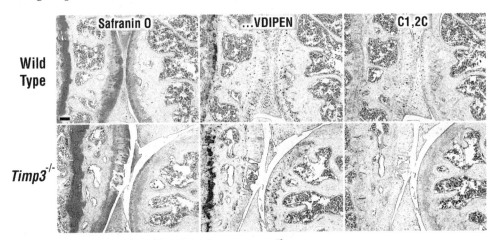

Fig. 3. Effect of increased MMP activity in mouse cartilage.
Hind joint sections of wild type and *Timp3-/-* 1-year-old FVB mice. Paraffin embedded samples were stained with Safranin O and Fast Green which identifies areas of fixed negative charge, or incubated with rabbit antibodies to either VDIPEN or the collagen epitope C1,2C, followed by a secondary horse radish peroxidase coupled system. Intense staining of the growth plate is visible on the left of the sections for glycosaminoglycans (Safranin O) and for the VDIPEN epitope indicating normal turnover of aggrecan. The magnification bar represents 100 μm.

Staining for the cleavage product for type II collagen by collagenases (the C1,2C epitope, Fig. 1) was also increased in the joints from *Timp3-/-* animals (Fig. 3) illustrating the broad inhibitory potential of TIMP-3.

Recently we have generated an antibody which is able to recognize and quantitate a cleavage product of type II collagen generated on the cleavage of the triple helical region by the action of cathepsin K (Dejica et al., 2008). Immunohistochemical studies demonstrated regions of cartilage reflecting cathepsin K activity (Fig. 4). Staining was dramatically increased in cartilage taken from osteoarthritis patients compared to that obtained from individuals with macroscopically normal tissue. The cleavage products are localized towards the articular surface in similar sites to those identified as due to the action of MMP collagenases as determined using the polyclonal antibody C1,2C which recognizes the C-terminal neoepitope of the 3/4 cleavage fragment (Wu et al., 2002). These areas of collagen degradation co-localize with the sites rich in cathepsin K (Konttinen et al., 2002; Vinardell et al., 2009).

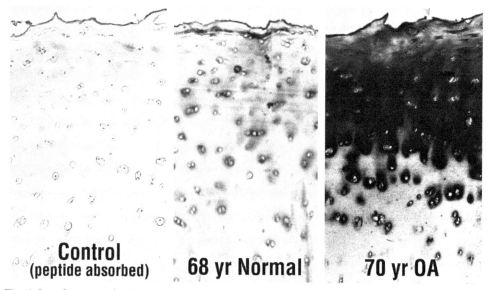

Control
(peptide absorbed)   **68 yr Normal**   **70 yr OA**

Fig. 4. Localization of cathepsin K generated type II cleavage products in cartilage from normal individuals and osteoarthritis (OA) patients.
Frozen sections were treated with chondroitinase ABC to remove glycosaminoglycans and stained using a rabbit antibody raised against the C2K epitope and a horse radish peroxidase labeled second step system. The reaction product was silver enhanced (Gallyas and Merchenthaler, 1988). A control section where the first step antibody was absorbed with the immunizing peptide is included.

The C2K epitope can be released from the tissue by digestion with chymotrypsin and quantitated using a competitive ELISA. Using this approach we demonstrated increased levels of cathepsin K-generated type II collagen fragments in cartilage from osteoarthritis patients relative to normal individuals. In addition, when cartilage was maintained in organ culture for two weeks in the presence of a specific cathepsin K inhibitor, a reduction in the levels of this epitope was observed, indicating that relatively short periods of cathepsin K activity produce detectable levels of this epitope (Dejica et al., 2008).

Together these results indicate that in addition to its critical role in bone resorption (Brömme and Lecaille, 2009; Tezuka et al., 1994), cathepsin K acts along with the MMPs and ADAMTS family members in the destruction of cartilage in osteoarthritis.

7. Acknowledgements

Work by the authors was supported by grants from the Canadian Arthritis Network of Centres of Excellence, the Canadian Institutes of Health Research and the Shriners of North America.

8. References

Aigner T.; Zien A.; Gehrsitz A.; Gebhard P.M. & McKenna L. (2001) Anabolic and catabolic gene expression pattern analysis in normal versus osteoarthritic cartilage using complementary DNA-array technology. *Arthritis Rheum.* Vol.44, pp. 2777-2789

Anway M.D.; Wright W.W.; Zirkin B.R.; Korah N.; Mort J.S. & Hermo L. (2004) Expression and location of cathepsin K in adult rat Sertoli cells. *Biol. Reprod.* Vol.70, pp. 562-569

Baragi V.M.; Becher G.; Bendele A.M.; Biesinger R.; Bluhm H.; Boer J.; Deng H.; Dodd R.; Essers M.; Feuerstein T.; Gallagher B.M., Jr.; Gege C.; Hochgurtel M.; Hofmann M.; Jaworski A.; Jin L.; Kiely A.; Korniski B.; Kroth H.; Nix D.; Nolte B.; Piecha D.; Powers T.S.; Richter F.; Schneider M.; Steeneck C.; Sucholeiki I.; Taveras A.; Timmermann A.; Van V.J.; Weik J.; Wu X. & Xia B. (2009) A new class of potent matrix metalloproteinase 13 inhibitors for potential treatment of osteoarthritis: Evidence of histologic and clinical efficacy without musculoskeletal toxicity in rat models. *Arthritis Rheum.* Vol.60, pp. 2008-2018

Barksby H.E.; Milner J.M.; Patterson A.M.; Peake N.J.; Hui W.; Robson T.; Lakey R.; Middleton J.; Cawston T.E.; Richards C.D. & Rowan A.D. (2006) Matrix metalloproteinase 10 promotion of collagenolysis via procollagenase activation: implications for cartilage degradation in arthritis. *Arthritis Rheum.* Vol.54, pp. 3244-3253

Bau B.; Gebhard P.M.; Haag J.; Knorr T.; Bartnik E. & Aigner T. (2002) Relative messenger RNA expression profiling of collagenases and aggrecanases in human articular chondrocytes in vivo and in vitro. *Arthritis Rheum.* Vol.46, pp. 2648-2657

Billinghurst R.C.; Dahlberg L.; Ionescu M.; Reiner A.; Bourne R.; Rorabeck C.; Mitchell P.; Hambor J.; Diekmann O.; Tschesche H.; Chen J.; Van Wart H. & Poole A.R. (1997) Enhanced cleavage of type II collagen by collagenases in osteoarthritic articular cartilage. *J. Clin. Invest.* Vol.99, pp. 1534-1545

Birkedal-Hansen H.; Moore W.G.I.; Bodden M.K.; Windor L.J.; Birkedal-Hansen B.; DeCarlo A. & Engler J.A. (1993) Matrix metalloproteinases: a review. *Crit. Rev. Oral Biol. Med.* Vol.4, pp. 197-250

Blaney Davidson E.N.; Vitters E.L.; van Lent P.L.; van de Loo F.A.; van den Berg W.B. & van der Kraan P.M. (2007) Elevated extracellular matrix production and degradation upon bone morphogenetic protein-2 (BMP-2) stimulation point toward a role for BMP-2 in cartilage repair and remodeling. *Arthritis Res. Ther.* Vol.9, pp. R102

Brömme D. & Lecaille F. (2009) Cathepsin K inhibitors for osteoporosis and potential off-target effects. *Expert Opin. Investig. Drugs* Vol.18, pp. 585-600

Burrage P.S.; Mix K.S. & Brinckerhoff C.E. (2006) Matrix metalloproteinases: role in arthritis. *Front. Biosci.* Vol.11, pp. 529-543

Büttner F.H.; Chubinskaya S.; Margerie D.; Huch K.; Flechtenmacher J.; Cole A.A.; Kuettner K.E. & Bartnik E. (1997) Expression of membrane type 1 matrix metalloproteinase in human articular cartilage. *Arthritis Rheum.* Vol.40, pp. 704-709

Cherney M.M.; Lecaille F.; Kienitz M.; Nallaseth F.S.; Li Z.; James M.N.G. & Brömme D. (2011) Structure-activity analysis of cathepsin K/chondroitin 4-sulfate interactions. *J. Biol. Chem.* Vol.286, pp. 8988-8998

Chung L.; Dinakarpandian D.; Yoshida N.; Lauer-Fields J.L.; Fields G.B.; Visse R. & Nagase H. (2004) Collagenase unwinds triple-helical collagen prior to peptide bond hydrolysis. *EMBO J.* Vol.23, pp. 3020-3030

Clegg P.D.; Burke R.M.; Coughlan A.R.; Riggs C.M. & Carter S.D. (1997a) Characterisation of equine matrix metalloproteinase 2 and 9; and identification of the cellular sources of these enzymes in joints. *Equine Vet. J.* Vol.29, pp. 335-342

Clegg P.D.; Coughlan A.R.; Riggs C.M. & Carter S.D. (1997b) Matrix metalloproteinases 2 and 9 in equine synovial fluids. *Equine Vet. J.* Vol.29, pp. 343-348

Cole A.A.; Chubinskaya S.; Schumacher B.; Huch K.; Cs-Szabo G.; Yao J.; Mikecz K.; Hasty K.A. & Kuettner K.E. (1996) Chondrocyte matrix metalloproteinase-8. Human articular chondrocytes express neutrophil collagenase. *J. Biol. Chem.* Vol.271, pp. 11023-11026

Collins-Racie L.A.; Flannery C.R.; Zeng W.; Corcoran C.; Annis-Freeman B.; Agostino M.J.; Arai M.; DiBlasio-Smith E.; Dorner A.J.; Georgiadis K.E.; Jin M.; Tan X.Y.; Morris E.A. & LaVallie E.R. (2004) ADAMTS-8 exhibits aggrecanase activity and is expressed in human articular cartilage. *Matrix Biol.* Vol.23, pp. 219-230

Dejica V.M.; Mort J.S.; Laverty S.; Percival M.D.; Antoniou J.; Zukor D.J. & Poole A.R. (2008) Cleavage of type II collagen by cathepsin K in human osteoarthritic cartilage. *Am. J. Pathol.* Vol.173, pp. 161-169

Doege K.J.; Coulter S.N.; Meek L.M.; Maslen K. & Wood J.G. (1997) A human-specific polymorphism in the coding region of the aggrecan gene. Variable number of tandem repeats produce a range of core protein sizes in the general population. *J. Biol. Chem.* Vol.272, pp. 13974-13979

Durigova M.; Soucy P.; Fushimi K.; Nagase H.; Mort J.S. & Roughley P.J. (2008) Characterization of an ADAMTS-5-mediated cleavage site in aggrecan in OSM-stimulated bovine cartilage. *Osteoarthritis Cartilage* Vol.16, pp. 1245-1252

Flannery C.R.; Lark M.W. & Sandy J.D. (1992) Identification of a stromelysin cleavage site within the interglobular domain of human aggrecan. Evidence for proteolysis at this site *in vivo* in human articular cartilage. *J. Biol. Chem.* Vol.267, pp. 1008-1014

Fosang A.J.; Last K.; Neame P.J.; Murphy G.; Knäuper V.; Tschesche H.; Hughes C.E.; Caterson B. & Hardingham T.E. (1994) Neutrophil collagenase (MMP-8) cleaves at the aggrecanase site E^{373}-A^{374} in the interglobular domain of cartilage aggrecan. *Biochem. J.* Vol.304, pp. 347-351

Fosang A.J.; Neame P.J.; Hardingham T.E.; Murphy G. & Hamilton J.A. (1991) Cleavage of cartilage proteoglycan between G1 and G2 domains by stromelysins. *J. Biol. Chem.* Vol.266, pp. 15579-15582

Fosang A.J.; Neame P.J.; Last K.; Hardingham T.E.; Murphy G. & Hamilton J.A. (1992) The interglobular domain of cartilage aggrecan is cleaved by PUMP, gelatinases, and cathepsin B. *J. Biol. Chem.* Vol.267, pp. 19470-19474

Fosang A.J. & Rogerson F.M. (2010) Identifying the human aggrecanase. *Osteoarthritis Cartilage* Vol.18, pp. 1109-1116

Freemont A.J.; Byers R.J.; Taiwo Y.O. & Hoyland J.A. (1999) In situ zymographic localisation of type II collagen degrading activity in osteoarthritic human articular cartilage. *Ann. Rheum. Dis.* Vol.58, pp. 357-365

Freemont A.J.; Hampson V.; Tilman R.; Goupille P.; Taiwo Y. & Hoyland J.A. (1997) Gene expression of matrix metalloproteinases 1, 3, and 9 by chondrocytes in osteoarthritic human knee articular cartilage is zone and grade specific. *Ann. Rheum. Dis.* Vol.56, pp. 542-549

Freije J.M.P.; Díez-Itza I.; Balbín M.; Sánchez L.M.; Blasco R.; Tolivia J. & López-Otín C. (1994) Molecular cloning and expression of collagenase-3, a novel human matrix metalloproteinase produced by breast carcinomas. *J. Biol. Chem.* Vol.269, pp. 16766-16773

Gallyas F. & Merchenthaler I. (1988) Copper-H_2O_2 oxidation strikingly improves silver intensification of the nickel-diaminobenzidine (Ni-DAB) end-product of the peroxidase reaction. *J. Histochem. Cytochem.* Vol.36, pp. 807-810

Garnero P.; Borel O.; Byrjalsen I.; Ferreras M.; Drake F.H.; McQueney M.S.; Foged N.T.; Delmas P.D. & Delaissé J.M. (1998) The collagenolytic activity of cathepsin K is unique among mammalian proteinases. *J. Biol. Chem.* Vol.273, pp. 32347-32352

Gebauer M.; Saas J.; Sohler F.; Haag J.; Soder S.; Pieper M.; Bartnik E.; Beninga J.; Zimmer R. & Aigner T. (2005) Comparison of the chondrosarcoma cell line SW1353 with primary human adult articular chondrocytes with regard to their gene expression profile and reactivity to IL-1beta. *Osteoarthritis Cartilage* Vol.13, pp. 697-708

Glasson S.S.; Askew R.; Sheppard B.; Carito B.; Blanchet T.; Ma H.L.; Flannery C.R.; Peluso D.; Kanki K.; Yang Z.; Majumdar M.K. & Morris E.A. (2005) Deletion of active ADAMTS5 prevents cartilage degradation in a murine model of osteoarthritis. *Nature* Vol.434, pp. 644-648

Gordon M.K. & Hahn R.A. (2010) Collagens. *Cell Tissue Res.* Vol.339, pp. 247-257

Harris E.D. & Krane S.M. (1974) Collagenases. *N. Engl. J. Med.* Vol.291, pp. 605-609

Hughes C.E.; Caterson B.; Fosang A.J.; Roughley P.J. & Mort J.S. (1995) Monoclonal antibodies that specifically recognize neoepitope sequences generated by 'aggrecanase' and matrix metalloproteinase cleavage of aggrecan: application to catabolism *in situ* and *in vitro*. *Biochem. J.* Vol.305, pp. 799-804

Imai K.; Ohta S.; Matsumoto T.; Fujimoto N.; Sato H.; Seiki M. & Okada Y. (1997) Expression of membrane-type 1 matrix metalloproteinase and activation of progelatinase A in human osteoarthritic cartilage. *Am. J. Pathol.* Vol.151, pp. 245-256

Imai K.; Yokohama Y.; Nakanishi I.; Ohuchi E.; Fujii Y.; Nakai N. & Okada Y. (1995) Matrix metalloproteinase 7 (matrilysin) from human rectal carcinoma cells. Activation of the precursor, interaction with other matrix metalloproteinases and enzymic properties. *J. Biol. Chem.* Vol.270, pp. 6691-6697

Janusz M.J.; Little C.B.; King L.E.; Hookfin E.B.; Brown K.K.; Heitmeyer S.A.; Caterson B.; Poole A.R. & Taiwo Y.O. (2004) Detection of aggrecanase- and MMP-generated catabolic neoepitopes in the rat iodoacetate model of cartilage degeneration. *Osteoarthritis Cartilage* Vol.12, pp. 720-728

Johnson A.R.; Pavlovsky A.G.; Ortwine D.F.; Prior F.; Man C.F.; Bornemeier D.A.; Banotai C.A.; Mueller W.T.; McConnell P.; Yan C.; Baragi V.; Lesch C.; Roark W.H.; Wilson M.; Datta K.; Guzman R.; Han H.K. & Dyer R.D. (2007) Discovery and characterization of a novel inhibitor of matrix metalloprotease-13 that reduces cartilage damage in vivo without joint fibroplasia side effects. *J. Biol. Chem.* Vol.282, pp. 27781-27791

Kafienah W.; Brömme D.; Buttle D.J.; Croucher L.J. & Hollander A.P. (1998) Human cathepsin K cleaves native type I and II collagens at the N-terminal end of the triple helix. *Biochem. J.* Vol.331, pp. 727-732

Kevorkian L.; Young D.A.; Darrah C.; Donell S.T.; Shepstone L.; Porter S.; Brockbank S.M.; Edwards D.R.; Parker A.E. & Clark I.M. (2004) Expression profiling of metalloproteinases and their inhibitors in cartilage. *Arthritis Rheum.* Vol.50, pp. 131-141

Knäuper V.; López-Otín C.; Smith B.; Knight C.G. & Murphy G. (1996) Biochemical characterization of human collagenase-3. *J. Biol. Chem.* Vol.271, pp. 1544-1550

Konttinen Y.T.; Mandelin J.; Li T.F.; Salo J.; Lassus J.; Liljestrom M.; Hukkanen M.; Takagi M.; Virtanen I. & Santavirta S. (2002) Acidic cysteine endoproteinase cathepsin K in the degeneration of the superficial articular hyaline cartilage in osteoarthritis. *Arthritis Rheum.* Vol.46, pp. 953-960

Koo B.H.; Longpre J.M.; Somerville R.P.T.; Alexander J.P.; Leduc R. & Apte S.S. (2007) Regulation of ADAMTS9 secretion and enzymatic activity by its propeptide. *J. Biol. Chem.* Vol.282, pp. 16146-16154

Koolwijk P.; Miltenburg A.M.M.; van Erck M.G.M.; Oudshoorn M.; Niedbala M.J.; Breedveld F.C. & van Hinsbergh V.W.M. (1995) Activated gelatinase-B (MMP-9) and urokinase-type plasminogen activator in synovial fluids of patients with arthritis. Correlation with clinical and experimental variables of inflammation. *J. Rheumatol.* Vol.22, pp. 385-393

Kuno K.; Kanada N.; Nakashima E.; Fujiki F.; Ichimura F. & Matsushima K. (1997) Molecular cloning of a gene encoding a new type of metalloproteinase-disintegrin family protein with thrombospondin motifs as an inflammation associated gene. *J. Biol. Chem.* Vol.272, pp. 556-562

Leco K.J.; Waterhouse P.; Sanchez O.H.; Gowing K.L.M.; Poole A.R.; Wakeham T.W.; Mak T.W. & Khokha R. (2001) Spontaneous air space enlargement in the lungs of mice lacking tissue inhibitor of metalloproteinases-3 (TIMP-3). *J. Clin. Invest.* Vol.108, pp. 817-829

Lee E.R.; Lamplugh L.; Kluczyk B.; Leblond C.P. & Mort J.S. (2009) Neoepitopes reveal the features of type II collagen cleavage and the identity of a collagenase involved in the transformation of the epiphyses anlagen in development. *Dev. Dyn.* Vol.238, pp. 1547-1563

Lee E.R.; Lamplugh L.; Leblond C.P.; Mordier S.; Magny M.-C. & Mort J.S. (1998) Immunolocalization of the cleavage of the aggrecan core protein at the Asn^{341}-Phe^{342} bond, as an indicator of the location of the metalloproteinases active in the lysis of the rat growth plate. *Anat. Rec.* Vol.252, pp. 117-132

Lee M.H. & Murphy G. (2004) Matrix metalloproteinases at a glance. *J. Cell Sci.* Vol.117, pp. 4015-4016

Li Z.; Hou W.S. & Brömme D. (2000) Collagenolytic activity of cathepsin K is specifically modulated by cartilage-resident chondroitin sulfates. *Biochemistry* Vol.39, pp. 529-536

Little C.B.; Barai A.; Burkhardt D.; Smith S.M.; Fosang A.J.; Werb Z.; Shah M. & Thompson E.W. (2009) Matrix metalloproteinase 13-deficient mice are resistant to osteoarthritic cartilage erosion but not chondrocyte hypertrophy or osteophyte development. *Arthritis Rheum.* Vol.60, pp. 3723-3733

Little C.B.; Mittaz L.; Belluoccio D.; Rogerson F.M.; Campbell I.K.; Meeker C.T.; Bateman J.F.; Pritchard M.A. & Fosang A.J. (2005) ADAMTS-1-knockout mice do not exhibit abnormalities in aggrecan turnover *in vitro* or *in vivo. Arthritis Rheum.* Vol.52, pp. 1461-1472

Lohmander L.S.; Brandt K.D.; Mazzuca S.A.; Katz B.P.; Larsson S.; Struglics A. & Lane K.A. (2005) Use of the plasma stromelysin (matrix metalloproteinase 3) concentration to predict joint space narrowing in knee osteoarthritis. *Arthritis Rheum.* Vol.52, pp. 3160-3167

Lohmander L.S.; Hoerrner L.A. & Lark M.W. (1993a) Metalloproteinases, tissue inhibitor, and proteoglycan fragments in knee synovial fluid in human osteoarthritis. *Arthritis Rheum.* Vol.36, pp. 181-189

Lohmander L.S.; Neame P.J. & Sandy J.D. (1993b) The structure of aggrecan fragments in human synovial fluid: evidence that aggrecanase mediates cartilage degradation in inflammatory joint disease, joint injury and osteoarthritis. *Arthritis Rheum.* Vol.36, pp. 1214-1222

Majumdar M.K.; Askew R.; Schelling S.; Stedman N.; Blanchet T.; Hopkins B.; Morris E.A. & Glasson S.S. (2007) Double-knockout of ADAMTS-4 and ADAMTS-5 in mice results in physiologically normal animals and prevents the progression of osteoarthritis. *Arthritis Rheum.* Vol.56, pp. 3670-3674

Malfait A.M.; Arner E.C.; Song R.H.; Alston J.T.; Markosyan S.; Staten N.; Yang Z.; Griggs D.W. & Tortorella M.D. (2008) Proprotein convertase activation of aggrecanases in cartilage in situ. *Arch. Biochem. Biophys.* Vol.478, pp. 43-51

Malfait A.M.; Liu R.Q.; Ijiri K.; Komiya S. & Tortorella M.D. (2002) Inhibition of ADAM-TS4 and ADAM-TS5 prevents aggrecan degradation in osteoarthritic cartilage. *J. Biol. Chem.* Vol.277, pp. 22201-22208

Maroudas A.I. (1976) Balance between swelling pressure and collagen tension in normal and degenerate cartilage. *Nature* Vol.260, pp. 808-809

Martel-Pelletier J.; Welsch D.J. & Pelletier J.P. (2001) Metalloproteases and inhibitors in arthritic diseases. *Best Pract. Res. Clin. Rheumatol.* Vol.15, pp. 805-829

Mehraban F.; Lark M.W.; Ahmed F.N.; Xu F. & Moskowitz R.W. (1998) Increased secretion and activity of matrix metalloproteinase-3 in synovial tissues and chondrocytes from experimental osteoarthritis. *Osteoarthritis Cartilage* Vol.6, pp. 286-294

Mitchell P.G.; Magna H.A.; Reeves L.M.; Lopresti-Morrow L.L.; Yocum S.A.; Rosner P.J.; Geoghegan K.F. & Hambor J.E. (1996) Cloning, expression, and type II collagenolytic activity of matrix metalloproteinase-13 from human osteoarthritic cartilage. *J. Clin. Invest.* Vol.97, pp. 761-768

Mittaz L.; Russell D.L.; Wilson T.; Brasted M.; Tkalcevic J.; Salamonsen L.A.; Hertzog P.J. & Pritchard M.A. (2004) Adamts-1 is essential for the development and function of the urogenital system. *Biol. Reprod.* Vol.70, pp. 1096-1105

Moldovan F.; Pelletier J.P.; Hambor J.; Cloutier J.M. & Martel-Pelletier J. (1997) Collagenase-3 (matrix metalloprotease 13) is preferentially localized in the deep layer of human arthritic cartilage in situ: in vitro mimicking effect by transforming growth factor beta. *Arthritis Rheum.* Vol.40, pp. 1653-1661

Mort J.S. & Billington C.J. (2001) Articular cartilage and changes in arthritis: matrix degradation. *Arthritis Res.* Vol.3, pp. 337-341

Mort J.S. & Buttle D.J. (1999) The use of cleavage site specific antibodies to delineate protein processing and breakdown pathways. *J. Clin. Pathol. :Mol. Pathol.* Vol.52, pp. 11-18

Mort J.S.; Flannery C.R.; Makkerh J.; Krupa J.C. & Lee E.R. (2003) The use of anti-neoepitope antibodies for the analysis of degradative events in cartilage and the molecular basis for neoepitope specificity. *Biochem. Soc. Symp.* Vol.70, pp. 107-114

Mosig R.A.; Dowling O.; DiFeo A.; Ramirez M.C.; Parker I.C.; Abe E.; Diouri J.; Aqeel A.A.; Wylie J.D.; Oblander S.A.; Madri J.; Bianco P.; Apte S.S.; Zaidi M.; Doty S.B.; Majeska R.J.; Schaffler M.B. & Martignetti J.A. (2007) Loss of MMP-2 disrupts skeletal and craniofacial development and results in decreased bone mineralization, joint erosion and defects in osteoblast and osteoclast growth. *Hum. Mol. Genet.* Vol.16, pp. 1113-1123

Murphy G.; Cockett M.I.; Ward R.V. & Docherty A.J.P. (1991) Matrix metalloproteinase degradation of elastin, type IV collagen and proteoglycan. A quantitative comparison of the activities of 95 kDa and 72 kDa gelatinases, stromelysins-1 and -2 and punctuated metalloproteinase (PUMP). *Biochem. J.* Vol.277, pp. 277-279

Nagase H. (1997) Activation mechanisms of matrix metalloproteinases. *Biol. Chem.* Vol.378, pp. 151-160

Nagase H. & Fushimi K. (2008) Elucidating the function of non catalytic domains of collagenases and aggrecanases. *Connect. Tissue Res.* Vol.49, pp. 169-174

Nagase H. & Woessner J.F. (1999) Matrix metalloproteinases. *J. Biol. Chem.* Vol.274, pp. 21491-21494

Naito S.; Shiomi T.; Okada A.; Kimura T.; Chijiiwa M.; Fujita Y.; Yatabe T.; Komiya K.; Enomoto H.; Fujikawa K. & Okada Y. (2007) Expression of ADAMTS4 (aggrecanase-1) in human osteoarthritic cartilage. *Pathol. Int.* Vol.57, pp. 703-711

Neuhold L.A.; Killar L.; Zhao W.; Sung M.L.; Warner L.; Kulik J.; Turner J.; Wu W.; Billinghurst C.; Meijers T.; Poole A.R.; Babij P. & DeGennaro L.J. (2001) Postnatal expression in hyaline cartilage of constitutively active human collagenase-3 (MMP-13) induces osteoarthritis in mice. *J. Clin. Invest.* Vol.107, pp. 35-44

Ohta S.; Imai K.; Yamashita K.; Matsumoto T.; Azumano I. & Okada Y. (1998) Expression of matrix metalloproteinase 7 (matrilysin) in human osteoarthritic cartilage. *Lab. Invest.* Vol.78, pp. 79-87

Okada Y.; Shinmei M.; Tanaka O.; Naka K.; Kimura A.; Nakanishi I.; Bayliss M.T.; Iwata K. & Nagase H. (1992) Localization of matrix metalloproteinase 3 (stromelysin) in osteoarthritic cartilage and synovium. *Lab. Invest.* Vol.66, pp. 680-690

Pei D. & Weiss S.J. (1995) Furin-dependent intracellular activation of the human stromelysin-3 zymogen. *Nature* Vol.375, pp. 244-247

Plaas A.; Osborn B.; Yoshihara Y.; Bai Y.; Bloom T.; Nelson F.; Mikecz K. & Sandy J.D. (2007) Aggrecanolysis in human osteoarthritis: confocal localization and biochemical characterization of ADAMTS5-hyaluronan complexes in articular cartilages. *Osteoarthritis Cartilage* Vol.15, pp. 719-734

Poole, AR (2001) Cartilage in health and disease. In Arthritis and Allied Conditions (Koopman, W. J., ed.), 226-284, Lippincott, Williams and Wilkins, Baltimore

Poole A.R.; Kojima T.; Yasuda T.; Mwale F.; Kobayashi M. & Laverty S. (2001) Composition and structure of articular cartilage: a template for tissue repair. *Clin. Orthop.* pp. S26-S33

Porter S.; Clark I.M.; Kevorkian L. & Edwards D.R. (2005) The ADAMTS metalloproteinases. *Biochem. J.* Vol.386, pp. 15-27

Pratta M.A.; Yao W.; Decicco C.; Tortorella M.D.; Liu R.Q.; Copeland R.A.; Magolda R.; Newton R.C.; Trzaskos J.M. & Arner E.C. (2003) Aggrecan protects cartilage collagen from proteolytic cleavage. *J. Biol. Chem.* Vol.278, pp. 45539-45545

Reboul P.; Pelletier J.P.; Tardif G.; Cloutier J.M. & Martel-Pelletier J. (1996) The new collagenase, collagenase-3, is expressed and synthesized by human chondrocytes but not by synoviocytes. A role in osteoarthritis. *J. Clin. Invest.* Vol.97, pp. 2011-2019

Roach H.I.; Yamada N.; Cheung K.S.; Tilley S.; Clarke N.M.; Oreffo R.O.; Kokubun S. & Bronner F. (2005) Association between the abnormal expression of matrix-degrading enzymes by human osteoarthritic chondrocytes and demethylation of specific CpG sites in the promoter regions. *Arthritis Rheum.* Vol.52, pp. 3110-3124

Rodriguez-Lopez J.; Mustafa Z.; Pombo-Suarez M.; Malizos K.N.; Rego I.; Blanco F.J.; Tsezou A.; Loughlin J.; Gomez-Reino J.J. & Gonzalez A. (2008) Genetic variation including nonsynonymous polymorphisms of a major aggrecanase, ADAMTS-5, in susceptibility to osteoarthritis. *Arthritis Rheum.* Vol.58, pp. 435-441

Rodríguez-Manzaneque J.C.; Westling J.; Thai S.N.M.; Luque A.; Knäuper V.; Murphy G.; Sandy J.D. & Iruela-Arispe M.L. (2002) ADAMTS1 cleaves aggrecan at multiple sites and is differentially inhibited by metalloproteinase inhibitors. *Biochem. Biophys. Res. Commun.* Vol.293, pp. 501-508

Salminen H.J.; Säämänen A.-M.K.; Vankemmelbeke M.N.; Auho P.K.; Perälä M.P. & Vuorio E.I. (2002) Differential expression patterns of matrix metalloproteinases and their inhibitors during development of osteoarthritis in a transgenic mouse model. *Ann. Rheum. Dis.* Vol.61, pp. 591

Sandy J.D.; Flannery C.R.; Neame P.J. & Lohmander L.S. (1992) The structure of aggrecan fragments in human synovial fluid. Evidence for the involvement in osteoarthritis of a novel proteinase which cleaves the Glu 373-Ala 374 bond of the interglobular domain. *J. Clin. Invest.* Vol.89, pp. 1512-1516

Sandy J.D.; Neame P.J.; Boynton R.E. & Flannery C.R. (1991) Catabolism of aggrecan in cartilage explants. Identification of a major cleavage site within the interglobular domain. *J. Biol. Chem.* Vol.266, pp. 8683-8685

Settle S.; Vickery L.; Nemirovskiy O.; Vidmar T.; Bendele A.; Messing D.; Ruminski P.; Schnute M. & Sunyer T. (2010) Cartilage degradation biomarkers predict efficacy of a novel, highly selective matrix metalloproteinase 13 inhibitor in a dog model of osteoarthritis: Confirmation by multivariate analysis that modulation of type ii collagen and aggrecan degradation peptides parallels pathologic changes. *Arthritis Rheum.* Vol.62, pp. 3006-3015

Shlopov B.V.; Lie W.R.; Mainardi C.L.; Cole A.A.; Chubinskaya S. & Hasty K.A. (1997) Osteoarthritic lesions: involvement of three different collagenases. *Arthritis Rheum.* Vol.40, pp. 2065-2074

Soder S.; Roach H.I.; Oehler S.; Bau B.; Haag J. & Aigner T. (2006) MMP-9/gelatinase B is a gene product of human adult articular chondrocytes and increased in osteoarthritic cartilage. *Clin. Exp. Rheumatol.* Vol.24, pp. 302-304

Somerville R.P.T.; Longpre J.M.; Jungers K.A.; Engle J.M.; Ross M.; Evanko S.; Wight T.N.; Leduc R. & Apte S.S. (2003) Characterization of ADAMTS-9 and ADAMTS-20 as a distinct ADAMTS subfamily related to *Caenorhabditis elegans* GON-1. *J. Biol. Chem.* Vol.278, pp. 9503-9513

Song R.H.; Tortorella M.D.; Malfait A.M.; Alston J.T.; Yang Z.; Arner E.C. & Griggs D.W. (2007) Aggrecan degradation in human articular cartilage explants is mediated by both ADAMTS-4 and ADAMTS-5. *Arthritis Rheum.* Vol.56, pp. 575-585

Song X.Y.; Zeng L.; Jin W.; Thompson J.; Mizel D.E.; Lei K.; Billinghurst R.C.; Poole A.R. & Wahl S.M. (1999) Secretory leukocyte protease inhibitor suppresses the inflammation and joint damage of bacterial cell wall-induced arthritis. *J. Exp. Med.* Vol.190, pp. 535-542

Stanton H.; Rogerson F.M.; East C.J.; Golub S.B.; Lawlor K.E.; Meeker C.T.; Little C.B.; Last K.; Farmer P.J.; Campbell I.K.; Fourie A.M. & Fosang A.J. (2005) ADAMTS5 is the major aggrecanase in mouse cartilage in vivo and in vitro. *Nature* Vol.434, pp. 648-652

Stremme S.; Duerr S.; Bau B.; Schmid E. & Aigner T. (2003) MMP-8 is only a minor gene product of human adult articular chondrocytes of the knee. *Clin. Exp. Rheumatol.* Vol.21, pp. 205-209

Sukhova G.K.; Shi G.P.; Simon D.I.; Chapman H.A. & Libby P. (1998) Expression of the elastolytic cathepsins S and K in human atheroma and regulation of their production in smooth muscle cells. *J. Clin. Invest.* Vol.102, pp. 576-583

Suzuki K.; Enghild J.J.; Morodomi T.; Salvesen G. & Nagase H. (1990) Mechanisms of activation of tissue procollagenase by matrix metalloproteinase 3 (stromelysin). *Biochemistry* Vol.29, pp. 10261-10270

Sztrolovics R.; White R.J.; Roughley P.J. & Mort J.S. (2002) The mechanism of aggrecan release from cartilage differs with tissue origin and the agent used to stimulate catabolism. *Biochem. J.* Vol.362, pp. 465-472

Tchetverikov I.; Lohmander L.S.; Verzijl N.; Huizinga T.W.; TeKoppele J.M.; Hanemaaijer R. & Degroot J. (2005) MMP protein and activity levels in synovial fluid from patients with joint injury, inflammatory arthritis, and osteoarthritis. *Ann. Rheum. Dis.* Vol.64, pp. 694-698

Tezuka K.; Tezuka Y.; Maejima A.; Sato T.; Nemoto K.; Kamioka H.; Hakeda Y. & Kumegawa M. (1994) Molecular cloning of a possible cysteine proteinase predominantly expressed in osteoclasts. *J. Biol. Chem.* Vol.269, pp. 1106-1109

Tortorella M.D.; Liu R.Q.; Burn T.; Newton R.C. & Arner E. (2002) Characterization of human aggrecanase 2 (ADAM-TS5): substrate specificity studies and comparison with aggrecanase 1 (ADAM-TS4). *Matrix Biol.* Vol.21, pp. 499-511

Tortorella M.D.; Malfait A.M.; Deccico C. & Arner E. (2001) The role of ADAM-TS4 (aggrecanase-1) and ADAM-TS5 (aggrecanase-2) in a model of cartilage degradation. *Osteoarthritis Cartilage* Vol.9, pp. 539-552

Tortorella M.D.; Pratta M.; Liu R.Q.; Austin J.; Ross O.H.; Abbaszade I.; Burn T. & Arner E. (2000) Sites of aggrecan cleavage by recombinant human aggrecanase-1 (ADAMTS-4). *J. Biol. Chem.* Vol.275, pp. 18566-18573

Turk V.; Turk B. & Turk D. (2001) Lysosomal cysteine proteases: facts and opportunities. *EMBO J.* Vol.20, pp. 4629-4633

van Lent P.L.E.M.; Grevers L.; Blom A.B.; Sloetjes A.; Mort J.S.; Vogl T.; Nacken W.; van den Berg W.B. & Roth J. (2008) Myeloid-related proteins S100A8/S100A9 regulate joint inflammation and cartilage destruction during antigen-induced arthritis. *Ann. Rheum. Dis.* Vol.67, pp. 1750-1758

Vinardell T.; Dejica V.; Poole A.R.; Mort J.S.; Richard H. & Laverty S. (2009) Evidence to suggest that cathepsin K degrades articular cartilage in naturally occurring equine osteoarthritis. *Osteoarthritis Cartilage* Vol.17, pp. 375-383

Vincenti M.P. & Brinckerhoff C.E. (2001) Early response genes induced in chondrocytes stimulated with the inflammatory cytokine interleukin-1β. *Arthritis Res.* Vol.3, pp. 381-388

Volk S.W.; Kapatkin A.S.; Haskins M.E.; Walton R.M. & D'Angelo M. (2003) Gelatinase activity in synovial fluid and synovium obtained from healthy and osteoarthritic joints of dogs. *Am. J. Vet. Res.* Vol.64, pp. 1225-1233

Wachsmuth L.; Bau B.; Fan Z.; Pecht A.; Gerwin N. & Aigner T. (2004) ADAMTS-1, a gene product of articular chondrocytes in vivo and in vitro, is downregulated by interleukin 1beta. *J. Rheumatol.* Vol.31, pp. 315-320

Wassilew G.I.; Lehnigk U.; Duda G.N.; Taylor W.R.; Matziolis G. & Dynybil C. (2010) The expression of proinflammatory cytokines and matrix metalloproteinases in the synovial membranes of patients with osteoarthritis compared with traumatic knee disorders. *Arthroscopy* Vol.26, pp. 1096-1104

Wu W.; Billinghurst R.C.; Pidoux I.; Antoniou J.; Zukor D.; Tanzer M. & Poole A.R. (2002) Sites of collagenase cleavage and denaturation of type II collagen in aging and osteoarthritic articular cartilage and their relationship to the distribution of matrix metalloproteinase 1 and matrix metalloproteinase 13. *Arthritis Rheum.* Vol.46, pp. 2087-2094

Yoshida M.; Tsuji M.; Funasaki H.; Kan I. & Fujii K. (2005) Analysis for the major contributor of collagenase to the primary cleavage of type II collagens in cartilage degradation. *Mod. Rheumatol.* Vol.15, pp. 180-186

2

Cartilage Extracellular Matrix Integrity and OA

Chathuraka T. Jayasuriya and Qian Chen
Alpert Medical School of Brown Universit, Rhode Island Hospital
United States of America

1. Introduction

Articular cartilage tissue is mostly composed of extracellular matrix (ECM) in which a sparse population of cells (chondrocytes) reside. These cells produce both anabolic and catabolic factors that perpetuate a homeostatic process of ECM breakdown and repair termed cartilage turnover. This balance between tissue anabolism and catabolism is characteristic of normal articular cartilage. However, during osteoarthritis (OA), this process is disrupted due to disregulation of chondrocyte function. Although articular cartilage is anatomically classified as a single tissue type, it is divided into four zones defined by their physiological position relative to the joint surface. Likewise, the populations of chondrocytes housed within these zones and their respective ECMs often differ from one another in both appearance and organization. The calcified zone lies directly on top of the subchondral bone, which the cartilage tissue shields from physical forces. This zone contains a very small population of chondrocytes that are slowly being replaced by bone forming cells (osteoblasts) continuously throughout life. When compared to other cartilage zones, the calcified zone ECM is highly mineralized and contains the sparsest chondrocyte population. Osteoblasts from the neighboring subchondral bone secrete bone morphogenic factor (BMPs), and other factors such as stromal cell derived factor 1 (SDF-1) which promote chondrocyte hypertrophy and mineralization. The deep zone cartilage layer lies directly above the calcified zone and contains small vertical aggregates of chondrocytes embedded within a uniquely organized ECM which histologically resemble columnar structures. The middle zone is by far the largest layer containing round bodied chondrocytes and a well hydrated and robust collagen ECM network. Chondrocyte content increases gradually from the subchondral bone towards the articular surface that is in direct contact with the joint synovium. The superficial zone (A.K.A. tangential zone) makes up the articular surface and therefore contains the largest number of chondrocytes of all four zones. OA can affect just one or all four of these cartilage zones depending on the severity and pathological stage of the disease. Given its anatomical position, the superficial zone is often the first cartilage tissue zone to be exposed to injury or wear-and-tear due to excessive joint loading. Therefore this zone often appears to be the initial point of OA pathogenesis. During early stage OA, a sustained injury to the articular surface initially induces a mild but chronic inflammatory response (Martel-Pelletier et al., 2008) that slowly manifests into the disruption of cartilage homeostasis due to disredulation of chondrocyte function (Goldring & Marcu, 2009). As the disease persists, continued homeostatic imbalances eventually cause the release of excessive amounts of catabolic enzymes that break down the ECM resulting in lesion formation within the articular cartilage tissue. Similarly, the disregulated release of anabolic factors such as BMPs and IHH by chondrocytes can result in chondrocyte hypertrophy and eventually calcification of the cartilage ECM. Such changes often lead to osteophyte (bone spur) formation on the otherwise smooth articular surface making normal movement painful and destructive to the connective tissue demonstrating the importance of ECM microenvironment to cartilage tissue health.

2. Structure and function of cartilage ECM molecules and their mutations in degenerative joint diseases

Articular cartilage is an avascular aneural connective tissue composed of chondrocytes that produce and maintain a robust ECM protein network. During early bone development, mesenchymal stem cells of the chondrogenic progeny undergo differentiation into chondrocytes which proliferate, mature, and eventually calcify and undergo cell death as they are replaced by bone. This process leaves behind a layer of articullar cartilage that covers the surfaces of bones providing a low friction surface that can act as a weight/shear stress-bearing coat allowing for smooth joint transition during movement. Articular cartilage tissue has high water content contributing to its near frictionless nature.

2.1 Collagens
Articular cartilage ECM is composed mainly of three kinds of macromolecules: (1) collagens, (2) proteoglycans and (3) non-collagenous matrix proteins. Several collagens are cartilage specific including type II, VI, IX, X, and XI. Table 1 lists the most common cartilage ECM proteins and human diseases that result from their mutation, including their association with chondrodysplasia and OA.

2.1.1 Collagen II
Type II collagen makes up approximately 80 to 90 percent of all collagen content found in normal healthy articular cartilage tissue. In OA, tissue degradation is predominantly caused by the breakdown of cartilage ECM due to the overabundance of reactive proteases, many of which cleave type II collagen containing fibrils resulting in tissue destabilization due to reduction in tensile strength. Type II collagen is initially synthesized as pro-alpha-chains that are assembled into a triple helical structure by the globular domains that exist at both its N and C terminal ends. Two forms of pro-collagen are found in cartilage: Type IIA (COL2A1) and Type IIB. These trimeric type II collagen molecules crosslink with other collagens (i.e. type IX and XI) to form large fibrils that compose a web-like network, which binds to various ECM molecules. The stability of the triple helical structure provides the strength required by cartilage to resist tensile stress and also prevents type II collagen from being easily degraded by most endogenous proteases found in the tissue. Due to its long half-life (over 100 years under physiological conditions) and relative stability, the type II collagen network is never completely broken down or remodeled during normal cartilage homeostatic processes. Type II collagen mutations can cause a plethora of mild to severe phenotypes depending on the nature and location of the mutation. While heterozygous deletion of this gene in mice show a minimal phenotype, complete homozygous deletion predictably causes severe cartilage tissue disorganization and death shortly after birth (Li et al., 1995). In addition to being linked to the development of degenerative joint diseases such

Protein	Gene(s)	Human diseases caused by mutations	Chondrodysplasia	OA causative
Type II collagen	COL2A1	Stickler syndrome	Yes (mild)	May
		Achondrogenesis (type II)	Yes	No evidence
		Hypochondrogenesis	Yes	No evidence
		Spondyloepiphyseal dysplasia	Yes	May
		Spondyloepimetaphyseal dysplasia	Yes	May
Type VI collagen	COL6A1, COL6A2, COL6A3	Ullrich congenital muscular dystrophy	No evidence	No evidence
		Bethlem myopathy	No evidence	No evidence
Type IX collagen	COL9A1, COL9A2, COL9A3	Multiple epiphyseal dysplasia	Yes	May
		Lumbar disk disease	No evidence	No evidence
		Premature OA	No evidence	Yes
Type X collagen	COL10A1	Schmid metaphyseal dysplasia	Yes	No evidence
		Spondylometaphyseal dysplasia	Yes	May
Type XI collagen	COL11A1, COL11A2	Stickler syndrome	Yes (mild)	May
		Spondylomegaepiphyseal dysplasia	Yes	May
		Premature OA	No evidence	Yes
Aggrecan	ACAN	Several chondrodysplasias	Yes	May
Matrilin-3	MATN3	Multiple epiphyseal dysplasia	Yes	May
		Spondyloepimetaphyseal dysplasia	Yes	May
		Premature OA	No evidence	Yes
Cartilage oligomeric matrix protein	COMP	Pseudoachondroplasia	Yes	May
		Multiple epiphyseal dysplasia	Yes	May
Lubricin	PRG4	Camptodactyly-arthropathy-coxa vara-pericarditis syndrome	No evidence	No evidence

Table 1. Cartilage matrix proteins and common human diseases associated with their mutation, including their association with chondrodysplasia and osteoarthritis (OA)

as familial OA, various mutations in this molecule can cause more severe phenotypes such as Stickler syndrome, and several major chondrogenic defects (Byers, 2001). A mutation in the alpha helical domain causing a substitution of a glycine codon with a larger amino acid has been shown to disrupt proper alpha helix formation of type II collagen leading to severe chondrodysplasias and a significant reduction in cartilage tissue stability (Kuivaniemi et al., 1997; Prockop et al., 1997). Similarly in the 1990s, particular families were discovered to have missense mutation (R519C) causing the production of abnormal type II collagen pro-alpha-chains. These alpha chains formed protein dimers leading to mild chondrodysplasia followed by a unique form of familial OA (Byers, 2001; Eyre et al., 1991; Pun et al., 1994; Bleasel et al., 1998).

2.1.2 Collagen XI

Type XI collagen is the second most abundant collagen (3% of all collagens) found in adult articular cartilage and it is a core component of collagen fibrils. It is a heterotrimeric molecule composed of three alpha-chains. Interestingly, the first two chains are coded by the COL11A1 and COL11A2 genes respectively while the third chain is coded by COL2A1 and uniquely post transcriptionally modified (Martel-Pelletier et al., 2008). Type XI collagen makes hydroxylysine-based aldehyde cross-links with type II collagen to form collagen fibrils that stabilize articular cartilage (Cremer et al., 1988) and it has been suggested that the ratio of type XI to type II determines collagen fibril diameter and tensile strength. Like COL2A1, mutations in the type XI collagen genes can cause Stickler syndrome. A study done in 1995 also discovered that a single base pair deletion in the type XI collagen gene creates a frame shift resulting in a premature stop codon which is functionally equivalent to knocking out the gene itself (Li et al., 1995). Mice that are homozygous for this nonsense mutation develop serious chondrodysplasia and die at birth. Missense mutations in the COL11A2 gene have also been associated with spondylo-megaepiphyseal dysplasia (OSMED) (Vikkula et al., 1995) and mutations in both COL11A1 and COL11A2 can cause premature development of OA (Rodriguez et al., 2004).

2.1.3 Collagen IX

Type IX collagen is normally co expressed with type II collagen in hyaline cartilage. In adults, this collagen makes up about 1% of the collagen content found in the articular cartilage. Similar to type VI collagen, type IX collagen molecules exist in heterotrimeric form composed of three alpha-chains. Each of these heterotrimers has seven sites with which to form cross-links with other collagen molecules. Type IX collagen is found to be covalently bonded through aldimine-derived crosslinks to the surface of large type II collagen fibrils (Wu et al., 1992) and it is believed to constrain the lateral expansion of these fibrils (Blaschke et al., 2000; Gregory et al., 2000). Missense mutations in the type IX collagen genes have been associated with lumbar disk disease (LDD) (Zhu et al., 2011) and multiple epiphyseal dysplasia (MED) (Jackson et al., 2010) which indirectly leads to the development of OA. Surprisingly, mice deficient in type IX collagen exhibit normal signs of skeletal and chondral development; however they are afflicted by early joint cartilage degradation that resemble the formation of OA-like lesions (Hu et al., 2006).

2.1.4 Collagen VI

Hyaline cartilage contains a relatively low content of type VI collagen (less than 2% of all articular cartilage tissue collagens) that is found in all cartilage zones within the pericellular regions around chondrocytes (Pullig et al., 1999). Type VI collagen molecules are of heterotrimeric organization as they are composed of three non-identical alpha chains. Each chain contains a triple helical domain allowing for the formation of dimers and tetramers with each other (Engel et al., 1985; Furthmayr et al., 1983). Type VI collagen interacts with non-collagenous matrix proteins forming a network in the pericellular regions. It has been previously demonstrated that type VI collagen content is increased in certain patients suffering from OA. However, it is suspected that disregulated tissue homeostasis causes excessive collagen anabolism and deposition (Pullig et al., 1999). Mutations in the genes that code for the three type VI collagen alpha chains have been associated with noncartilage-specific abnormalities such as muscular dystrophy (Pace et al., 2008) and Bethlem myopathy (Lamandé et al., 1998). And a study conducted in 2009 demonstrated that COL6A1 homozygous knockout mice display lower bone mineral density and develop OA more rapidly than wild-type mice of the same genetic background (Alexopoulos et al., 2009).

2.1.5 Collagen X
Chondrocytes only express type X collagen within the hypertrophic zone of the growth plate (Linsenmayer et al., 1988). It is a homotrimer composed of three pro-alpha-chains each containing a C terminal alpha helical domain which allows these chains to assemble into short triple helices (Wagner et al., 2000). It has been demonstrated that type X collagen expression and distribution is altered during OA such that these molecules are found among the noncalcified regions of the articular cartilage implying the occurrence of premature chondrocyte hypertrophy in these zones (von der Mark et al., 1992). Abnormalities in type X collagen can cause spinal and metaphyseal dysplasias (i.e. Schmid MCD) due to improper enchondral ossification (Bignami et al., 1992). A heterozygous missence mutation (Gly595Glu) in the COL10A1 gene was also previously found to correlate with spondylometaphyseal dysplasia (SMD) within a certain family (Ikegawa et al., 1998). And transgenic mice with deletions in the triple-helical domain of type X collagen develop SMD (Jacenko et al., 1993).

2.2 Proteoglycans
The second major structural components of articullar cartilage tissue are proteoglycans of which aggrecan is the most common. These ECM proteins predominantly help cartilage tissue to retain water and withstand compressive force during joint transition and loading.

2.2.1 Aggrecan
Aggrecan is a large chondroitin sulfate proteoglycan that consists of a 220 kDa protein core containing three globular domains (G1, G2 and G3) which allow it to form covalent bonds with its glycosaminoglycan (GAG) side chain components (Doege et al., 1991). Each GAG side chain is composed of a single keratin sulfate and two chondroitin sulfate domain regions all of which are adjacent to the G2 and G3 globular domains. The G1 domain is attached to a link protein that enables multiple aggrecan subunits to bind to a long nonsulfated glycosaminoglycan backbone known as hyluronic acid (HA). Thus aggrecan becomes trapped within the collagen network where some suspect that it acts to physically shield type II collagen from proteolytic cleavage (Pratta et al., 2003). Due to its overall negative charge, aggrecan draws water into the cartilage ECM allowing the tissue to swell. This swelling gives the tissue a spring-like quality helping it to withstand compressive

forces that are applied to the joint during movement. Proteolytic cleavage of this vital ECM protein is mediated by proteases known as aggrecanases. During OA, the disregulation of aggrecanase synthesis and release causes much damage to aggrecan molecules and the cartilage tissue loses the ability to retain water as it suffers from a reduction in overall stability. As is the case with type II collagen and other major cartilage ECM proteins, deletions/mutations in aggrecan lead to severe chondrodysplasia which can often cause premature OA.

2.2.2 Hyaluronic acid

HA is a nonsulfated GAG that is covalently linked to aggrecan monomers and allows these subunits to aggregate in the cartilage ECM. HA species can have varying molecular mass depending on the length of the GAG. Their masses can range from as small as fifty to larger than thousands of Kilodaltons. The molecular weight of HA decreases during normal aging due to proteolytic cleavage and the cartilage tissue of young individuals tends to have larger species of HA compared to that of the elderly. In addition to the cartilage ECM, HA is also largely found in synovial fluid and contributes to its viscoelasticity. HA recognizes and specifically binds several different cell surface receptors (i.e. CD44, ICAM-1 and RHAMM) where it remains as a major component of the pericellular network surrounding chondrocytes. Due to its large size, HA can shield cells from coming into contact with inflammatory mediators such as cytokines and chemokines. It has also been suggested that HA can regulate collagenase and aggrecanase expression from chondrocytes and synovial cells. Previous studies have demonstrated that higher molecular mass species of HA can inhibit IL-1 mediated stimulation of certain MMPs and ADAMTS-4 by interacting with CD44 (Julovi et al., 2004; Wang et al., 2006; Theuns et al., 2008) while the opposite effect has been found to occur in the presence of smaller mass species (20 kDa) of this proteoglycan. Additionally, these larger species can also inhibit proteoglycan release from cartilage tissue ECM. HA is currently used as an intra-articularly therapy via joint injection for knee OA as this long proteoglycan is believed to decrease OA associated joint pain by increasing both the viscoelastic properties of synovial fluid and the lubrication of the articular surface preventing tissue tearing due to the friction generated during joint transition. (Moreland, 2003; Wobig et al., 1998; Altman & Moskowitz, 1998). Its efficacy in relieving OA related pain has been reported to be depend on the molecular mass of the HA chains as species of larger molecular mass were found to have a greater effect in reducing joint pain. Although the exact biological mechanism with which HA relieves OA associated joint pain remains to be elucidated, it is believed that this large proteoglycan supplements the natural synovial fluid increasing its viscoelasticity and reducing the friction generated during joint movement.

2.2.3 Leucine-rich small proteoglycans

Articullar cartilage also consists of a group of small proteoglycans classified for having seven to eleven leucine-rich repeats (SLRPs). The major cartilage SLRPs are decorin, biglycan, fibromodulin, lumican and epiphycan in the order of decreasing abundance. These small proteoglycans have several roles in maintaining cartilage tissue ECM organization and homeostasis such as interacting with various collagen species to strengthen the ECM network and protecting collagen fibrils from proteolytic cleavage by collagenases. The SLRPs decorin and biglycan are similar in structure as both consist of a leucine-rich core protein linked to either one (in the case of decorin) or two (in the case of biglycan) chondroitin/dermatan sulfate containing GAG chain(s). Previous literature has suggested that decorin can alter the cell cycle by modulating growth factor (i.e. TGF-β and EGF) signaling and it is currently studied in cancer research. Although similar in structure to decorin, biglycan has a different physiological role in ECM. It has been suggested that this proteoglycan modulates BMP-4 signaling during osteoblast differentiation (Chen et al., 2004). Biglycan is essential during skeletal development to maintain normal bone mineral density. Fibromodulin and lumican are SLRPs that competitively bind the same region of collagen fibrils helping to regulate fibril diameter and ECM network assembly (Svensson et al. 2000). Epiphycan is a dermatan sulfate proteoglycan with seven leucine-rich repeats believed to maintain joint integrity, yet little is known about its function and the biological mechanism with which it protects tissue. Mutations and/or deletions in SLRP genes are associated primarily with connective tissue and eye disorders. One recent study demonstrated that biglycan and epiphycan double knockout mice are normal at birth but develop several skeletal abnormalities later in life along with premature OA (Nuka et al., 2010). But there have yet to be more studies that suggest abnormalities in these genes are linked to degenerative joint diseases. Given the importance of SLRPs in regulating tissue homeostasis and matrix organization, this is quite surprising.

2.3 Non-collagenous matrix proteins
Other important non-collagenous matrix proteins found in articular cartilage include the matrilins (matrilin-1 and -3), the cartilage oligomeric matrix protein (COMP), and the lubricating protein predominantly secreted by chondrocytes of the superficial zone: lubricin.

2.3.1 Matrilins
The matrilins are a family of noncollagenous oligomeric ECM proteins that are found in a broad range of tissues including articular cartilage and bone (Deak et al., 1999; Wagener et al., 1997; Piecha et al., 1999; Klatt et al., 2001). There are currently four known members within this family. MATN1 and MATN3 are cartilage specific while MATN2 and MATN4 are found in many connective tissue types (van der Weyden et al. 2006; Wu et al., 1998; Piecha et al., 2002). It has been demonstrated that matrilins form a filamentous network pericellularly in the cartilage ECM (Klatt et al., 2000). Structurally, MATN1 consists of two Von Willebrand Factor A (vWFA) domains, one epidermal growth factor-like (EGF) domain, so named because they share a forty amino-acid long residue commonly found in epidermal growth factor protein, and one alpha helical coil-coiled oligomerization domain. Each vWFA domain contains a metal ion-dependant adhesion site (MIDAS) and previous studies have demonstrated that its mutation can abolish filamentous network formation resulting in abnormal ECM assembly (Chen et al., 1999). Its coil-coiled oligomerization domain allows it to form homotrimers with other MATN1 molecules or hetero-oligomers with MATN3. MATN1 is expressed by post proliferative chondrocytes that constitute the zone of maturation within the growth plate. MATN1 interacts with both type II collagen and aggrecan playing a role in organizing fibril formation. MATN1 knockout mice exhibit abnormal fibrillogenesis as their collagen fibrils become aggregated in a uniform directional orientation as opposed to the normal matrix network-like organization observed in wild-type animals.

Although mutations of MATN1 have not been associated with the development of degenerative joint diseases, MATN3 is the smallest and most recently discovered member of the matrilin family of ECM proteins. MATN3 contains a single vWFA domain, four EGF-like domains, and one alpha-helical oligomerization domain which allows it to form homo-oligomers with other MATN3 peptides and hetero-oligomers with MATN1 (Klatt et al., 2000). MATN3 is naturally found in the articular cartilage in its tetrameric form composed of four single oligomers covalently bound together by their alpha-helical oligomerization domains. Several known MATN3 mutations can lead to developmental abnormalities in articular cartilage and bone. These mutations can eventually either lead to OA directly, in the case of hand OA (Aeschlimann et al., 1993; Cepko et al., 1992) or indirectly, in the case of MED, which manifests with joint pain and early onset OA (Chen et al., 1992; Chen et al., 1993). A threonine to methionine missense mutation (T298M) in the first EGF-like domain of MATN3 has been found to correlate with the development of hand OA (Stefánsson et al., 2003) while a cystine to serine (C299S) missense mutation in this same region is common to many patients suffering from spondylo-epi-metaphyseal dysplasia (SEMD), which is a condition often leading to vertebral, epiphyseal/metaphyseal anomalies during development (Borochowitz et al., 2004). Likewise, an arginine to tryptophan missense mutation (R116W) in the vWFA domain has been associated with MED. It was discovered that this particular mutation prevents normal secretion of MATN3 from chondrocytes due to a dominant negative interaction between mutant and normal MATN3 quickly leading to an increase in MATN3 retention within the endoplasmic reticulum of these cells (Otten et al., 2005). Consequently, this reduction in the secretion of functional MATN3 is believed to contribute to MED. Interestingly, during advanced stages of OA, joint synovial fluid contains higher levels of cleaved ECM proteins including MATN3 oligomers due to the proteolysis of articular cartilage. One study has even shown that MATN3 mRNA is upregulated in some OA patients suggesting that the body may produce an excess of the protein (Pullig et al., 2002). Matrilin proteins are relatively well conserved between mice and humans making them ideal proteins to investigate in the mouse model. Complete homozygous deletion of the MATN3 gene in mice surprisingly results in no gross skeletal deformities at birth, but it does however result in the development of OA much earlier in life. MATN3 knockout mice were maintained in a C57BL/6J background and developed several signs of enhanced OA including osteophyte formation and the presence of large lesions in the superficial zone of the articular cartilage, which is the layer that is in direct contact with the knee joint synovium. Additionally, these knockout mice appear to have a higher bone mineral density (BMD) and lower overall cartilage proteoglycan content when compared to wild-type mice of the same genetic background. Perhaps the increase in BMD leads to over-loading of diarthroidial joints, which eventually manifests in the form of enhanced cartilage damage. Tentatively, MATN3's ability to prevent OA-like lesion formation in articular cartilage may also be related to its regulatory functions. The complete biological mechanism with which this ECM protein acts chondroprotectively remains to be elucidated.

2.3.2 COMP

Cartilage oligomeric matrix protein (COMP) is another non-collagenous ECM protein found in articular cartilage with a function that is not yet completely understood. It is a pentameric molecule which consists of five glycoprotein subunits held to one another by disulfide bonds.

Each subunit contains an EGF-like domain and a thrombospondin-like domain. Previous studies have shown that COMP can stimulate type II collagen fibrillogenesis (Rosenberg et al., 1998). In cartilage, COMP is found bound to types I, II, and IX collagen molecules. While COMP knockout mice exhibit normal chondral and skeletal development, various missense mutation in the COMP gene have been shown to cause severe chondrodysplasias such as pseudoachondroplasia (PSACH) and MED, which is accompanied by premature OA development. COMP is also used as a marker of OA pathogenesis because its concentration is commonly elevated in OA patients (Williams & Spector et al., 2008)

2.3.3 Lubricin

Lubricin is a large soluble proteoglycan that is highly expressed by synoviocytes and chondrocytes of superficial zone articular cartilage. It is found in the synovial fluid and it covers articular surfaces of joints acting as a lubricant that prevents friction induced tissue wear and tear during joint transition. Lubricin consists of a central core protein containing heavily glycosylated oligosaccharide side chains. The core protein contains two somatomedin B-like (SMB) domains, a single a hemopexin-like domain (PEX), and two glycosylated mucin-like domains (Rhee et al., 2005). It is coded by the PGR4 gene, which when knocked out results in cartilage degradation and synovial cell hyperplasia in mice. Mutations in this gene can cause camptodactyly-arthropathy-coxa vara-pericarditis syndrome (CACP), which is an autosomal recessive disease that causes synovial hyperplasia and joint degredation similar to the phenotype of mice that are completely deficient in this protein (Rhee et al., 2005).

3. Extracellular matrix breakdown during osteoarthritis

During cartilage turnover, ECM molecules are slowly broken down via proteolysis and replaced by newly synthesized ECM proteins secreted from nearby chondrocytes. The catabolic and anabolic processes of this turnover are balanced in normal cartilage so that the rate of proteolysis and ECM loss matches the rate of ECM synthesis. However, in OA cartilage, this balance is often observed to be shifted towards catabolism. Proteases act to degrade the ECM network by cleaving excessive amounts collagen and proteoglycans. These cleaved fragments are released into the cartilage matrix and some can even trigger further tissue catabolism by both known and unknown biological mechanisms. The degeneration of the joint cartilage is further enhanced by the lackluster process of tissue repair due to disregulated anabolism. During OA, the disregulation of common anabolic growth factors native to the articular cartilage (i.e. TGF-β, FGF and IGF) prevents adequate protection against the catabolic effects induced by proteases ultimately leading to an imbalanced cartilage turnover process that favors degradation.

3.1 Activation of matrix proteases: MMPs, ADAMTS family

OA is clinically characterized by its degenerative effect on major articular cartilage ECM components such as collagen fibrils and proteoglycans by proteolysis (Takaishi et al., 2008). This enhancement of articular cartilage ECM catabolism is mediated mostly by the matrix metalloproteinase (MMP) family of collagenases and the ADAMTS family of aggrecanases, which are often expressed by chondrocytes in response to inflammatory cytokines such as IL-1β (Martel-Pelletier et al., 2008; Glasson et al. 2005; Stanton et al.,

2005). MMPs are neutral zinc-dependent endoproteinases that, when activated, cleave and degrade ECM components during normal tissue turnover. The MMP family is divided into several categories based on their enzymatic activity: collagenases, gelatinases, stromelysins, and membrane-type MMPs (MT-MMPs). MMPs commonly involved in cartilage homeostasis are collagenases and gelatinases. Most MMPs are initially secreted as inactive pro-MMP proteins (zymogens) which are then activated by proteolytic cleavage themselves. Because of their catabolic activity, this family of proteases has received much attention in arthritis research. Both mRNA expression and enzymatic activity of certain metalloproteinase are increased in cartilage tissue during OA pathogenesis including: MMP-1 (Drummond et al., 1999), MMP-2 (Imai et al., 1997; Mohtai et al., 1993), MMP-3 (Okada et al., 1992), MMP-7 (Ohta et al., 1998), MMP-8 (Drummond et al., 1999), MMP-9 (Mohtai et al., 1993), MMP-10 and MMP-13 (Mitchell et al., 1996). Table 2 lists OA associated catabolic proteases and the matrix protein targets that they cleave.

OA associated proteinase	Matrix Substrate
MMP-1	Types I, II, III, VII, VIII, X collagen Aggrecan
MMP-2	Types IV, V, VII, X collagen Aggrecan, decorin
MMP-3	Types II, III, IV, V, IX, X collagen Aggrecan, decorin
MMP-7	Types IV, X collagen Aggrecan, versican
MMP-8	Types I, II, III collagen Aggrecan
MMP-9	Types IV, V collagen Decorin
MMP-10	Types III, IV, V collagen Aggrecan
MMP-13	Types II, III, IV, IX, X collagen Aggrecan
ADAMTS-4	Aggrecan Matrilin-3
ADAMTS-5	Aggrecan Brevican, matrilin-3

Table 2. Osteoarthritis (OA) associated MMPs and their cartilage extracellular matrix substrates.

3.1.1 MMP-1

MMP-1 is classified as a collagenase that shows preference for cleaving type III and type X collagens (Martel-Pelletier et al., 2008; Nwomeh et al., 2002) which, while not a major component of ECM, is still present in articular cartilage tissue. MMP-1 is stoichiometrically inhibited by tissue inhibitor of metalloproteinase (TIMP) 1 and 2.

3.1.2 MMP-2

MMP-2 (gelatinase A) is one of two gelatinases found in human tissues. It further degrades a broad range of collagen and proteoglycan species after these substrates have been initially cleaved by other protyolitic enzymes (i.e. collagenases and aggrecanases). During OA, most of the cartilage tissue damage caused by this metalloproteinase comes from its breakdown of aggrecan, decorin, type IV and X collagen. Active MMP-2 is present in superficial and transition zones of OA cartilage (Imai et al., 1997).

3.1.3 MMP-3

Similarly, MMP-3 is upregulated in early OA but mRNA levels subside during later stages. Immunohistochemical studies have previously demonstrated that MMP-3 is expressed primarily in the superficial and transition zone in early stage OA cartilage and MMP-3 staining positively correlates with tissue Mankin scores. In addition to degrading type IX collagen and certain proteoglycans (Martel-Pelletier et al., 2008; Okada et al., 1989), MMP-3 initiates a cascade that ultimately cleaves and activates pro-MMP-1.

3.1.4 MMP-7

Like MMP-2 and MMP-3, MMP-7 is mainly found in the superficial and transition zones of OA cartilage (Ohta et al., 1998). This metalloproteinase cleaves type IV and X collagens as well as various proteoglycans including aggrecan and versican. Additionally MMP-7 is involved in cleavage and activation of MMP-1, MMP-2, MMP-8 and MMP-9 pro-protein precursors (Dozier et al., 2006).

3.1.5 MMP-8

Unlike other OA associated metalloproteinases, MMP-8 is a collagenase that is produced by neutrophils in response to inflammatory cytokines. Although chondrocytes themselves produce very little of this catabolic enzyme (Stremme et al., 2003), inflammation of the synovium can cause the migration of neutrophils that synthesize and secrete it into and around the superficial zone of cartilage contributing to tissue destruction. MMP-8 cleaves type I, II, and III collagen species as well as various proteoglycans including aggrecan.

3.1.6 MMP-9

The second gelatinase common to human tissue is MMP-9 (gelatinase B) which prefers denatured collagen, mostly type IV and V, as a substrate for its catabolic activity (Okada et al., 1992). Its mRNA expression is minimal in normal articular cartilage but it is greatly elevated in fibrillated areas of OA cartilage.

3.1.7 MMP-10

MMP-10 is a collagenase that degrades collagens types III, IV, V and aggrecan (Nicholson et al., 1989; Fosang et al., 1991; Rechardt et al., 2000). It can also cleave and activate pro-MMP-1, -7, -8 and -9 (Nakamura et al., 1998).

3.1.8 MMP-13

Although many members of the MMP family are involved in cartilage ECM catabolism, no other MMP is as damaging to cartilage tissue during OA as is the collagenase MMP-13. Type

II collagen is the primary structural component of the articular cartilage ECM for which MMP-13 shows digestive preference over any other collagen type (Okada et al., 1992; Ohta et al., 1998). For this reason, it is the collagenase that causes the most cartilage ECM destruction during OA. In addition to type II collagen, it also cleaves type III, IV, IX and X collagen species endogenous to cartilage tissue. MMP-13 is normally expressed in many different tissues including skin, bone, muscle, and cartilage. Its expression normally coincides with type X collagen expression in cartilage undergoing hypertrophic differentiation (Kamekura et al., 2005). In normal healthy cartilage, the primary role of MMP-13 is to enable hypertrophic zone expansion as it denatures pre-existing type II collagen fibrils of the ECM. However, it has been shown that overexpression of MMP-13 in articular chondrocytes also induces OA phenotypic changes (Mitchell et al., 1996). Previous studies have attempted to use MMP-13 inhibitors such as pyrimidinetrione analogs (Drummond et al., 1999) and benzofuran (Blagg et al., 2005) to remedy OA induced cartilage damage. However, their responsiveness was found to be dose dependant and often caused unwanted musculoskeletal side effects (Wu et al., 2005).

3.1.9 Aggrecanases
Aggrecanase-1 (ADAMTS-4) and aggrecanase-2 (ADAMTS-5) are known to be the two most active aggrecanases that lead to articular cartilage ECM catabolism during both OA and rheumatoid arthritis (RA) (Tortorella et al., 1999; Abbaszade et al., 1999). ADAMTS-4 and -5 act on a specific cleavage site (Glu 373/Ala 374) truncating these large proteoglycan chains (Kuno et al. 2000; Rodrı´quez-Manzaneque et al., 2002). In addition to their primary activity of aggrecan cleavage, they have also been shown to cleave MATN3 tetramers at the alpha-helical oligomerization domain releasing MATN3 monomers into the extracellular space (Ahmad et al., 2009; Tahiri et al., 2008). Interestingly, a meniscal transaction induced OA model in mice showed that ADAMTS-5 KO mice sustain less damage to their articular cartilage than wild-type mice (Glasson et al., 2005) linking the expression of this aggrecanase to diminishing cartilage integrity.

3.2 Release and function of cleaved matrix proteins
Proteolytic cleavage of cartilage matrix constituents releases small oligomeric protein fragments into the extracellular space where they can mediate further tissue degradation. The release of oligomeric fragments produced during cleavage of ECM components such as fibronectin, HA, and type II collagen has previously been implicated in the enhancement of cartilage catabolism. Increasing concentrations of such fragments in synovial fluid samples of patients have been found to positively correlate with increasing grade of OA.

3.2.1 Fibronectin cleavage fragments
Fibronectin is a large (450 kDa) adhesive glycoprotein found in many tissues throughout the body including articular cartilage. While native fibronectin normally plays a role in cell-to-cell adhesion and migration, its smaller cleavage fragments (Fn-fs) have different properties and function. Due to enhanced proteolytic cleavage that characteristically occurs during OA and RA, elevated levels of Fn-fs (30 – 200 kDa) are commonly found in articular cartilage tissue and synovial fluid samples. Interestingly, injecting Fn-fs (but not native full length fibronectin) into the knees of rabbits causes up to a 50% depletion of total proteoglycan content in articular cartilage (Homandberg et al., 1993). These Fn-fs enhance the release of

the catabolic cytokines: IL-1α/β, TNF-α, and IL-6, which greatly enhance the release of pro-MMP-2 and pro-MMP-3, while simultaneously suppressing the expression of aggrecan (Bewsey et al., 1996). The exact biological mechanism by which Fn-fs stimulate these catabolic effects is currently unknown however, the Fn-fs found in synovial fluid appear to bind and penetrate the articular cartilage surface of the superficial zone where they may then bind the fibronectin receptors of chondrocytes activating a cascade of events that result in the release of the aforementioned inflammatory cytokines (Xie & Homandberg, 1993). This is further supported by the finding that competitive inhibition of Fn-fs binding to the fibronectin receptor prevents Fn-fs associated catabolic activity (Homandberg & Hui, 1994).

3.2.2 Hyaluronan cleavage fragments
As previously discussed, injection of large molecular mass species of HA into the joint space of OA patients have been deemed therapeutic due to their pain relieving capabilities. However, cleavage of large HA species into smaller HA fragments (HA-fs) by proteolysis or oxidation generates oligomers that potentially have different properties than the original macromolecule (Soltés et al., 2007). CD44 is the primary cell membrane receptor that binds native HA. Adhesion to cells through CD44 allows HA to remain pericellular to chondrocytes where HA bound aggrecan aggregates can gather to draw water into the cartilage ECM giving the tissue compressive resistance required to withstand forces generated during joint loading and movement. However, HA-fs can competitively inhibit the interaction between CD44 and native high molecular weight HA species causing depletion of this (and other) proteoglycans within the cartilage ECM. Low mass (< 5 kDa) HA-fs can also induce MMP-3 and MMP-13 via Nf-kB activation by an unknown biological mechanism in explant culture experiments causing damage to cartilage tissue similar to the effect of Fn-fs. Additionally, HA-fs, but not native high molecular mass HA, have been known to activate iNOS in articular chondrocytes leading to enhanced production of NO ultimately causing further joint degredation.

3.2.3 Collagen cleavage fragments
During the normal pathophysiology of degenerative joint disease, type II collagen is also cleaved and partially degraded to produce smaller protein fragments with novel regulatory functions contributing to further tissue catabolism, as is the case with fibronectin and HA.
Both the C-terminal and N-terminal ends of type II collagen monomers can be cleaved through proteolysis producing fragments termed CT and NT peptides, respectively. Such fragments have been shown to penetrate cartilage tissue and greatly enhance the mRNA expression of MMP-2, 3, 9, and 13 (Fichter et al., 2006) through MAPK p38 and NFκB signaling causing ECM breakdown and proteoglycan depletion (Guo et al., 2009). Similar to the way that HA-fs competitively inhibit HA interaction with CD44, it is surmised that type II collagen fragments can also bind chondrocyte cell membrane integrins preventing these receptors from interacting with type II collagen fibrils, thereby disrupting collagen network integrity. Annexin V is another chondrocyte cell membrane receptor that commonly interacts with native type II collagen. This interaction is vital for matrix vesicle mediated cartilage calcification. Like native type II collagen, the NT peptide can also regulate calcification by binding and activating this receptor. In high concentration, the NT peptide may potentially be responsible for pathological mineralization of the cartilage tissue as commonly seen in OA.

4. Extracellular matrix repair during osteoarthritis

In addition to ECM degradation due to the presence of reactive proteases, as well as their catabolic by-products (such as cleaved matrix protein fragments), OA is also characterized by a disregulation of important structural proteins as well as several important growth factors and their respective antagonists. This altered anabolism is most likely a compensatory reaction by chondrocytes attempting to repair OA induced tissue damage. However, the enhanced expression of some anabolic factors can trigger significant changes to cartilage homeostasis exacerbating the situation.

4.1 Altered expression of structural proteins

While proteolytic processing of collagens is a common characteristic of OA, some of these structural proteins exhibit increased expression and synthesis during disease pathogenesis. Type II, and VI collagens are both highly expressed in OA cartilage. The increase in these native collagen species also provide substrates for proteolysis which generates collagen fragments that have catabolic properties that ultimately results in MMP and NO release followed by proteoglycan depletion, as discussed previously. It is understandable how such events can mediate further tissue degradation during OA.   Additionally, the expression and spatial distribution of type X collagen also changes in the OA joint. While typically type X collagen expression is only localized to the calcified zone, which lies right above the subchondral bone, this marker is also expressed by middle zone cartilage during OA pathogenesis.   The appearance of type X collagen is often indicative of calcification, which seems to corroborate the increased tissue mineralization characteristic of later stages of this disease.

Although aggrecan expression is initially increased during early stage OA, during later stages of OA, its expression is downregulated in cartilage. Thus aggrecan depletion from cartilage tissue is not simply a result by ECM breakdown but it is also due to altered gene regulation. While the biological mechanism responsible for such alterations in gene regulation is not completely understood, it is at least partly due to cytokines and growth factors that are produced by chondrocytes, synoviocytes, and tissue localized immune cells during OA pathogenesis.

4.2 Altered expression of growth factors

The disregulation of potent growth factors during OA can significantly change tissue morphology.

4.2.1 BMPs & TGF-β

While members of the bone morphogenic protein (BMP) family are present in low amounts in normal articular cartilage, their expression is altered during OA. Normally, BMP-2, 4, 6, 7, 9, and 13 are expressed in articular cartilage. These growth factors stimulate chondrocytes to synthesize ECM constituents such as aggrecan and type II collagen to undergo chondrogenic differentiation. They play a role in cartilage repair and help to maintain joint integrity. Some members of the family such as BMP-7 can even inhibit inflammatory cytokine induced MMP synthesis in chondrocytes and synoviocytes. This family of growth factors also has endogenous inhibitors known as BMP antagonists. BMP antagonists are a group of proteins that function by directly binding BMPs as to prohibit them from interacting with their cognate receptors. This effectively prevents BMP signaling. During

OA, only BMP-2 is reported to be upregulated. However, BMP antagonists are also highly expressed in this disease. These antagonists alter normal cartilage homeostasis by inhibiting ECM anabolism mediated by all BMPs and significantly hindering cartilage tissue repair. The expression and protein synthesis of the transforming growth factor beta (TGF-β) family are also altered during OA pathogenesis. Normal cartilage contains small amounts of these growth factors as they promote chondrocyte proliferation and chondrogenic differentiation. Similar to BMPs, they stimulate synthesis of ECM constituent proteins type II collagen and aggrecan. Additionally, TGF-β inhibits the expression and synthesis of MMP-1 and MMP-9. However, the exact function of TGF-β in the joint is still somewhat controversial due to its strong stimulation of MMP-13 and ADAMTS-4 expression in chondrocytes. OA cartilage displays a greater abundance of TGF-β than seen in normal non-diseased cartilage. This is consistent with the increase of both MMP-13 and ADAMTS-4 observed during disease progression. Inhibition of TGF-β has also been shown effective in preventing osteophyte formation in OA cartilage explants suggesting that this growth factor may play a role in inhibiting chondrocyte hypertrophy and premature ossification characteristic of OA (Scharstuhl et al., 2002).

4.2.2 IGFs, FGFs & HGF

Insulin-like growth factors (IGFs) and fibroblast growth factors (FGFs) are also two important proteins that are disregulated during OA. There are two types IGFs: IGF-1 and IGF-2. Both IGFs are present at higher levels in OA cartilage than normal. IGFs regulate homeostatic processes in many tissue types. In articular cartilage it promotes cell division, growth, and proteoglycan synthesis. A family of insulin-like growth factors binding proteins (IGFBPs) can modulate IGF activity by direct interaction. Out of the seven currently known IGFBPs (IGFBP-1 to 7), IGFBP-3 is the most common protein to modulate IGF activity. It has been shown that IGFBP-3 can inhibit the activity of both IGF-1 and IGF-2 in a dose dependant manner (Devi et al., 2001). In articular cartilage, IGFBP-3 has been found to increase in abundance with age. During OA pathogenesis, IGFBP-3 levels are increased even further potentially hindering the process of tissue repair. Like IGFs, FGFs are also upregulated during OA. This family of proteins includes 22 currently identified members. In cartilage biology, the most studied members are FGF-2, FGF-9, and FGF-18 due to their strong stimulation of matrix synthesis and tissue repair. However, the role of these growth factors during OA progression remains to be elucidated. Hepatocyte growth factor (HGF) is another potent multifunctional mitogenic protein that is disregulated in OA cartilage. Deep zone cartilage tissue normally contains two different truncated HGF isoforms (NK1 and NK2) (Guévremont et al., 2003). Although full length HGF is not produced by chondrocytes, osteoblasts from the subchondral bone produce HGF which may be processed in the nearby tissue generating these truncated peptides which diffuse into the calcified and deep zones of cartilage. MMP-13 expression is enhanced by chondrocytes and synoviocytes that come into contact with HGF. Its increasing abundance in OA cartilage can potentially enhance collagen fibril catabolism. Interestingly, HGF is also known for its ability to induce angiogenesis. It is unclear whether this function directly exacerbates the inflammation commonly characteristic of degenerative joint diseases.

5. Effect of major OA associated cytokines and chemokines on cartilage ECM

Unlike RA, OA is not traditionally classified an inflammatory arthropathy. It is unclear if the inflammation is intrinsic to osteoarthritis or a manifestation of associated crystal (e.g., calcium pyrophosphate or hydroxyapatite) arthritis complicating the osteoarthritis. It is characterized by mild yet chronic inflammation that indirectly plays a significant role in disease progression and tissue destruction. Pro-inflammatory cytokine and chemokine production by mononuclear cells, cells of the synovial membrane, and articular chondrocytes can disrupt normal cartilage homeostasis favoring proteoglycan depletion and tissue destruction. The two main pro-inflammatory cytokines noted for their destructive effects during OA are IL-1β and TNF-α.

5.1 IL-1β

IL-1β is expressed and released mainly by synoviocytes and mononuclear cells during joint inflammation, but studies have shown that articular chondrocytes of OA cartilage too upregulate its expression and synthesis. IL-1β exerts several significant catabolic and anti-anabolic effects that make it the most disease causative cytokine in OA. It induces expression of the collagenases, especially MMP-1, MMP-3, MMP-9 and MMP-13, which are believed to contribute significantly to the enhancement of articular cartilage catabolism that occurs during OA (Martel-Pelletier et al., 2008). The IL-1β pathway ultimately activates nuclear factor-κB (NFκB), which is necessary for the transcription of many genes relevant to OA and joint inflammation including MMPs (Park et al., 2004). It has been shown in murine articular cartilage explants that suppressing MMP production via IκB kinase inhibitiors is sufficient to reduce the degredation of both type II collagen and aggrecan (Pattoli et al., 2005).

The ability of IL-1β to downregulate the expression of type II collagen and aggrecan, the two main structural components of the articular cartilage ECM, further illustrates how this pathway can potentially hinder ECM repair in OA pathogenesis. It has been previously demonstrated that IL-1β induces a greater than twofold downregulation of both type II collagen and aggrecan expression in human chondrocytes (Toegal et al., 2008; Goldring et al., 1988). The production of type II collagen and aggrecan are important to the process of chondrogenesis during which mesenchymal stem cells of the chondrocyte lineage secrete the ECM protein components necessary to constitute articular cartilage. Even though chondrogenesis occurs primarily during development in humans, it can also be induced as a result of damage sustained to existing cartilage (as in the case of OA) (van Beuningen et al., 2000). IL-1β can inhibit chondrogenesis (Murakami et at., 2000) by downregulating the transcription factor SOX9 (Wehrli et al., 2003), which is a master regulator of the chondrogenesis pathway. Similarly, IL-1β downregulates the expression of certain TIMPs that normally bind and inhibit active MMPs (Martel-Pelletier et al., 2008). It is also known that the IL-1 receptor (IL-1RI) expression is higher in OA cartilage than in normal cartilage (Jacques et al., 2006) indicating the possibility that the IL-1β pathway is more active in OA chondrocytes. IL-1RI KO mice are resistant to the early development of OA (Jacques et al., 2006). All evidence point to IL-1β stimulation as a potential cause of articular cartilage ECM breakdown during OA. This is why it may be possible to regulate IL-1β activity, perhaps through endogenous pathway inhibition, to slow down OA development/progression.

5.1.1 IL-1RI and IL-1RA

The IL-1β pathway has several endogenous inhibitors (Martel-Pelletier et al., 2008; Arend et al., 2000). Normal signal transduction of this pathway is initiated upon ligand binding to the IL-1 receptor (IL-1RI). The ligand binding event enables IL-1RI to associate with another cell membrane bound protein known as the interleukin-1 receptor accessory protein (IL-1RAcP), which is necessary for pathway activation (Wesche et al., 1997). The association of these two membrane bound proteins allows for cross phosphorylation to occur in their transmembrane signaling domains initiating the signaling cascade that eventually leads to transcription of the proteases and cytokines described previously. Interleukin-1 receptor II (IL-1RII) is a cell membrane bound protein which competes with IL-1RI for IL-1 ligand binding (Gabay et al., 2010). IL-1RII is an IL-1RI protein mimic that does not contain a transmembrane signaling domain therefore it will not initiate signal transduction of the pathway and it is classified as an IL-1β pathway inhibitor. Two other endogenous inhibitors of this pathway are known as soluble interleukin-1 receptor II (sIL-1RII) and soluble interleukin-1 receptor accessory protein (sIL-1RAcP) (Gabay et al., 2010). These proteins mimic IL-1RI and IL-1RAcP respectively. sIL-1RII competes with IL-1RI to bind IL-1β, similarly sIL-1RAcP competes with IL-1RAcP to bind the IL-1RI.

The fifth, and arguable the most effective, inhibitor of this pathway is the IL-1RA. This protein is an IL-1α/β protein mimic and binds IL-1RI with a much higher affinity than does either IL-1α or IL-1β. IL-1RA bound IL-1RI cannot associate with IL-1RAcP and therefore is unable to initiate signal transduction of the IL-1β pathway. The IL-1RA gene can be alternatively spliced to form different isoforms. Currently four isoforms are known to exist in humans and two in mice. In humans, there are three intracellular isoforms of IL-RA (icIL-RA1, icIL-RA2, icIL-RA3) and one cell secreted isoform (sIL-1RA). The intracellular isoforms tend to be cell associated and stays in contact with the cell membrane of the cell from which it was produced. The secreted form of IL-1RA, however, can move into the extracellular space and proceed to inhibit the IL-1β signal transduction of cells that are further away. Several of these isoforms can be easily distinguished form one another due to their varying size: icIL-RA1/ icIL-RA2 (18-kDa), icIL-RA3 (16-kDa), and sIL-1RA (17-kDa) (Gabay et al., 2010).

IL-1RA is produced by many cell types including articular chondrocytes. It has been established that chondrocyte produced/secreted IL-1RA protein helps sustain articular cartilage integrity during both RA and OA induced inflammation. The later was demonstrated when chondrocytes taken from OA cartilage, which was transduced with IL-1RA, protected against IL-1-induced cartilage degradation in organ culture experiments (Baragi et al., 1995). Further support for the idea that IL-1RA is chondroprotective comes from IL-1RA knockout mice of multiple genetic backgrounds, which have been shown to develop early arthritis compared to wild-type mice of the same background (Arend et al., 2000). IL-RA knockout mice bred in both BALB/cA and MFIx129 backgrounds developed severe inflammatory arthritis. Additionally, IL-1β protein levels where elevated as high as three fold in these IL-1RA knock-out mice of both backgrounds while detectable levels of B-cells and T-cells remained constant between IL-1RA knock-out and wild-type mice (Nicklin et al., 2000).

In 1999, *in vivo* IL-1RA gene transfer experiments done in rabbits also demonstrated its potential to reduce OA severity. In these experiments, OA was artificially induced in the animals via meniscectomy after which local IL-1RA gene therapy by intra-articular plasmid injection was performed at 24 hour intervals 4 weeks post surgery. The animals were sacrificed exactly 4 weeks after the first injection and the joint synoviums were dissected and stained for IL-1RA. The level of IL-1RA present in the synoviums of these rabbits positively correlated with a reduction in articular cartilage lesions that resulted from OA indicating that IL-1RA was chondroprotective (Fernandes et al., 1999). A more recent study in 2005 looked at the levels of several potential chondrodestructive (IL-1α, IL-1β, TNF-α, etc.) as well as chondroprotective cytokines, one of which was sIL-1RA, in 31 patients who are at a higher risk of developing OA in one of their knees due to chronic anterior cruciate ligament (ACL) deficiency. This study found concentrations of IL-1β and TNF-α to be significantly higher in the ACL deficient vs. normal knees while the concentration of sIL-1RA decreased with increasing grades of articular chondral damage (Marks et al., 2005). Finally, a 2008 randomized double-blinded cohort study done in 167 patients with knee OA looked at the symptomatic effect of chromium sulfate induced autologous IL-1RA production and found a significant reduction of OA induced pain in the treated patients based on Knee injury and Osteoarthritis Outcome Score (KOOS) and Knee Society Clinical Rating System .

It is important to note that the chondroprotective effects of IL-1RA during OA are only observable when the protein is consistently present in the joint synovium of the arthritic joint. This explains why short-lived drugs such as AnikinRA (Cohen, 2004), which only last 4 hours post-intraarticular injection into human patients (as determined by serum analysis) have limited efficacy in treating OA progression (Chevalier et al., 2009). This is also most likely the underlying reason behind the success of longer lasting treatment options such as gene therapy and other methods aimed at increasing autologous IL-1RA production within the synovium of the OA joint.

5.2 TNF-α

Second only to IL-1β, TNF-α is a potent pro-inflammatory cytokine responsible for initiating much joint destruction during OA and other such joint degenerative diseases. TNF-α is currently looked on as a potential target for late stage OA therapy as its appearance in the joint is a telltale sign of advanced severity of the disease. In late stage OA, both TNF-α and its p55 receptor undergoes increased expression by articular chondrocytes and synoviocytes enhancing TNF-α pathway signaling. This leads to increased production of NO, ECM degrading enzymes, especially the highly catabolic collagenases MMP-3 and MMP-13, and other inflammatory cytokines like IL-1 and IL-6, which overall off-balances tissue homeostasis favoring ECM destruction. TNF-α also enhances the synthesis and release of the prostaglandin PGE2, which inhibits chondrocyte differentiation and maturation while simultaneously promoting MMP production and IL-6 expression. Additionally, circulating mononuclear cells that are localized to areas of inflammation that have undergone OA induced tissue injury also release TNF-α worsening joint inflammation and ultimately further favoring catabolism. Although commercially available TNF-α inhibitors are most efficacious for relieving of RA associated joint inflammation, it has been demonstrated that certain inhibitors, such as infliximab and etanercept, can suppress NO production in human cartilage (Vuolteenaho et al., 2002) making them potentially effective for treating OA. Despite these findings, only a handful of clinical studies have delved into testing the efficacy of this approach to OA treatment.

5.3 SDF-1

Recently, SDF-1 has received attention in arthritis research. Patients suffering from OA and RA display an increase of this chemokine in their synovial fluid. Although no evidence suggests that chondrocytes produce SDF-1, superficial and deep zone chondrocytes do however express the SDF-1 receptor (CXCR4) (Kanbe et al., 2002). Both synovial fibroblasts and osteoblasts from the subchondral bone produce SDF-1 and so it is also found in the deep zone of cartilage tissue. During OA pathogenesis, macrophages and lymphoid cells that have been localized to the inflamed synovium and/or joint cartilage will produce this chemokine. Since SDF-1 is known for its strong chemotactic abilities attracting lymphocytes to the site of joint inflammation, it has been implicated in enhancing cartilage tissue catabolism. In addition to its chemotactic ability, SDF-1 also stimulates the production of MMP-3 and MMP-13 by interacting with the CXCR4 receptors of articular chondrocytes (Kanbe et al., 2002; Chiu et al., 2007) contributing to collagen and proteoglycan cleavage.

6. Conclusion and future prospects in ECM biology and OA treatment

There are no FDA approved drugs specific for the treatment of OA. Currently, the most effective interventions merely alleviate OA symptoms. The three main interventions available are: (1) Supplements that attempt to enhance the body's endogenous cartilage regenerative capabilities, (2) Drugs that attempt to reduce OA associated pain, and (3) Surgical interventions such as total joint replacement, which is currently the most effective form of relieving the pain and inflammation occuring during the more severe later stages of this degenerative joint disease. Today, total joint replacement is a commonly performed routine surgery. It offers significant and permanent pain relief that other alternative therapies cannot provide, but it remains to be the last resort for late stage OA sufferers.

The use of anti-cytokine therapy to prevent cartilage tissue destruction has recently received attention in OA research. As previously discussed, OA induced ECM destruction most closely associates with induction of the IL-1β and TNF-α pathways. These major inflammatory cytokines stimulate mononuclear cells, synovial fibroblasts, and articular chondrocytes to release IL-6, NO, and chemokines that enhance joint damage. They additionally disregulate the release of anabolic growth factors and tissue destructive proteolytic enzymes from chondrocytes causing major alteration in the process of cartilage homeostasis. Numerous *in vitro* and *in vivo* studies conducted in animal models show that using IL-1Ra protein to inhibit IL-1β pathway activation has promise for preventing OA induced ECM degradation and inflammation. However, in human studies, the efficacy of IL-1 pathway inhibition for the purpose of OA therapy has been somewhat less successful. A paper published in 2009 reported the short-term efficacy of treating OA patients with recombinant IL-1Ra protein (Anakinra), which is a anti-inflammatory drug initially approved by the FDA for the treatment of RA. In this randomized double-blinded study, 160 knee OA sufferers were given 50 to 150 mg of Anakinra via intra-articular injection and their status was monitored for 4 weeks. During this time, knee joint pain was graded using the WOMAC pain index. Although there was no observable difference in cartilage destruction between the 150 mg Anakinra and placebo injected groups, Anakinra did prove to reduce OA associated knee joint pain on the fourth day after treatment. However, given the short half-life of this recombinant protein (approximately 5 hours), it did not have a significant beneficial effect after the fourth day (Chevalier et al., 2009). Similarly, inhibition of IL-1β and IL-1 receptor expression using a synthetic anti-inflammatory analgesic molecule named Diacerein has proved to have similar pain relieving effects with the additional benefit of preventing ECM catabolism to some degree. This drug also seems to have longer lasting therapeutic effects than Anakinra due to its relative stability (Pelletier et al., 2000).

As previously discussed, the intra-articular (or joint) injection of disease modifying ECM proteins such as lubricin and HA have been somewhat effective in reducing inflammation and tissue destruction. Similar use of various growth factors to repair OA induced ECM damage may be another promising avenue that warrants further investigation. Recent studies using "Preparations rich in growth factors" (PRGF), commonly consisting of platelet rich plasma (PRP), have demonstrated the efficacy of combining anabolic and anti-catabolic proteins to deliver a dual beneficial effect that reduces proteolytic ECM breakdown and promotes tissue repair in OA joints. Several studies conducted in the past decade have demonstrated that PRDF treatment reduces joint pain up to 5 weeks post injection while also showing signs that it may enhance regenerative capabilities of cartilage tissue. However, some of anabolic proteins used in these growth factor cocktails (i.e. TGF-β, IGF) are known to already be increased during OA pathogenesis. More studies need to be conducted in order to understand the mode by which such therapies are chondroprotective. Currently the use of PRP for the treatment of knee OA is in Phase 2 of clinical trials.

Localized intra-articular gene therapy is a very exciting and novel approach for treating degenerative joint diseases such as OA and RA. It provides a controlled method to sustain production of potentially therapeutic gene products that cannot be matched by more transient methods such as simple intra-articular injection. Sites of localized gene transfer include the synovium (most common target in past studies) as well as articular cartilage tissue itself. Thus far, gene candidates used for this approach include those that can potentially enhance ECM synthesis and repair and/or prevent ECM breakdown. IL-1Ra is an example of a chondroprotective gene that has been successfully utilized for gene transfer experiments in several animal models. These studies clearly show positive outcomes correlating with its expression within the joint including reduced inflammation and decreased tissue destruction (Calich et al., 2010). IGF-1 is another gene candidate that has been introduced into the knee joints of rabbits via adenovirus mediated gene transfer. These animals experienced enhanced ECM synthesis by the articular cartilage in their knee joints under both normal and inflamed conditions (Mi et al., 2000). The use of gene therapy for the treatment of OA has presented much promise; however, due to issues involving the practicality of its use, we are still a long time away from utilizing its full potential.

7. References

Abbaszade, I., Liu, RQ., Yang, F., Rosenfeld, SA., Ross, OH., Link, JR., et al. (1999). Cloning and characterization of ADAMTS11, an aggrecanase from the ADAMTS family. *J. Biol. Chem.*, Vol. 274, No. 33, (August 1999), pp. 23443–23450. ISSN 0021-9258

Aeschlimann, D., Wetterwald, A., Fleisch, H. & Paulsson, M. (1993). Expression of tissue transglutaminase in skeletal tissues correlates with events of terminal differentiation of chondrocytes. *Journal of Cell Biology*. Vol. 120, No. 6, (March 1993), pp. 1461-70, ISSN 0021-9525

Ahmad, R., Sylvester, J., Ahmad, M. & Zafarullah, M. (2009) Adaptor proteins and Ras synergistically regulate IL-1-induced ADAMTS-4 expression in human chondrocytes. *J. Immunol.*, Vol. 182, No.8 (April 2009), pp. 5081-5087, ISSN 1550-6606

Alexopoulos, LG., Youn, I., Bonaldo, P. & Guilak F. (2009). Developmental and osteoarthritic changes in Col6a1-knockout mice: biomechanics of type VI collagen in the cartilage pericellular matrix. *Arthritis Rheum.*, Vol. 60, No. 3, (March 2009), pp. 771-9, ISSN 0004-3591

Altman, RD. & Moskowitz, R. (1998). Intraarticular sodium hyaluronate (Hyalgan) in the treatment of patients with osteoarthritis of the knee: a randomized clinical trial. Hyalgan Study Group. *J Rheumatol.* Vol. 25, No. 11, (November 1998), pp. 2203-2212. ISSN 0315-162X

Arend, WP. & Gabay, C. (2000) Physiologic role of interleukin-1 receptor antagonist. *Arthritis Res.*, Vol. 2, No. 4, (May 2000), pp. 245-248, ISSN 1465-9905

Baragi, VM., Renkiewicz, RR., Jordan, H., Bonadio, J., Hartman, JW. & Roessler, BJ. (1995).Transplantation of transduced chondrocytes protects articular cartilage from interleukin 1-induced extracellular matrix degradation. *J. Clin. Invest.*, Vol. 96, No. 5, (November 1995), pp. 2454-2460, ISSN 0021-9738

Bewsey, KE., Wen, C., Purple, C. & Homandberg, GA. (1996). Fibronectin fragments induce the expression of stromelysin-1 mRNA and protein in bovine chondrocytes in monolayer culture. *Biochim Biophys Acta.*, Vol. 1317, No. 1, (October 1996), pp. 55-64, ISSN 0006-3002

Bignami, A., Asher, R. & Perides, G. (1992). The extracellular matrix of rat spinal cord: a comparative study on the localization of hyaluronic acid, glial hyaluronate-binding protein, and chondroitin sulfate proteoglycan. *Exp Neurol.*, Vol. 117, No. 1, (July 1992), pp. 90-3, ISSN 0014-4886

Blagg, JA., Noe, MC., Wolf-Gouveia, LA., Reiter, LA., Laird, ER., Chang, SP., et al. (2005) Potent pyrimidinetrione- based inhibitors of MMP-13 with enhanced selectivity over MMP-14. Bioorg. *Med. Chem. Lett.*, Vol. 15, No. 7 (April 2005), pp. 1807-1810, ISSN 0960-894X

Blaschke, UK., Eikenberry, EF., Hulmes, DJ., Galla, HJ. & Bruckner, P. (2000). Collagen XI nucleates self-assembly and limits lateral growth of cartilage fibrils. *J Biol Chem.* Vol. 275, No. 14, (April 2000), pp. 10370-10378, ISSN 0021-9258

Bleasel ,JF., Holderbaum, D., Brancolini, V., Moskowitz, RW., Considine, EL., Prockop, DJ., et al. (1998). Five families with arginine 519-cysteine mutation in COL2A1: evidence for three distinct founders. *Hum Mutat.* Vol. 12, No. 3, (October 1998), pp. 172-176, ISSN 1059-7794

Borochowitz, ZU., Scheffer, D., Adir, V., Dagoneau, N., Munnich, A. & Cormier-Daire, V. (2004) Spondylo-epi-metaphyseal dysplasia (SEMD) matrilin 3 type: homozygote matrilin 3 mutation in a novel form of SEMD. *J. Med. Genet.*, Vol. 41, No. 5, (May 2004), pp. 366–372, ISSN 1468-6244

Byers, PH. (2001). Folding defects in fibrillar collagens. *Philos Trans R Soc Lond B Biol Sci.*, Vol. 356, No. 1406, (February 2001), pp. 151-158, ISSN 0962-8436

Calich, AL., Domiciano, DS. & Fuller, R. (2010). Osteoarthritis: can anti-cytokine therapy play a role in treatment? *Clin Rheumatol.* Vol. 29, No. 5, (January 2010), pp. 451-455, ISSN 1434-9949

Cepko, C. L. Transduction of genes using retrovirus vectors. In: Current Protocols in Molecular Biology, edited by A. F.M., R. Brent, R. Kingston, D. D. Moore, J. G. Seidman, J. A. Smith and K. Struhl. New York: Greene Publishing Associates, 1992, p. 9.10-9.14.

Chen, Q., Fitch, JM., Linsenmayer, C. & Linsenmayer, TF. (1992) Type X collagen: covalent crosslinking to hypertrophic cartilage-collagen fibrils. *Bone & Mineral.* Vol. 17, No. 2, (May 1992), pp. 223-7, ISSN 0169-6009

Chen, Q., Fitch, JM., Gibney, E. & Linsenmayer, TF. (1993). Type II collagen during cartilage and corneal development: immunohistochemical analysis with an anti- telopeptide antibody. *Developmental Dynamics.* Vol. 196, No. 1, (January 1993), pp. 47-53, ISSN 1058-8388

Chen, Q., Zhang, Y., Johnson, DM. & Goetinck, PF. (1999). Assembly of a novel cartilage matrix protein filamentous network: molecular basis of differential requirement of von Willebrand factor A domains. *Mol Biol Cell.* Vol. 10, No. 7, (July 1999) pp. 2149-2162. ISSN 1059-1524

Chen, XD., Fisher, LW., Robey, PG. & Young, MF. (2004). The small leucine-rich proteoglycan biglycan modulates BMP-4-induced osteoblast differentiation. *FASEB J.,* Vol. 18, No. 9, (June 2004), pp. 948-58, ISSN 1530-6860

Chevalier, X., Goupille, P., Beaulieu, AD., Burch, FX., Bensen, WG., Conrozier, T. et al. (2009). Intraarticular injection of anakinra in osteoarthritis of the knee: a multicenter, randomized, double-blind, placebo-controlled study. *Arthritis Rheum.* Vol. 61, No. 3, (March 2009), pp. 344-352, ISSN 0004-3591

Chiu, YC., Yang, RS., Hsieh, KH., Fong, YC., Way, TD. & Lee, TS., (2007). Stromal cell-derived factor-1 induces matrix metalloprotease-13 expression in human chondrocytes. *Mol Pharmacol.,* Vol. 72, No. 3, (September 2007), pp. 695-703, ISSN 0026-895X

Cohen, SB. (2004) The use of anakinra, an interleukin-1 receptor antagonist, in the treatment of rheumatoid arthritis. *Rheum. Dis. Clin. N. Am.,* Vol. 30, No. 2 (May 2004), pp. 365-380, ISSN 0889-857X

Cremer, MA., Rosloniec, EF. & Kang AH. (1988). The cartilage collagens: a review of their structure, organization, and role in the pathogenesis of experimental arthritis in animals and in human rheumatic disease. *J Mol Med.,* Vol. 76, No. 3-4, (March 1988), pp. 275-88, ISSN 0946-2716

Deak, F., Wagener, R., Kiss, I. & Paulsson, M. (1999). The matrilins: a novel family of oligomeric extracellular matrix proteins. *Matrix Biol.,* Vol. 18, No. 1, (February 1999), pp.55–64, ISSN 0945-053X

Devi, GR., Graham, DL., Oh, Y. & Rosenfeld, RG. (2001). Effect of IGFBP-3 on IGF- and IGF-analogue-induced insulin-like growth factor-I receptor (IGFIR) signaling. *Growth Horm IGF Res.,* Vol. 11, No. 4, (August 2001), pp. 231-9, ISSN 1096-6374

Doege, KJ., Sasaki, M., Kimura, T. & Yamada, Y. (1991). Complete coding sequence and deduced primary structure of the human cartilage large aggregating proteoglycan, aggrecan. Human-specific repeats, and additional alternatively spliced forms. *J Biol Chem.,* Vol. 266, No. 2, (January 1991), pp. 894-902, ISSN 0021-9258

Dozier S., Escobar GP. & Lindsey ML. (2006) Matrix metalloproteinase (MMP)-7 activates MMP-8 but not MMP-13. *Med Chem.* Vol. 2, No. 5, (September 2006), pp. 523-526, ISSN 1573-4064

Drummond, AH., Beckett, P., Brown, PD., Bone, EA., Davidson, AH., Galloway, WA., et al. (1999). Preclinical and clinical studies of MMP inhibitors in cancer. *Ann N Y Acad Sci.,* Vol. 878, (June 1999), pp. 228-235, ISSN 0077-8923

Engel, J., Furthmayr, H., Odermatt, E., von der Mark, H., Aumailley, M., Fleischmajer, R., et al. (1985). Structure and macromolecular organization of type VI collagen. *Ann N Y Acad Sci.*, Vol. 460, (December 1985), pp. 25-37, ISSN 0077-8923

Eyre, DR., Weis, MA., & Moskowitz, RW. (1991). Cartilage expression of a type II collagen mutation in an inherited form of osteoarthritis associated with a mild chondrodysplasia. *J Clin Invest.*, Vol. 87, No. 1, (January 1991), pp. 357-361, ISSN 0021-9738

Fernandes, J., Tardif, G., Martel-Pelletier, J., Lascau-Coman, V., Dupuis, M., Moldovan, F., et al. (1999) In vivo transfer of interleukin-1 receptor antagonist gene in osteoarthritic rabbit knee joints: prevention of osteoarthritis progression. *Am. J. Pathol.*, Vol. 154, No. 4, (April 1999), pp.1159-1169, ISSN 0002-9440

Fichter, M., Korner, U., Schomburg, J., Jennings, L., Cole, AA., & Mollenhauer, J. (2006). Collagen degradation products modulate matrix metalloproteinase expression in cultured articular chondrocytes. *J Orthop Res.* Vol. 24, No. 1, (January 2006), pp. 63-70, ISSN 0736-0266

Fosang, AJ., Neame, PJ., Hardingham, TE., Murphy, G. & Hamilton, JA. (1991). Cleavage of cartilage proteoglycan between G1 and G2 domains by stromelysins. *J Biol Chem.* Vol. 266, No. 24, (August 1991), pp. 15579-15582, ISSN 0021-9258

Furthmayr, H., Wiedemann, H., Timpl, R., Odermatt, E. & Engel, J. (1983). Electron-microscopical approach to a structural model of intima collagen. *Biochem J. Vol.* 211, No. 2, (May 1983), pp. 303-311, ISSN 0264-6021

Gabay, C., Lamacchia, C. & Palmer, G. (2010). IL-1 pathways in inflammation and human diseases. Nat. Rev. *Rheumatol.*, Vol. 6, No. 4, (April 2010), pp. 232-41, ISSN 1759-4804

Glasson, SS., Askew, R., Sheppard, B., Carito, B., Blanchet, T., Ma, HL., et al. (2005) Depletion of active ADAMTS5 prevents cartilage degradation in murine model of osteoarthritis. *Nature.* Vol. 434, No. 7033 (March 2005), pp. 644-648, ISSN 1476-4687

Goldring, MB., Birkhead, J., Sandell, LJ., Kimura, T. & Krane, SM. (1988) Interleukin 1 suppresses expression of cartilage-specific types II and IX collagens and increases types I and III collagens in human chondrocytes. *J. Clin. Invest.*,Vol. 82, No. 6, (December 1988), pp. 2026-2037, ISSN 0021-9738

Goldring, MB. & Marcu, KB. (2009). Cartilage homeostasis in health and rheumatic diseases. *Arthritis Res Ther.* Vol. 11, No. 3, (May 2009), pp. 224, ISSN 1478-6362

Gregory, KE., Oxford, JT., Chen, Y., Gambee, JE., Gygi, SP., Aebersold, R., et al. (2000). Structural organization of distinct domains within the non-collagenous N-terminal region of collagen type XI. *J Biol Chem.* Vol. 275, No. 15, (April 2000), pp. 11498-11506, ISSN 0021-9258

Guévremont, M., Martel-Pelletier, J., Massicotte, F., Tardif, G., Pelletier, JP., Ranger, P., et al. (2003). Human adult chondrocytes express hepatocyte growth factor (HGF) isoforms but not HgF: potential implication of osteoblasts on the presence of HGF in cartilage. *J Bone Miner Res.*, Vol. 18, No. 6, (June 2003), pp. 1073-81, ISSN 0884-0431

Guo, D., Ding, L. & Homandberg, GA. (2009). Telopeptides of type II collagen upregulate proteinases and damage cartilage but are less effective than highly active fibronectin fragments. *Inflamm Res.*, Vol. 58, No. 3, (March 2009), pp. 161-9, ISSN 1420-908X

Homandberg, GA., Meyers, R. & Williams, JM. (1993). Intraarticular injection of fibronectin fragments causes severe depletion of cartilage proteoglycans in vivo. *J Rheumatol.* Vol. 20, No. 8, (August 1993), pp. 1378-1382, ISSN 0315-162X

Homandberg, GA. & Hui, F. (1994). Arg-Gly-Asp-Ser peptide analogs suppress cartilage chondrolytic activities of integrin-binding and nonbinding fibronectin fragments. *Arch Biochem Biophys.* Vol. 310, No. 1, (April 1994), pp. 40-48, ISSN 0003-9861

Hu, K., Xu, L., Cao, L., Flahiff, CM., Brussiau, J., Ho, K., et al. (2006). Pathogenesis of osteoarthritis-like changes in the joints of mice deficient in type IX collagen. *Arthritis Rheum.* Vol. 54, No. 9, (September 2006), pp. 2891-2900, ISSN 0004-3591

Ikegawa, S., Nishimura, G., Nagai, T., Hasegawa, T., Ohashi, H., Nakamura, Y. et al. (1998). Mutation of the type X collagen gene (COL10A1) causes spondylometaphyseal dysplasia. *Am J Hum Genet.*, Vol. 63, No. 6, (December 1998), pp. 1659-62, ISSN 0002-9297

Imai, K., Ohta, S., Matsumoto, T., Fujimoto, N., Sato, H., Seiki, M., et al. (1997). Expression of membrane-type 1 matrix metalloproteinase and activation of progelatinase A in human osteoarthritic cartilage. *Am. J. Pathol.*, Vol. 15, No. 1, (July 1997), pp. 245-256, ISSN 0002-9440

Jacenko O, LuValle PA & Olsen BR. (1993). Spondylometaphyseal dysplasia in mice carrying a dominant negative mutation in a matrix protein specific for cartilage-to-bone transition. *Nature.* Vol. 365, No. 6441, (September 1993), pp. 56-61, ISSN 0028-0836

Jackson, GC., Marcus-Soekarman, D., Stolte-Dijkstra, I., Verrips, A., Taylor, JA. & Briggs, MD. (2010). Type IX collagen gene mutations can result in multiple epiphyseal dysplasia that is associated with osteochondritis dissecans and a mild myopathy. *Am J Med Genet A.*, Vol. 152A, No. 4, (April 2010), pp. 863-9, ISSN 1552-4833

Jacques, C., Gosset, M., Berenbaum, F. & Gabay, C. (2006). The role of IL-1 and IL-1Ra in joint inflammation and cartilage degradation. *Vitam. Horm.*, Vol. 74, (December 2006), pp. 371-403, ISSN 0083-6729

Julovi, SM., Yasuda, T., Shimizu, M., Hiramitsu, T., & Nakamura, T. (2004). Inhibition of interleukin-1beta-stimulated production of matrix metalloproteinases by hyaluronan via CD44 in human articular cartilage. *Arthritis Rheum.* Vol. 50, No. 2, (February 2004), pp. 516-525, ISSN 0004-3591

Kamekura, S., Hoshi, K., Shimoaka, T., Chung, U., Chikuda, H., Yamada, T., et al. (2005) Osteoarthritis development in novel experimental mouse models induced by knee joint instability. *Osteoarthritis Cartil.*, Vol. 13, No. 7 (July 2005), pp. 632-641, ISSN 1063-4584

Kanbe, K., Takagishi, K. & Chen, Q. (2002). Stimulation of matrix metalloprotease 3 release from human chondrocytes by the interaction of stromal cell-derived factor 1 and CXC chemokine receptor 4. *Arthritis Rheum.*, Vol. 46, No. 1, (January 2002), pp. 130-7, ISSN 0004-3591

Klatt, AR., Nitsche, DP., Kobbe, B., Mörgelin, M., Paulsson, M. & Wagener, R. (2000) Molecular structure and   tissue distribution of matrilin-3, a filament-forming extracellular matrix protein expressed during skeletal   development. *Journal of Biological Chemistry.* Vol. 275, No. 6, (February 2000), pp. 3999-4006, ISSN 0021-9258

Klatt, AR., Nitsche, DP., Kobbe, B., Macht, M., Paulsson, M. & Wagener, R. (2001). Molecular structure, processing, and tissue distribution of matrilin-4. *J. Biol. Chem.*, Vol. 276, No. 20, (May 2001), pp. 17267-17275, ISSN 0021-9258

Kuivaniemi, H., Tromp, G., & Prockop, DJ. (1997). Mutations in fibrillar collagens (types I, II, III, and XI), fibril-associated collagen (type IX), and network-forming collagen (type X) cause a spectrum of diseases of bone, cartilage, and blood vessels. *Hum Mutat.*, Vol. 9, No. 4, (June 1997), pp. 300-315, ISSN 1059-7794

Kuno, K., Okada, Y., Kawashima, H., Nakamura, H., Miyasaka, M., Ohno, H., et al. (2000) ADAMTS-1 cleaves a cartilage proteoglycan, aggrecan. *FEBS Lett.*, Vol. 478, No. 3 (August 2000), pp. 241–245, ISSN 0014-5793

Lamandé, SR., Bateman, JF., Hutchison, W., McKinlay Gardner, RJ., Bower, SP., Byrne E., et al. (1998). Reduced collagen VI causes Bethlem myopathy: a heterozygous COL6A1 nonsense mutation results in mRNA decay and functional haploinsufficiency. *Hum Mol Genet.*, Vol. 7, No. 6 (June 1998), pp. 981-9, ISSN 0964-6906

Li, SW., Prockop, DJ., Helminen, H., Fässler, R., Lapveteläinen, T., Kiraly, K., et al. (1995). Transgenic mice with targeted inactivation of the Col2 alpha 1 gene for collagen II develop a skeleton with membranous and periosteal bone but no endochondral bone. *Genes Dev.*, Vol. 9, No. 22, (November 1995), pp. 2821-2830, ISSN 0890-9369

Li, Y., Lacerda, DA., Warman, ML., Beier, DR., Yoshioka, H., Ninomiya, Y., et al. (1995). A fibrillar collagen gene, Col11a1, is essential for skeletal morphogenesis. *Cell*, Vol. 80, No. 3, (February 1995), pp. 423-30, ISSN 0092-8674

Linsenmayer, TF., Eavey, RD. & Schmid, TM. (1988). Type X collagen: a hypertrophic cartilage-specific molecule. *Pathol Immunopathol Res.*, Vol. 7, No. 1-2, (1988), pp. 14-9, ISSN 0257-2761

Marks, PH. & Donaldson, ML. (2005) Inflammatory cytokine profiles associated with chondral damage in the anterior cruciate ligament-deficient knee. *Arthroscopy.* Vol. 21, No. 11, (November 2005), pp.1342-1347, ISSN 1526-3231

Martel-Pelletier, J., Boileau, C., Pelletier, JP. & Roughley, PJ. (2008). Cartilage in normal and osteoarthritis conditions. *Best Pract Res Clin Rheumatol.* Vol. 22, No. 2, (April 2008), pp. 351-384, ISSN 1521-6942

Mi, Z., Ghivizzani, SC., Lechman, ER., Jaffurs, D., Glorioso, JC., Evans, CH. et al. (2000). Adenovirus-mediated gene transfer of insulin-like growth factor 1 stimulates proteoglycan synthesis in rabbit joints. *Arthritis Rheum.* Vol. 43, No. 11, (November 2000), pp. 2563-2570, ISSN 0004-3591

Mitchell, PG., Magna, HA., Reeves, LM., Lopresti-Morrow, LL., Yocum, SA., Rosner, PJ., et al. (1996) Cloning, expression, and type II collagenolytic activity of matrix metalloproteinase-13 from human osteoarthritic cartilage. *J. Clin. Invest.*, Vol. 97, No. 3 (February 1996), pp. 761-768, ISSN 0021-9738

Mohtai,M., Smith, RL., Schurman, DJ., Tsuji, Y., Torti, FM., Hutchinson, NI., et al. (1993). Expression of 92-kD type IV collagenase/gelatinase (gelatinase B) in osteoarthritic cartilage and its induction in normal human articular cartilage by interleukin 1. *J. Clin. Invest.*, Vol. 92, No. 1, (July 1993), pp. 179-185, ISSN 0021-9738

Moreland, LW . (2003). Intra-articular hyaluronan (hyaluronic acid) and hylans for the treatment of osteoarthritis: mechanisms of action. *Arthritis Res Ther.* Vol 5, No. 2, (January 2003), pp. 54-67. ISSN 1478-6362

Murakami ,S., Lefebvre, V. & de Crombrugghe, B. (2000). Potent Inhibition of the Master Chondrogenic FactorSox9 Gene by Interleukin-1 and Tumor Necrosis Factor-α. *J. Biol. Chem.*, Vol. 275, No. 5, (February 2000), pp. 3687-92 , ISSN 0021-9258

Nakamura, H., Fujii, Y., Ohuchi, E., Yamamoto, E. & Okada, Y. (1998). Activation of the precursor of human stromelysin 2 and its interactions with other matrix metalloproteinases. *Eur J Biochem.* Vol. 253, No. 1, (April 1998), pp. 67-75, ISSN 0014-2956

Nicholson, R., Murphy, G. & Breathnach R. (1989). Human and rat malignant-tumor-associated mRNAs encode stromelysin-like metalloproteinases. *Biochemistry.* Vol. 28, No. 12, (June 1989), pp. 5195-5203, ISSN 0006-2960

Nicklin, MJ., Hughes, DE., Barton, JL., Ure, JM. & Duff, GW. (2000) Arterial inflammation in mice lacking the interleukin 1 receptor antagonist gene. *J. Exp. Med.*, Vol. 191, No. 2 (January 2000), pp. 303-312, ISSN 0022- 1007

Nuka, S., Zhou, W., Henry, SP., Gendron, CM., Schultz, JB., Shinomura, T., et al. (2010). Phenotypic characterization of epiphycan-deficient and epiphycan/biglycan double-deficient mice. *Osteoarthritis Cartilage.* Vol. 18, No. 1, (January 2010), pp. 88-96, ISSN 1522-9653

Nwomeh, BC., Liang, HX., Diegelmann, RF., Cohen, IK. & Yager, DR. (2002) Dynamics of the matrix metalloproteinases MMP-1 and MMP-8 in acute open human dermal wounds. *Wound Repair and Regeneration.* Vol. 6, No. 2, (March-April 2002), pp. 127-134, ISSN 1067-1927

Ohta, S., Imai, K., Yamashita, K., Matsumoto, T., Azumano, I. & Okada, Y. (1998) Expression of matrix metalloproteinase 7 (matrilysin) in human osteoarthritic cartilage. *Lab. Invest.*, Vol. 78, No. 1, (January 1998), pp. 79-87, ISSN 0023-6837

Okada, Y., Konomi, H., Yada, T., Kimata, K., and Nagase, H. (1989). Degradation of type IX collagen by matrix metalloproteinase 3 (stromelysin) from human rheumatoid synovial cells. FEBS Lett., Vol. 244, No. 2, (February 1989), pp. 473-476, ISSN 0014-5793

Okada, Y., Shinmei, M., Tanaka, O., Naka, K., Kimura, A., Nakanishi, I., et al. (1992). Localization of matrix metalloproteinase 3 (stromelysin) in osteoarthritic cartilage and synovium. *Lab. Invest.*, Vol. 66, No. 6, (June 1992), pp. 680-690, ISSN 0023-6837

Otten, C., Wagener, R., Paulsson, M. & Zaucke, F. (2005) Matrilin-3 mutations that cause chondrodysplasias interfere with protein trafficking while a mutation associated with hand osteoarthritis does not. *J. Med. Genet.*, Vol. 42, No. 10, (October 2005), pp. 774-779, ISSN 1468-6244

Pace, RA., Peat, RA., Baker, NL., Zamurs, L., Mörgelin, M., Irving, M., et al. (2008). Collagen VI glycine mutations: perturbed assembly and a spectrum of clinical severity. *Ann Neurol.*, Vol. 64, No. 3, (September 2008), pp. 294-303, ISSN 1531-8249

Park, MY., Jang, HD., Lee, SY., Lee, KJ. & Kim, E. (2004). Fas-associated factor-1 inhibits nuclear factor-kappaB (NF-kappaB) activity by interfering with nuclear translocation of the RelA (p65) subunit of NF-kappaB. *J Biol Chem.* Vol. 279, No. 4, (January 2004), pp. 2544-2549, ISSN 0021-9258

Pattoli, MA., MacMaster, JF., Gregor, KR. & Burke, JR. (2005) Collagen and aggrecan degradation is blocked in interleukin-1-treated cartilage explants by an inhibitor of

IkappaB kinase through suppression of metalloproteinase expression. *J. Pharmacol. Exp. Ther.*, Vol. 315, No. 1, (October 2005), pp. 382-388, ISSN 0022-3565

Pelletier, JP., Yaron, M., Haraoui, B., Cohen, P., Nahir, MA., Choquette, D. et al. (2000). Efficacy and safety of diacerein in osteoarthritis of the knee: a double-blind, placebo-controlled trial. The Diacerein Study Group. *Arthritis Rheum.* Vol. 43, No. 10, (October 2000), pp. 2339-2348, ISSN 0004-3591

Piecha, D., Muratoglu, S., Mörgelin, M., Hauser, N., Studer, D., Kiss, I. et al. (1999) Matrilin-2, a large, oligomeric matrix protein, is expressed by a great variety of cells and forms fibrillar networks. *J. Biol. Chem.*, Vol. 274, No. 19, (May 1999), pp. 13353-13361, ISSN 0021-9258

Piecha, D., Hartmann, K., Kobbe, B., Haase, I., Mauch, C., Krieg, T., et al. (2002) Expression of Matrilin-2 in Human Skin. *Journal of Investigative Dermatology.* Vol. 119, No. 1 (July 2002), pp. 38-43. ISSN 0022-202X

Pratta, MA., Yao, W., Decicco, C., Tortorella, MD., Liu, RQ., Copeland, RA., et al. (2003). Aggrecan protects cartilage collagen from proteolytic cleavage. *J Biol Chem.*, Vol. 278, No. 46, (November 2003), pp. 45539-45, ISSN 0021-9258

Prockop, DJ., Ala-Kokko, L., McLain, DA., & Williams, C. (1997). Can mutated genes cause common osteoarthritis? *Br J Rheumatol.*, Vol. 36, No. 8, (August 1997), pp. 827-829, ISSN 0263-7103

Pullig, O., Weseloh, G. & Swoboda, B. (1999). Expression of type VI collagen in normal and osteoarthritic human cartilage. *Osteoarthritis Cartilage*, Vol. 7, No. 2, (March 1999), pp. 191-202, ISSN 1063-4584

Pullig, O., Weseloh, G., Klatt, AR., Wagener, R. & Swoboda, B. (2002) Matrilin-3 in human articular cartilage: increased expression in osteoarthritis. *Osteoarthritis Cartilage.*, Vol. 10 No. 4, (April 2002) pp. 253-263, ISSN 1063-4584

Pun, YL., Moskowitz, RW., Lie, S., Sundstrom, WR., Block, SR., McEwen, C., et al. (1994). Clinical correlations of osteoarthritis associated with a single-base mutation (arginine519 to cysteine) in type II procollagen gene. A newly defined pathogenesis. *Arthritis Rheum.* Vol. 37, No. 2, (February 1994), pp. 264-269, ISSN 0004-3591

Rechardt, O., Elomaa, O., Vaalamo, M., Pääkkönen, K., Jahkola, T., Höök-Nikanne, J., et al. (2000). Stromelysin-2 is upregulated during normal wound repair and is induced by cytokines. *J Invest Dermatol.* Vol. 115, No. 5, (November 2000), pp. 778-787, ISSN 0022-202X

Rhee, DK., Marcelino, J., Al-Mayouf, S., Schelling, DK., Bartels, CF., Cui, Y., et al. (2005). Consequences of disease- causing mutations on lubricin protein synthesis, secretion, and post-translational processing. *J Biol Chem.*, Vol. 280, No. 35, (September 2005), pp. 31325-32, ISSN 0021-9258

Rodriguez, RR., Seegmiller, RE., Stark, MR. & Bridgewater, LC. (2004). A type XI collagen mutation leads to increased degradation of type II collagen in articular cartilage. *Osteoarthritis Cartilage*, Vol. 12, No. 4, (April 2004), pp. 314-20, ISSN 1063-4584

Rodríguez-Manzaneque, JC., Westling, J., Thai, SN., Luque, A., Knauper, V., Murphy, G., et al. (2002) ADAMTS1 cleaves aggrecan at multiple sites and is differentially inhibited by metalloproteinase inhibitors. *Biochem. Biophys. Res. Commun.*, Vol. 293, No. 1, (April 2002), pp. 501-508, ISSN 0006-291X

Rosenberg ,K., Olsson, H., Mörgelin, M. & Heinegård, D. (1998). Cartilage oligomeric matrix protein shows high affinity zinc-dependent interaction with triple helical collagen. *J Biol Chem.*, Vol. 273, No. 32, (August 1998), pp. 20397-403, ISSN 0021-9258

Scharstuhl, A., Glansbeek, HL., van Beuningen, HM., Vitters, EL., van der Kraan, PM. & van den Berg, WB. (2002). Inhibition of endogenous TGF-beta during experimental osteoarthritis prevents osteophyte formation and impairs cartilage repair. *J Immunol.*, Vol. 169, No. 1, (July 2002), pp. 507-14, ISSN 0022-1767

Soltés, L., Kogan, G., Stankovska, M., Mendichi, R., Rychlý, J., Schiller, J., et al. (2007). Degradation of high-molar-mass hyaluronan and characterization of fragments. *Biomacromolecules.*, Vol. 8, No. 9, (September 2007), pp. 2697-705, ISSN 1525-7797

Stanton, H., Rogerson, FM., East, CJ., Golub, SB., Lawlor, KE., Meeker, CT., et al. (2005) ADAMTS5 is the major aggrecanase in mouse cartilage in vivo and in vitro. *Nature.* Vol. 434, No. 7033, (March 2005), pp. 648-652, ISSN 1476-4687

Stefánsson, SE., Jónsson, H., Ingvarsson, T., Manolescu, I., Jónsson, HH., Olafsdóttir, G., et al. (2003) Genomewide scan for hand osteoarthritis: a novel mutation in matrilin-3. *Am. J. Hum. Genet.*, Vol. 72, No. 6, (June 2003), pp.1448–1459, ISSN 0002-9297

Stremme, S., Duerr, S., Bau, B., Schmid, E. & Aigner, T. (2003). MMP-8 is only a minor gene product of human adult articular chondrocytes of the knee. *Clin Exp Rheumatol.*, Vol. 21, No. 2, (March-April 2003), pp. 205-9, ISSN 0392-856X

Svensson, L., Närlid, I. & Oldberg, A. (2000). Fibromodulin and lumican bind to the same region on collagen type I fibrils. *FEBS Lett.*, Vol. 470, No. 2, (March 2000), pp. 178-82, ISSN 0014-5793

Tahiri, K., Korwin-Zmijowska, C., Richette, P., Héraud, F., Chevalier, X., Savouret, JF., et al. (2008) Natural chondroitin sulphates increase aggregation of proteoglycan complexes and decrease ADAMTS-5 expression in interleukin 1 beta-treated chondrocytes. *Ann. Rheum. Dis.*, Vol. 67, No. 5, (May 2008), pp. 696-702, ISSN 1468-2060

Takaishi, H., Kimura, T., Dalal, S., Okada, Y. & D'Armiento, J. (2008) Joint diseases and matrix metalloproteinases: a role for MMP-13. *Current Pharm. Biotech.*, Vol. 9, No. 1 (February 2008), pp. 47-54, ISSN 1873-4316

Theuns, DA., Rivero-Ayerza, M., Goedhart, DM., Miltenburg, M. & Jordaens, LJ. (2008). Morphology discrimination in implantable cardioverter-defibrillators: consistency of template match percentage during atrial tachyarrhythmias at different heart rates. *Europace.*, Vol. 10, No. 9, (September 2008), pp. 1060-6, ISSN 1532-2092

Toegel, S., Wu, SQ., Piana, C., Unger, FM., Wirth, M., Goldring, MB., et al. (2008) Comparison between chondroprotective effects of glucosamine, curcumin, and diacerein in IL-1β-stimulated C-28/I2 chondrocytes. *Osteoarthritis and Cartilage.* Vol. 16, No. 10, (October 2008), pp. 1205-1212, ISSN 1522-9653

Tortorella, MD., Burn, TC., Pratta, MA., Abbaszade, I., Hollis, JM., Liu ,R., et al. (1999) Purification and cloning of aggrecanase-1: amember of the ADAMTS family of proteins. *Science.*Vol. 284, No. 5420, (June 1999), pp.1664–1666, ISSN 0036-8075

van Beuningen, HM., Glansbeek, HL., van der Kraan, PM. & van den Berg, WB. (2000) Osteoarthritis-like changes in the murine knee joint resulting from intra-articular transforming growth factor-beta injections. *Osteoarthritis and Cartilage.* Vol. 8, No. 1, (January 2000), pp. 25-33, ISSN 1063-4584 van der Weyden, L., Wei, L., Luo, J., Yang, X., Birk, DE., Adams, DJ., et al. (2006) Functional knockout of the matrilin- 3 gene causes premature chondrocyte maturation to hypertrophy and increases bone mineral density and osteoarthritis. *American Journal of Pathology*. Vol. 169, No. 2, (August 2006), pp. 515-527, ISSN 0002-9440

Vikkula, M., Mariman, EC., Lui, VC., Zhidkova, NI., Tiller, GE., Goldring, MB., et al. (1995). Autosomal dominant and recessive osteochondrodysplasias associated with the COL11A2 locus. *Cell*. Vol. 80, No. 3, (February 1995), pp. 431-437, ISSN 0092-8674

von der Mark, K., Kirsch, T., Nerlich, A., Kuss, A., Weseloh, G., Glückert, K., et al. (1992). Type X collagen synthesis in human osteoarthritic cartilage. Indication of chondrocyte hypertrophy. *Arthritis Rheum.*, Vol. 35, No. 7, (July 1992) pp. 806- 11, ISSN 0004-3591

Vuolteenaho, K., Moilanen, T., Hämäläinen, M., & Moilanen, E. (2002). Effects of TNFalpha-antagonists on nitric oxide production in human cartilage. *Osteoarthritis Cartilage*, Vol. 10, No. 4, (April 2002), pp. 327-32, ISSN 1063-4584

Wagener, R., Kobbe, B., & Paulsson, M. (1997). Primary structure of matrilin-3, a new member of a family of extracellular matrix proteins related to cartilage matrix protein (matrilin-1) and von Willebrand factor. *FEBS Lett.*, Vol. 413, No. 1, (August 1997), pp. 129–134, ISSN 0014-5793

Wagner, K., Pöschl, E., Turnay, J., Baik, J., Pihlajaniemi, T., Frischholz, S., et al. (2000). Coexpression of alpha and beta subunits of prolyl 4-hydroxylase stabilizes the triple helix of recombinant human type X collagen. *Biochem J.*, Vol. 352, No. 3 (December 2000), pp. 907-11, ISSN 0264-6021

Wang, CT., Lin, YT., Chiang, BL., Lin, YH. & Hou, SM. (2006). High molecular weight hyaluronic acid down-regulates the gene expression of osteoarthritis- associated cytokines and enzymes in fibroblast-like synoviocytes from patients with early osteoarthritis. *Osteoarthritis Cartilage*. Vol. 14, No 14, (December 2006), pp. 1237-1247, ISSN 1063-4584

Wehrli, BM., Huang, W., De Crombrugghe, B., Ayala, AG. & Czerniak, B. (2003) Sox9, a master regulator of chondrogenesis, distinguishes mesenchymal chondrosarcoma from other small blue round cell tumors. *Hum. Pathol.*, Vol. 34, No. 3, (March 2003), pp. 263-269, ISSN 0046-8177

Wesche, H., Korherr, C., Kracht, M., Falk, W., Resch, K., & Martin, MU. (1997). The interleukin-1 receptor accessory protein (IL-1RAcP) is essential for IL-1-induced activation of interleukin-1 receptor-associated kinase (IRAK) and stress-activated protein kinases (SAP kinases). *J. Biol. Chem.*, Vol. 272, No. 12, (March 1997), pp. 7727-31, ISSN 0021-9258

Williams, FM. & Spector, TD. (2008). Biomarkers in osteoarthritis. *Arthritis Res Ther.* Vol. 10, No. 1, (January 2008), pp. 101, ISSN 1478-6362

Wobig, M., Dickhut, A., Maier, R. & Vetter, G. (1998) Viscosupplementation with hylan G-F 20: a 26-week controlled trial of efficacy and safety in the osteoarthritic knee. *Clin Ther.* Vol. 20, No. 3, (June 1998), pp. 410-423. ISSN 0149-2918

Wu, J., Rush, TS 3rd., Hotchandani, R., Du, X., Geck, M., Collins, E., et al. (2005) Identification of potent and selective MMP-13 inhibitors. *Bioorg. Med. Chem. Lett.*, Vol. 15, No. 18, (September 2005), pp. 4105-4109, 0960-894X

Wu, JJ., Woods, PE. & Eyre, DR. (1992). Identification of cross-linking sites in bovine cartilage type IX collagen reveals an antiparallel type II-type IX molecular relationship and type IX to type IX bonding. *J Biol Chem.*, Vol. 267, No. 32, (November 1992), pp. 23007-14, ISSN 0021-9258

Wu, JJ. & Eyre, DR. (1998) Matrilin-3 forms disulfide-linked oligomers with matrilin-1 in bovine epiphyseal cartilage. *J. of Biol. Chem.* Vol. 273, No. 28, (July 1998), pp. 17433-17438 ISSN 0021-9258

Xie, D. & Homandberg, GA. (1993). Fibronectin fragments bind to and penetrate cartilage tissue resulting in proteinase expression and cartilage damage. *Biochim Biophys Acta.* Vol. 1182, No. 2, (September 1993), pp. 189-196, ISSN 0006-3002

Zhu, Y., Wu, JJ., Weis, MA., Mirza, SK. & Eyre, DR. (2011). Type IX Collagen Neo-Deposition in Degenerative Discs of Surgical Patients Whether Genotyped Plus or Minus for COL9 Risk Alleles. *Spine* (Phila Pa 1976)., Epub ahead of print. (February 2011), ISSN 1528-1159

3

Simple Method Using Gelatin-Coated Film for Comprehensively Assaying Gelatinase Activity in Synovial Fluid

Akihisa Kamataki[1], Wataru Yoshida[1], Mutsuko Ishida[1],
Kenya Murakami[1], Kensuke Ochi[2] and Takashi Sawai[1]
[1]Iwate Medical University,
[2]Kawasaki Municipal Kawasaki Hospital
Japan

1. Introduction

Rheumatoid arthritis (RA) is a chronic inflammatory disease that leads to the irreversible destruction of cartilage and bone. An important step in the destruction of tissue is the degradation of extracellular matrix (ECM), whose major components are type II collagen and aggrecan in cartilage, and type I collagen in bone. The synovial fluid of RA patients often contains high concentrations of proteinases, such as those of the matrix metalloproteinase (MMP) and a disintegrin-like and metalloproteinase with thrombospondin type 1 motif (ADAMTS) families, which induce ECM degradation either directly or indirectly and participate in joint destruction. MMP-1, MMP-8, and MMP-13, which function as collagenases, have proteolytic activity towards type I and type II collagen (Chakraborti et al., 2003; Murphy & Nagase, 2008). MMP-2 and MMP-9, termed gelatinases, degrade denatured collagen, while MMP-3 degrades several ECM proteins (Chakraborti et al., 2003). All of them have the gelatinase activity. ADAMTS-4 and ADAMTS-5 are major enzymes involved in the degradation of aggrecan (Arner, 2002) and have low levels of gelatinase activity (Gendron et al., 2007; Lauer-Fields et al., 2007).

The concentration and activity of MMP and ADAMTS enzymes in synovial fluid and serum are measurable using ELISA or enzyme-specific substrates. In particular, MMP-3 is often the target of laboratory tests as a biomarker for disease progression. However, for the elucidation of actual RA progression, it is important to measure the comprehensive activity of all enzymes.

In situ zymography is a method for assessing endogenous protease activity in tissue section (Yan & Blomme, 2003). Film *in situ* zymography (FIZ) using gelatin-coated film is a useful method for assessing the enzymes involved in arthritis (Yoshida et al., 2009). In this method, a frozen tissue section is adhered onto a gelatin-coated film and gelatin degradation loci on the film are then analyzed after a suitable incubation period. A locus of gelatin degradation represents an area where comprehensive enzymatic activity is high. This chapter describes a method for assaying the comprehensive gelatinase activity in synovial fluid using gelatin-coated films for FIZ.

2. Method for synovial fluid analysis using gelatin-coated film

2.1 Synovial fluid samples

Synovial fluid samples were obtained from RA patients, osteoarthritis (OA) patients. Patients provided written consent for collection of synovial fluid samples before the procedure. All RA patients fulfilled the American College of Rheumatology criteria for the classification of RA. OA was diagnosed according to clinical findings. All the OA samples we examined were grade III or IV according to the Kellgren/Lawrence radiographic grading system. This study were approved by the ethics committees at Iwate Medical University

2.2 Method

Gelatin-coated film (Zymo-film; Fuji Film Co., Tokyo, Japan) is adhered onto a slide glass and a silicon gasket with 12 wells (flexi PERM; Greiner Bio-One GmbH, Frickenhausen, Germany) is then attached onto the film using Vaseline (Fig. 1). Two-hundred microliters of a two-fold serial dilution of synovial fluid sample is added into each well. To prevent the sample from evaporating, a lid is placed on the gasket and a moist chamber is used for the incubation period. After overnight incubation at 37 °C, the gelatin-coated film is washed twice with PBS, stained with a 0.2% Ponceau S solution, and then dried at room temperature (Fig. 2).

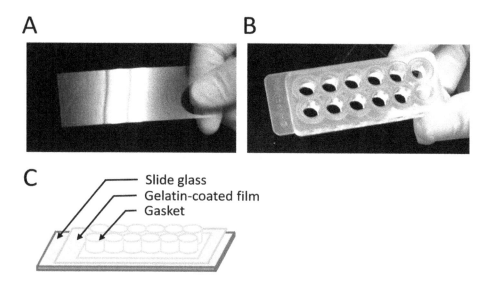

A: gelatin-coated film, B: gasket, C: illustration of the assembled detection system

Fig. 1. Gelatin-coated film and gasket

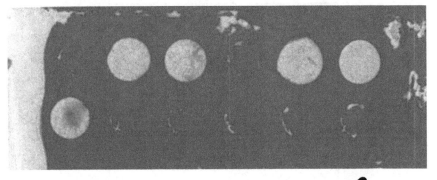

Gelatin-degraded spots are optically transparent. In this case, gelatinase activity was detected in the synovial fluid samples diluted up to 1:4.

Fig. 2. Ponceau S stained gelatin-coated film

PBS is used as a negative control, and a trypsin solution (1 and 10 μg/ml) is used as a positive control. To lower the viscosity of the synovial fluid, 15 units/μl hyaluronidase from *Streptomyces hyalyticus* (Sigma-Aldrich, St. Louis, MO, USA) is added to the synovial fluid samples. As p-aminophenylmercuric acetate (APMA) activates MMPs (Nagase et al., 1990, 1991), APMA is also added to the samples.

We demonstrated that six synovial fluid samples obtained from RA patients did not show gelatin degradation without APMA treatment (Fig. 3A, left, and Fig. 3B). However, treatment of the same samples with a final concentration of 1 mM APMA resulted in gelatin degradation (Fig. 3A, right, and Fig. 3B).

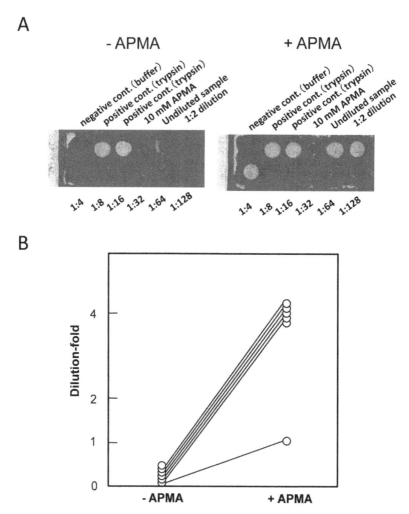

A. Gelatin-coated film incubated with synovial fluid treated with (right) and without (left) APMA. Without APMA treatment, even undiluted sample did not degrade the coated gelatin. With APMA treatment, samples diluted up to 1:4 showed gelatinase activity.

B. Change of gelatinase activity for six synovial fluid samples from RA patients following APMA treatment. The vertical axis shows the highest dilution-fold of samples that was positive for gelatinase activity. Zero indicates negative gelatinase activity.

Fig. 3. Gelatinase activity in synovial fluid samples with or without APMA treatment.

The optimal incubation time for the detection of gelatinase activity was determined by incubating synovial fluid samples for 3, 6, 12, 18, and 24 h on the gelatin-coated film. Only low levels of degradation levels were detected at 3 and 6 h (data not shown). The degradation levels at 18 and 24 h were constant for many samples (Fig. 4). In only one of seven samples, the degradation levels were elevated from 18 to 24 h. In the following experiments, the incubation time was fixed at 24 h.

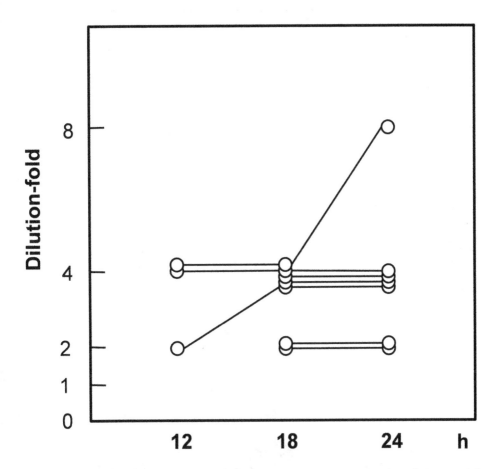

The vertical axis shows the highest dilution-fold of samples that was positive for gelatinase activity. Zero indicates negative gelatinase activity. Gelatin-coated films with synovial fluid samples were incubated for 12, 18, and 24 h.

Fig. 4. Gelatin degradation levels at various incubation times.

3. Comparison of gelatinase activity of RA and OA synovial fluid

Osteoarthritis (OA) is a disease of the joints and is caused by mechanical stress and an imbalance between catabolic and anabolic activities for cartilage (Sun, 2010). Although OA has a different etiology from RA, their mechanisms of pathogenesis are partly shared, with MMPs and ADAMTSs also playing a role in the development of OA (Huang & Wu, 2008; Murphy & Nagase, 2008; Sun, 2010). Therefore, the gelatinase activities of synovial fluid from RA and OA patients were analyzed and compared using the gelatin-coated film assay method. The synovial fluid from RA patients displayed higher proteinase activity than that from OA patients (Fig. 5), a result that is consistent with a previous study (Mahmoud et al., 2005).

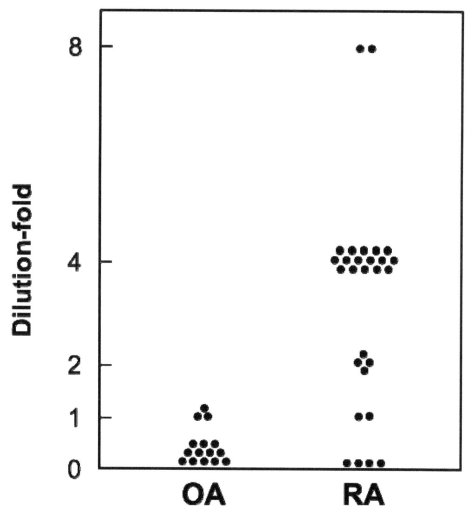

The vertical axis indicates the highest dilution-fold of sample that was positive for gelatinase activity. A value of zero indicates negative gelatinase activity. While only 3 of 15 (20%) samples from OA patients exhibited gelatinase activity, activity was detected in 24 of 28 (86%) samples from RA patients. Gelatinase activity was detected in two samples from RA patients diluted 1:8.

Fig. 5. Gelatinase activity of synovial fluid from OA and RA patients.

4. Correlation between gelatinase activity and biological marker

The concentration of proteases in serum and synovial fluid often correlates with that of biological markers. For example, MMP-3 levels significantly correlate with those of C-reactive protein (CRP) (Posthumus et al., 2003; Wassilew et al., 2010). On comparison of gelatinase activity with biological markers, it was demonstrated that samples with high gelatinase activity tended to have high CRP levels (Fig. 6).

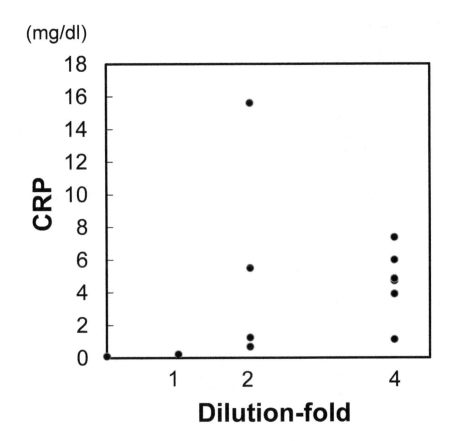

The horizontal axis represents the highest dilution-fold of synovial fluid sample that was positive for gelatinase activity from RA patients. The vertical axis indicates the CRP level.

Fig. 6. Correlation between gelatinase activity and CRP levels.

5. Conclusions

The protease MMP-3, which degrades several ECM proteins and activates a number of MMPs, is often a useful predictor of joint destruction (Mamehara et al., 2010; Yamanaka et al., 2000). However, other proteases present in synovial fluid are also involved in cartilage destruction and warrant measurement. Our method using gelatin coated-film allows the comprehensive assay of gelatinase activity, including MMP-3 and other proteases, and is thought to accurately reflect the pathological condition of RA and OA and serve as a useful tool for the prediction of joint destruction. Notably, the observed gelatinase activities of the synovial fluid from RA and OA patients assayed by this method were consistent with a previous report. Gelatinase activity measured by this method also correlated with CRP levels.

The benefits of this assay method include the capability to measure comprehensive enzyme activity and simplicity, as special instruments are not required. Despite these advantages, the detection sensitivity of the proposed method is not sufficient to detect the enzyme activities of many OA samples. Improvement of the detection sensitivity is the most important issue to address, and will provide detailed information about the gelatinase activity in synovial fluid and more closely reflect clinical conditions.

The developed assay method is expected to be a useful tool for predicting the effect of therapy for not only RA, but also OA.

6. Abbreviations

The abbreviations used are: RA, rheumatoid arthritis; OA, osteoarthritis; ECM, extracellular matrix; MMP, matrix metalloproteinase; ADAMTS, a disintegrin-like and metalloproteinase with thrombospondin type 1 motif; FIZ, film in situ zymography; APMA, p-Aminophenylmercuric acetate; CRP, C-reactive protein.

7. References

Arner EC. (2002). Aggrecanase-mediated cartilage degradation. Curr Opin Pharmacol. Vol. 2, No. 3, (Jun 2002) pp. 322-9. ISSN: 1471-4892

Chakraborti S, Mandal M, Das S, Mandal A, Chakraborti T. (2003). Regulation of matrix metalloproteinases: an overview. *Mol Cell Biochem*, Vol. 253, No. 1-2, (Nov 2003) pp. 269-85. ISSN: 0300-8177

Gendron C, Kashiwagi M, Lim NH, Enghild JJ, Thøgersen IB, Hughes C, Caterson B, Nagase H. (2007). Proteolytic activities of human ADAMTS-5: comparative studies with ADAMTS-4. *J Biol Chem*, Vol. 282, No. 25, (Jun 2007) pp. 18294-306. ISSN: 0021-9258

Huang K, Wu LD. (2008). Aggrecanase and aggrecan degradation in osteoarthritis: a review. J Int Med Res. Vol. 36, No. 6, (Nov-Dec 2008) pp. 1149-60. ISSN: 0300-0605

Lauer-Fields JL, Minond D, Sritharan T, Kashiwagi M, Nagase H, Fields GB. (2007). Substrate conformation modulates aggrecanase (ADAMTS-4) affinity and sequence specificity. Suggestion of a common topological specificity for functionally diverse proteases. *J Biol Chem*, Vol. 282, No. 1, (Jan 2007) pp. 142-50. ISSN: 0021-9258

Mahmoud RK, El-Ansary AK, El-Eishi HH, Kamal HM, El-Saeed NH. (2005). Matrix metalloproteinases MMP-3 and MMP-1 levels in sera and synovial fluids in patients with rheumatoid arthritis and osteoarthritis. *Ital J Biochem*, Vol. 54, No. 3-4, (Sep-Dec 2005) pp. 248-57, ISSN: 0021-2938

Mamehara A, Sugimoto T, Sugiyama D, Morinobu S, Tsuji G, Kawano S, Morinobu A, Kumagai S. (2010). Serum matrix metalloproteinase-3 as predictor of joint destruction in rheumatoid arthritis, treated with non-biological disease modifying anti-rheumatic drugs. *Kobe J Med Sci*, Vol. 56, No. 3, (Sep 2010) pp. E98-107. ISSN: 0023-2513

Murphy G, Nagase H. (2008). Reappraising metalloproteinases in rheumatoid arthritis and osteoarthritis: destruction or repair? *Nat Clin Pract Rheumatol*, Vol. 4, No. 3, (Mar 2008) pp. 128-35. ISSN: 1745-8382

Nagase H, Enghild JJ, Suzuki K, Salvesen G. (1990). Stepwise activation mechanisms of the precursor of matrix metalloproteinase 3 (stromelysin) by proteinases and (4-aminophenyl) mercuric acetate. *Biochemistry*, Vol. 29, No. 24 (Jun 1990) pp. 5783-9. ISSN: 0006-2960

Nagase H, Suzuki K, Enghild JJ, Salvesen G. (1991). Stepwise activation mechanisms of the precursors of matrix metalloproteinases 1 (tissue collagenase) and 3 (stromelysin). *Biomed Biochim Acta*, Vol. 50, No. 4-6, (1991) pp. 749-54. ISSN: 0232-766X

Posthumus MD, Limburg PC, Westra J, van Leeuwen MA, van Rijswijk MH. (2003). Serum matrix metalloproteinase 3 levels in comparison to C-reactive protein in periods with and without progression of radiological damage in patients with early rheumatoid arthritis. *Clin Exp Rheumatol*, Vol. 21, No. 4, (Jul-Aug 2003) pp. 465-72, ISSN: 0392-856X

Sun HB. (2010). Mechanical loading, cartilage degradation, and arthritis. *Ann N Y Acad Sci*, Vol. 1211, (Nov 2010) pp. 37-50. ISSN: 0077-8923

Wassilew GI, Lehnigk U, Duda GN, Taylor WR, Matziolis G, Dynybil C. (2010). The expression of proinflammatory cytokines and matrix metalloproteinases in the synovial membranes of patients with osteoarthritis compared with traumatic knee disorders. *Arthroscopy*, Vol. 26, No. 8, (Aug 2010) pp. 1096-104. ISSN: 0749-8063

Yamanaka H, Matsuda Y, Tanaka M, Sendo W, Nakajima H, Taniguchi A, Kamatani N. (2000). Serum matrix metalloproteinase 3 as a predictor of the degree of joint destruction during the six months after measurement, in patients with early rheumatoid arthritis. *Arthritis Rheum*, Vol. 43, No. 4, (Apr 2000) pp. 852-8, ISSN: 0004-3591

Yan SJ, Blomme EA. (2003). In situ zymography: a molecular pathology technique to localize endogenous protease activity in tissue sections. *Vet Pathol*, Vol. 40, No. 3 (May 2003) pp. 227-36. ISSN: 0300-9858

Yoshida W, Uzuki M, Nishida J, Shimamura T, Sawai T. (2009). Examination of in vivo gelatinolytic activity in rheumatoid arthritis synovial tissue using newly developed in situ zymography and image analyzer. *Clin Exp Rheumatol*, Vol. 27, No. 4, (Jul-Aug 2009) pp. 587-93. ISSN: 0392-856X

4

Biochemical Mediators Involved in Cartilage Degradation and the Induction of Pain in Osteoarthritis

Michael B. Ellman[1,2], Dongyao Yan[1], Di Chen[1] and Hee-Jeong Im[1,2,3]
1Department of Biochemistry,
2Department of Orthopedic Surgery,
3Department of Internal Medicine,
Section of Rheumatology, Rush University Medical Center, Chicago, IL,
USA

1. Introduction

Osteoarthritis, a debilitating degenerative joint disease predominantly found in elderly individuals, has become the principal source of physical disability resulting in increased health care costs and impaired quality of life in the United States. The pathogenesis of osteoarthritis (OA) involves the progressive deterioration of cartilage tissue, but many of the underlying biochemical and pathophysiological mechanisms involved in cartilage degradation and the induction of pain in this process remain largely unknown. Recent literature has focused on understanding many of these processes, with the intention of developing novel therapies aimed at slowing and/or reversing cartilage degradation and inducing symptomatic relief. This chapter provides an overview of several biochemical mediators involved in OA, with an emphasis on reviewing pertinent factors mediating cartilage breakdown and the induction of pain in degenerative conditions.

2. Anatomy

Articular cartilage lines the surfaces of joints and serves several important functions, including the provision of a smooth, low-friction surface, joint lubrication, and stress distribution with load bearing (1, 2). The components of articular cartilage include an elaborate mixture of water (65-80% of wet weight), collagen (10-20% of wet weight), proteoglycans (PGs; 10-15% of wet weight), and chondrocytes (5% of wet weight) (1). The extracellular matrix (ECM) includes collagen and PGs, principally aggrecan, with other proteins and glycoproteins in lesser amounts. This matrix allows normal cartilage to form the resilient, low-friction surface capable of absorbing shock with high impact mechanical loading (3).

Within the ECM, collagen fibers provide form, shape, and tensile strength to cartilage. The principal collagen fibers present in articular cartilage are type II fibers, with smaller quantities of types V, VI, IX, X, and XI (1). Collagen interacts to form fibrils that interact with and trap large aggregates of PGs, principally aggrecan. PGs bind water and help distribute stresses throughout the porous-permeable ECM under compressive loads. Aggrecan, the most abundant PG found in articular cartilage, is composed of a protein backbone bound by negatively-charged chondroitin sulfate and keratin sulfate groups. It binds with hyaluronic acid (HA) to form complexes within the ECM. Due to negatively-charged sulfated groups, these complexes electrostatically interact with cations, ultimately forming ion-dipole interactions with water, allowing cartilage to function as a hydrated tissue that resists compression.

The cellular makeup of cartilage consists of articular chondrocytes. Chondrocytes maintain and produce the components of the ECM that regulate cartilage homeostasis. They are mesenchymal in origin, few in number within the matrix, have a low rate of cell turnover, and receive nutrients and oxygen from the surrounding synovial fluid by means of diffusion (1). Further, they respond to a variety of factors, including matrix proteins, mechanical load, and soluble mediators such as growth factors and cytokines.

3. Metabolic disruption of cartilage homeostasis in osteoarthritis

Under normal conditions, chondrocytes maintain a dynamic equilibrium between synthesis and degradation of ECM components. In osteoarthritic states, however, there is a disruption of matrix equilibrium leading to progressive loss of cartilage tissue, clonal expansion of cells in the depleted regions, induction of oxidative states in a stressful cellular environment, and eventually, apoptosis of chondrocytes (2, 4). With progression, there is usually an increase in both degradation and synthesis within the joint, with an overall shift toward catabolism over anabolism. Chondrocyte metabolism is unbalanced due to excessive production of inflammatory cytokines and matrix-degrading enzymes, in conjunction with a downregulation of anabolic factors, eventually leading to destruction of the ECM and subsequent cartilage degradation. Oxidative stress elicited by reactive oxygen species (ROS) further disturbs cartilage homeostasis and promotes catabolism via induction of cell death, breakdown of matrix components, upregulation of latent matrix-degrading enzyme production, inhibition of ECM synthesis, and oxidation of intracellular and extracellular molecules (2).

One approach to slow or reverse catabolism involves attempts to downregulate the expression of catabolic factors and/or matrix-degrading enzymes, including matrix metalloproteases (MMPs) and a disintegrin-like and metalloprotease with thrombospondin motifs (ADAMTS family, aka aggrecanases)(5). In particular, MMP-13 is the most potent collagen type II-degrading enzyme in human articular cartilage (6). The regulation of matrix-degrading enzyme expression is stimulated by pro-inflammatory cytokines, growth factors, and metabolites, including lipopolysaccharide (LPS) (7), interleukin-1 (IL-1) (8), tumor necrosis factor-alpha (TNF-α) (8), fibroblast growth factor-2 (FGF-2, otherwise known as basic FGF) (9), and ROS (10). Equally important are attempts to upregulate anabolic factors in matrix homeostasis, including ECM components (e.g., aggrecan, collagen type II), growth factors (e.g. transforming growth factor (TGF)-β, bone morphogenetic proteins (BMPs), and insulin-like growth factor-1 (IGF-1)), and/or anti-destructive enzymes [e.g., tissue inhibitor of metalloproteases (TIMPs)] to prevent cartilage degradation.

4. Catabolic mediators in OA

Healthy articular chondrocytes and synoviocytes constitutively synthesize and secret a wide array of mediators to maintain their delicate homeostasis. When inappropriately regulated, a subset of mediators will drive detrimental catabolic processes in both cell populations, resulting in cartilage degeneration and chronic synovial inflammation. This section will summarize our current understanding of these key catabolic factors in OA pathogenesis.

4.1 Inflammatory mediators

Typical inflammatory mediators in OA include pro-inflammatory members from the interleukin family (IL-1, IL-6, and IL-17), TNF-α, and prostaglandin E2 (PGE2). The roles of these mediators have been extensively studied in arthritic tissues secondary to their high concentrations in degenerative states. Each of these mediators not only stimulates the production of cartilage-degrading proteases, but also upregulates other destructive factors via paracrine or autocrine mechanisms, thus perpetuating disease progression.

4.1.1 IL-1β

IL-1β is thought to play a prominent role in OA development. It demonstrates potent bioactivities in inhibiting ECM synthesis and promoting cartilage breakdown. Independent studies have shown that IL-1β represses the expression of essential ECM components, aggrecan and collagen type II, in chondrocytes (11-13). IL-1β also strikingly induces a spectrum of proteolytic enzymes, including collagenases (MMP-1 and MMP-13) and ADAMTS-4, in both chondrocytes and synovial fibroblasts. Aside from these direct effects, IL-1β induces a panel of cytokines, including IL-6, IL-8, and leukemia inducing factor (LIF), which produce additive or synergistic effects in the catabolic cascade (14). Further, IL-1β has been implicated in OA pathogenesis in numerous observational studies. Although less pronounced than what has been observed in rheumatoid arthritis patients, OA synovial fluids contains significantly higher levels of IL-1β compared to normal synovial fluid (15). Immunohistochemical analyses also reveal increased expression of IL-1β in OA cartilage and synovium (16, 17). Moreover, osteoarthritic chondrocytes exhibit heightened sensitivity to IL-1β stimulation, in part due to augmented IL-1 receptor type I expression (18). This pathological change renders OA chondrocytes even more susceptible to deleterious IL-1β attack. The significance of IL-1β in OA was further corroborated by *in vivo* studies and pharmaceutical efforts using IL-1 receptor antagonist (IL-1ra) as a potential therapeutic factor to prevent cartilage degeneration. As an inhibitory molecule of IL-1β, IL-1ra not only showed efficacy in OA animal models, but also improved clinical outcomes (19).

4.1.2 IL-6

Another constitutively expressed cytokine in human articular chondrocytes is IL-6 (20), yet only a fraction of OA patients contains increased IL-6 levels in arthritic cartilage and synovial fluid, suggesting that IL-6 may not be the ultimate driving force in this disease (21, 22). Nevertheless, *in vitro* studies demonstrate catabolic effects of IL-6 as this cytokine inhibits PG synthesis in chondrocytes, and this effect is potentiated by addition of soluble IL-6 receptor (sIL-6R) (23, 24). Combination treatment with IL-6 and sIL-6R has been shown to enhance aggrecanase-mediated PG depletion in cartilage (25). IL-6 also suppresses collagen type II expression (26), and to a lesser extent than IL-1β, dysregulates enzymatic antioxidant defense mechanisms in chondrocytes *via* modulation of key enzymes (27). Therefore, it is surprising that male IL-6-/- mice displayed more severe OA phenotypes compared with wild-type mice (28). In this report, de Hooge *et al* suggest that IL-6 exerted joint protection in aging murine OA joints. However, their findings differ qualitatively from those provided by Ryu *et al*, who reported that IL-6 promotes joint destruction in an instability-induced OA model (29). Further *in vivo* experiments are warranted to clarify such contradictions. Interestingly, a recent study suggested a mechanistic link between obesity and OA, based on the observation that the infrapatellar fat pad actively synthesizes IL-6 and sIL-6R in knee OA patients (30).

4.1.3 IL-17
The pro-inflammatory role of IL-17 is well-established in rheumatoid arthritis, but less so in OA. IL-17 is reported to exert stimulatory effects on MMP-3, MMP-13 and ADAMTS-4 expression in chondrocytes (31, 32). It directly inhibits PG synthesis, augments nitric oxide production, and triggers angiogenic factor release (33-35). Further, the IL-17 response can be amplified dramatically when other destructive cytokines, such as IL-1β and TNF-α, are present. In chondrocytes, IL-17-mediated type II collagen breakdown and MMP expression is synergistically enhanced by IL-1, IL-6, or TNF-α co-treatment (36). Likewise, synergy in nitric oxide production was observed when chondrocytes were treated with IL-17 and TNF-α (37). IL-17 also synergizes with IL-1β or TNF-α in PGE2 production in OA menisci *ex vivo* (38). Cytokine induction serves as a secondary mechanism in IL-17-mediated effects. In chondrocytes and synovial fibroblasts, IL-17 induces certain pro-inflammatory cytokines and chemokines, such as IL-1β, IL-6, and IL-8 (39, 40). In macrophages, IL-17 effectively upregulates IL-1 and TNF-α expression, which may contribute to chronic synovial inflammation observed in some OA patients (41). By way of adenovirus-mediated IL-17 overexpression, Koenders *et al.* showed that IL-17 is capable of causing joint inflammation and bone erosion by itself, and also synergizes with TNF-α (42). Conversely, IL-17 deficiency markedly mitigates the arthritic phenotype in a collagen-induced arthritis model, but whether IL-17 ablation also provides similar protection in OA models awaits investigation (43).

4.1.4 TNF-α
The relevance of TNF-α to OA pathogenesis is supported by the observation that TNF-α receptor expression is significantly upregulated in OA cartilage (44, 45). TNF-α concentration in synovial fluid also increases in patients with anterior cruciate ligament injury, suggesting this cytokine may play a role in OA development (46). Similar to IL-1β, TNF-α also promotes PG depletion (47-49). The induction of proteolytic enzymes MMP-3, MMP-9, and MMP-13 by TNF-α in chondrocytes may account for such an action (50, 51). TNF-α potently induces IL-6 and PGE2, which possibly results in secondary inflammatory events in the joint (47, 48, 52, 53). Another important process mediated by TNF-α is cell death. It appears that excessive exposure to TNF-α can elicit chondrocyte apoptosis, which will lead to local secondary necrosis and eventually a catabolic cascade due to absence of phagocytes in cartilage (54, 55). Consistent with these findings, TNF-α transgenic mice exhibit spontaneous cartilage damage and conspicuous occurrence of arthritis (54).

4.1.5 PGE2
PGE2 is yet another significant player in chondrocyte metabolism. Upregulated in OA, PGE2 inhibits PG and type II collagen synthesis with the highest cellular sensitivity among all prostanoids produced by chondrocytes (56, 57). Mechanistically, PGE2 appears to signal through the EP2 receptor to exert such inhibitory effects (58). Furthermore, EP4 receptor

activation increases MMP-13 and ADAMTS-5 expression, thus promoting ECM degradation (59). Interestingly, some evidence suggests that specific EP2 activation enhances cartilage regeneration in rabbit models, indicating species differences in PGE2 responses (60). PGE2 also mediates or sensitizes chondrocytes to apoptosis (61, 62). Both IL-1 and TNF-α induce PGE2 production, with the former being more potent (63-65), and the involvement of PGE2 in IL-1β-induced MMP-3 and MMP-13 expression is demonstrated in PGE synthase-1 knockout chondrocytes. In these modified cells, the catabolic effects of IL-1β are dramatically reduced (66). However, another group claims that PGE2 acts as a secretagogue of IGF-1, which in turn mediates anabolism in chondrocytes (67). Whether this induction brings any benefit to OA cartilage is questionable, because IGF-1 non-responsiveness has been reported in OA chondrocytes (68).

4.2 Oxidative stress mediators, growth factors and glycoproteins
4.2.1 Nitric oxide
Nitric oxide (NO), a member of ROS, mediates the destructive actions of IL-1β and TNF-α in cartilage, including suppression of PG and collagen synthesis, as well as stimulation of MMPs (69-73). Spontaneous overproduction of NO produces similar effects in chondrocytes (73, 74), and prolonged exposure to NO together with other ROS can lead to apoptosis of articular cell types (62, 75, 76). NO is also partially responsible for the insensitivity of OA chondrocytes to IGF-1 (77). As a mediator downstream of IL-1, NO also inhibits BMP-2-mediated PG synthesis (78).

Inducible nitric oxide synthase (iNOS) is the major enzyme responsible for NO generation in articular cartilage. OA chondrocytes in the superficial zone express higher levels of iNOS (79, 80). Several destructive cytokines, including IL-1 and TNF-α, induce iNOS expression in articular cell types (81, 82). Forced expression of iNOS inhibits matrix synthesis in chondrocytes (74). Futher, in OA cartilage, iNOS inhibition gives rise to IL-10 induction and MMP-10 repression in the presence of IL-1β (83). More recently, iNOS was found to function as a crucial mediator downstream of the advanced glycation end products pathway and the leptin pathway in chondrocytes (84, 85). Pelletier *et al* provided compelling evidence regarding the importance of iNOS in OA progression. In their canine OA model, selective inhibition of iNOS resulted in marked attenuation of joint destruction (86). Intra-articular delivery of an iNOS inhibitor counteracts the acute effects mediated by IL-1β, reaffirming the catabolic role of iNOS in OA progression (87).

4.2.2 FGF-2
A series of studies have demonstrated that FGF-2 (otherwise known as basic FGF) acts as a catabolic growth factor in addition to its well-established mitogenic role in articular cartilage. Despite its positive effect on proliferation, FGF-2 inhibits IGF-1/BMP-7-enhanced PG deposition in human articular chondrocytes, and negatively affects the physical properties of normal cartilage (88, 89). FGF-2 alters the ratio of type II to type I collagen in articular chondrocytes, thus possibly leading to the formation of fibrocartilage, a poor substitute for hyaline cartilage (90, 91). In porcine chondrocytes, FGF-2 antagonizes IGF-1/TGF-β-mediated decorin and type II collagen production (92). Moreover, FGF-2 promotes cartilage degeneration *ex vivo* (93). A mechanistic explanation of FGF-2-mediated effects lies in its ability to upregulate MMP-13 and ADAMTS-5 (94, 95). FGF-2 orchestrates the MAPK, NFκB, and substance P signaling pathway to induce MMP-13 (5, 93, 94). It has also been

shown that activation of FGF receptor 1 (FGFR1) is required for FGF-2-mediated MMP-13 and ADAMTS-5 induction (95).

Results acquired from comparative analyses suggest the biological relevance of FGF-2 to OA. FGF-2 levels in OA synovial fluids are significantly elevated compared to those in normal specimens (94). FGFR3 expression is markedly diminished in OA chondrocytes, which results in altered FGFR1 to FGFR3 ratios and may account for the inhibition of anabolism in the disease state (95). It should be noted that other studies indicate a chondroprotective role of FGF-2 in cartilage biology (96, 97). The discrepancies may arise from differences in cell origin (i.e. species, age, severity of OA, etc), and render future clarifications necessary.

4.2.3 Fibronectin

Fibronectin (Fn) is an adhesive glycoprotein found in cartilage and synovial membrane tissue (98). Evidence shows that Fn level is increased in OA cartilage as well as OA synovial fluid (99, 100). Heightened proteolytic activities in OA joints lead to the generation of Fn fragments (Fn-fs) of different sizes. Specifically, ADAMTS-8 was characterized as a fibronectinase in OA chondrocytes (101). Indeed, Fn-fs are found with increased abundance in OA synovial fluids and cartilage (99, 102). A 40-kDa collagen-binding Fn-f induces sustained PG degradation in both normal and OA cartilage (103). Furthermore, Fn-f stimulates type II collagen cleavage in an MMP-13-dependent manner (104). Preceding collagen disintegration, Fn-f disrupts the ECM by promoting the release of cartilage oligomeric matrix protein (COMP) and chondroadherin (105). Fn-f also augments cytokine, ROS, MMP and aggrecanase production in cartilage *ex vivo* and *in vitro* (10, 106-109). Stimulation of IL-1 leads to enhanced production of Fn-f, which exerts prolonged destructive effects (99).

4.2.4 Osteopontin

Osteopontin, a phosphorylated glycoprotein with cell and matrix binding affinities, has been characterized as a facilitator of osteoclast adhesion and an initiator of osteoid mineralization (110). Osteopontin deposition in cartilage exhibits a spatial pattern, based on the fact that it is mainly detected in chondrocytes residing in the upper deep zone (111). Comparative analyses reveal that, in contrast with healthy chondrocytes, OA chondrocytes express notable levels of osteopontin (111). Moreover, an apparent correlation exists between osteopontin level and the severity of OA lesions (111-113).

Nevertheless, the role of osteopontin in cartilage remains controversial. Osteopontin promotes calcium pyrophosphate dehydrate (CPPD) crystal formation in articular cartilage, suggesting that elevated osteopontin production in OA may be detrimental (114). Yet this stimulatory effect seems to depend on osteopontin concentration, because other studies demonstrate the opposite using higher concentrations of this protein (115). Another independent study also showed that osteopontin inhibits IL-1β-induced NO and PGE2 production in OA cartilage, suggesting an anti-catabolic role in cartilage homeostasis (116). Osteopontin deficiency exacerbates aging-induced and instability-induced OA in mice (117). Based on these apparently contradictory activities, it raises the possibility that osteopontin elicits different biological effects depending on the stages of OA.

4.2.5 Osteonectin
Osteonectin is a non-collagenous glycoprotein linking collagen fibrils to mineral in bone. It is also present in mineralizing chondroid bone (118). Articular chondrocytes synthesize osteonectin, and this process is regulated by endogenous stimuli. IL-1, TNF-α, and FGF-2, but not IL-6, greatly inhibit osteonectin expression (119, 120). IL-1 also impairs the glycosylation of osteonectin (120). On the other hand, TGF-β, PDGF, and IGF-1 upregulate osteonectin synthesis, even in the presence of IL-1 (119, 120). Osteonectin is localized to the superficial and middle zones of OA cartilage, while normal cartilage does not display such a pattern (120, 121). Osteonectin synthesis is also enhanced in OA synovial fibroblasts (120). Osteonectin induces collagenase expression in this cell type, which may contribute to cartilage damage (122).

4.3 Protective mediators in OA
In contrast to the aforementioned catabolic mediators in OA, several growth factors take on important anabolic roles in the joint, thus serving as potential targets for future therapeutic growth factor therapy in practice. While the literature has only begun to explore the *in vitro*, *in vivo*, and clinical effects of many of these factors, there is potential for these mediators to be major players in the treatment of degenerative joint diseases in the future. Multiple cytokines exert protection in articular joints, including IL-1 receptor antagonist (IL-1ra), IL-4, IL-10, IL-11, and IL-13. Perhaps the most well-studied anabolic factors to date include TGF-β, BMP-2, BMP-7, and IGF-1 (Table 1). We will also discuss two factors elucidated in our laboratory to have potent anabolic and anti-catabolic effects in human articular cartilage: resveratrol (RSV) and bovine lactoferricin (LfcinB).

4.3.1 Interleukins
The antagonistic effect of IL-1ra on IL-1 has been well established. By directly competing against IL-1 for its cognate receptor, IL-1ra effectively inhibits IL-1-mediated responses in chondrocytes, including PG depletion, MMP induction, and cytokine induction (123-125). IL-1ra expression is repressed by NO, which may blunt its action in OA cartilage (126). Not surprisingly, forced expression of IL-1ra confers resistance to IL-1 challenge in chondrocytes (127, 128). Both gene delivery and IL-1ra intra-articular injection have been shown to impede OA progression, indicating anti-IL-1 therapy is a viable option in OA disease modification (19, 129).

Protective roles of anti-inflammatory cytokines have also been linked to OA. An array of cytokines, including IL-4, IL-10, IL-11, and IL-13, has been shown to block the actions of catabolic cytokines *via* different mechanisms. IL-4 suppresses MMP-13, cathepsin B, and iNOS when cyclic tensile stress is applied on chondrocytes (130, 131). IL-4 has potent inhibitory effects on cartilage degradation in the presence of IL-1 and TNF-α (132). In synoviocytes, IL-4 downregulates apoptosis (133). IL-4 gene therapy appears to dampen inflammation in chondrocytes (134). Moreover, intra-articular injection of IL-4 results in notable amelioration of cartilage degenerative status (131).

IL-10 is upregulated in OA chondrocytes, and this phenomenon may represent a reparative effort (135). IL-10 suppresses IL-1 and TNF-α production (136). Compared to IL-1ra, IL-10 gene delivery into synoviocytes elicits moderate yet still significant protection on cartilage (137).

IL-1β	-: ↓ PG synthesis; ↓ type II collagen synthesis; ↑ MMPs; ↑ ADAMTS-4; ↑ ROS; ↑ IL-6; ↑ IL-8; ↑ LIF; ↑ synovial inflammation
IL-6	-: ↓ PG synthesis; ↓ type II collagen synthesis; ↑ PG depletion; dysregulation of antioxidant defense
IL-17	-: ↓ PG synthesis; ↑ type II collagen breakdown; ↑ MMPs; ↑ ADAMTS-4; ↑ NO; ↑ IL-1β; ↑ IL-6; ↑ IL-8; ↑ PGE2 (in menisci); ↑ TNF-α (in macrophage)
TNF-α	-: ↑ PG depletion; ↑ MMPs; ↑ IL-6; ↑ PGE2; ↑ chondrocyte apoptosis
PGE2	-: ↓ PG synthesis; ↓ type II collagen synthesis; ↑ MMPs; ↑ ADAMTS-5; ↑ chondrocyte apoptosis
NO	-: ↓ PG synthesis; ↓ type II collagen synthesis; ↑ MMPs; ↓ IGF-1 sensitivity; ↑ apoptosis
FGF-2	-: ↓ PG deposition; ↓ ratio of type II to type I collagen; ↑ MMP-13; ↑ ADAMTS-5
Fn-f	-: ↑ PG degradation; ↑ type II collagen cleavage; ↑ COMP and chondroadherin release; ↑ MMPs; ↑ aggrecanases; ↑ destructive cytokines
Osteopontin	-: ↑ CPPD formation +: ↓ NO; ↓ PGE2 (concentration-dependent)
Osteonectin	-: ↑ collagenases (in synovial fibroblasts)

(-) = Catabolic effects; (+) = Anabolic or anti-catabolic effects

Table 1. Effects of Catabolic Mediators in Articular Cartilage

IL-1ra	+: ↓ IL-1-mediated responses
IL-4	+: ↓ MMP-13; ↓ cathepsin B; ↓ iNOS; ↓ synovial fibroblast apoptosis; ↓ IL-1/TNF-α-mediated cartilage degradation
IL-10	+: ↓ IL-1; ↓ TNF-α; ↑ cartilage protection
IL-11	+: ↑ TIMP-1; ↓ pro-inflammatory cytokines; ↓ NO; ↓ TNF-α responses (synovial fibroblast)
IL-13	+: ↓ MMPs; ↓ IL-1β; ↓ TNF-α; ↑ IL-1ra; ↓ PGE2 and COX-2 (synovial fibroblasts); ↓ synoviocyte apoptosis
TGF-β	+: ↑ chondrocyte activity, ↑ PG synthesis, ↑ ECM synthesis; ↓IL-1, ↓ROS - : Osteophyte formation and synovial inflammation with prolonged exposure
BMP-2	+: ↑ ECM synthesis, ↑ collagen II expression - : +/- aggrecan degradation?
BMP-7	+: ↑ chondrocyte activity, ↑ PG synthesis, ↑ ECM synthesis; ↓cell proliferation; age-independent, ↑activity of other anabolic factors (IGF-1, BMPs), ↓MMPs, ↓IL-1 and IL-6; ↑ cartilage repair in vivo (sheep, rabbits) - : Unknown
IGF-1	+: ↑ ECM synthesis, ↑ PG synthesis; ↓apoptosis; + synergism with BMP-7 - : ↓effect with ↑ age and on OA cartilage
RSV	+: ↑ ECM synthesis, ↑ PG (aggrecan) synthesis; ↑ collagen II expression; ↓IL-1 & FGF-2 effects, + synergism with BMP-7 - : preliminary data; no in vivo studies
LfcinB	+: ↑ ECM synthesis, ↑ PG (aggrecan) synthesis; ↑ collagen II expression; ↓IL-1 & FGF-2 effects, + synergism with BMP-7 - : preliminary data; no in vivo studies

Table 2. Effects of Protective Mediators in Articular Cartilage

IL-11, an IL-6 family member, is believed to exert anti-catabolic and anti-inflammatory effects in articular joints, but remains poorly defined. IL-11 produced by articular chondrocytes stimulates the production of tissue inhibitor of metalloproteinase (TIMP) (138). IL-11 also downregulates pro-inflammatory cytokines and NO production (139). In OA synovial fibroblasts, IL-11 alone had no impact on PGE2 release, but shows anti-inflammatory properties in conjunction with TNF-α (140). In RA synovium, IL-11 directly inhibits MMP-1 and MMP-3 production, upregulates TIMP-1, and inhibits TNF-α production in the presence of soluble IL-11 receptor (141). Importantly, systemic treatment with IL-11 leads to a significant reduction in clinical and histological severity of established collagen-induced arthritis (CIA), suggesting an active role of IL-11 in joint homeostasis (142). IL-11 level is greatly increased in OA synovial fluid (143). However, IL-11 action is likely to be blunted due to the observation that the IL-11 receptor is markedly downregulated in OA chondrocytes (Im et al., unpublished data).

IL-13 downregulates MMP-13 expression in OA chondrocytes (144). Combined with IL-4, IL-13 abolishes IL-17 expression in RA synovial tissue (145). A more detailed study revealed that IL-13 represses IL-1β, TNF-α, and MMP-3, and simultaneously induces IL-1ra (146). IL-13, as well as IL-4 and IL-10, reduces TNF-α-induced PGE2 release and cyclooxygenase 2 (COX-2) in OA synovial fibroblasts (147). Similar to IL-4, IL-13 also inhibits synoviocyte apoptotic events (133). Nonetheless, IL-13 levels were found to be low in OA tissues (148). Whether IL-13 holds significance to OA pathogenesis needs to be further determined, especially in animal models.

4.3.2 TGF-β/BMP Superfamily

The TGF-β superfamily is composed of over 35 structurally-related members, with the majority of these members playing fundamental roles in development and homeostasis. In articular cartilage, three members of the TGF-β superfamily have been shown to play a significant role in cartilage homeostasis: TGF-β, BMP-2, and BMP-7. BMPs are structurally related to the transforming growth factor-β (TGF-β) superfamily and have wide-ranging biological activities, including the regulation of cellular proliferation, apoptosis, differentiation and migration, embryonic development and the maintenance of tissue homeostasis during adult life (149-151). It is now clear that they are expressed in a variety of tissues including adult articular cartilage.

4.3.2.1 TGF-β

Several studies demonstrate an anabolic role of TGF-β in articular cartilage. TGF-β has been shown to upregulate chondrocyte synthetic activity and suppress the catabolic activity of IL-1 (152, 153). *In vitro*, TGF-β stimulates chondrogenesis of synovial lining and bone marrow-derived mesenchymal stem cells (154). Additionally, asporin inhibits TGF-β-mediated stimulation of cartilage matrix genes such as collagen type II and aggrecan, and inhibits accumulation of PGs (155). In both Japanese (155) and Han Chinese (156) populations, patients with an asporin polymorphism demonstrated increased prevalence of arthritic conditions, presumably via inhibition of TGF-β expression, suggesting a protective role of TGF-β in articular cartilage. These findings were corroborated in knockout mice, as mice deficient for TGF-β or Smad3 (downstream mediator of TGF-β) developed cartilage degeneration resembling human OA (157, 158). Other studies demonstrate a vital role of TGF-β in the suppression of NO and other ROS levels (159), as well as the upregulation of PG synthesis in calf-cartilage explants in a dose-dependent manner (152, 160).

However, the literature also suggests that TGF-β demonstrates nondesirable side effects in joint tissues. For example, upon sustained exposure to in the joint, TGF-β can actually induce the formation of OA-like tissue pathology via stimulation of osteophyte formation, stimulation of synovial inflammation and fibrosis, and attraction of inflammatory leukocytes to the synovial lining (152, 153, 161, 162). These contradictory findings warrant further investigation, and recent research efforts are focused on downstream receptor usage to help provide further clues (152). Nevertheless, given its deleterious effects not seen in other growth factor-based strategies, TGF-β therapy is not presently a viable option for use in articular cartilage repair or regeneration.

4.3.2.2 BMP-2

Several studies have analyzed the role of BMP-2 in cartilage and found promising results. The effect of BMP-2 on mesenchymal stem cells is similar to that of TGF-β, with increased production of ECM and decreased expression of collage type 1, theoretically suppressing the formation of fibrocartilage (149, 154). *In vitro* analysis reveals that BMP-2 stimulates matrix synthesis and reverses chondrocyte dedifferentiation as indicated by an increase in synthesis of cartilage-specific collagen type II in OA chondrocytes (163). In rabbit knees, BMP-2-impregnated collagen sponges implanted into full-thickness cartilage defects enhance cartilage repair compared with empty defects or defects filled with collagen sponge alone, with this effect remaining at one year after implantation (164). Interestingly, however, in an IL-1-induced cartilage degeneration model in mice, BMP-2 stimulated matrix production via increased collagen type II and aggrecan expression (anabolic activity), but also increased aggrecan degradation as well, revealing a possible catabolic or self-regulatory role (165). Further studies are indeed warranted to further elucidate the effects of BMP-2 on cartilage repair.

4.3.2.3 BMP-7

BMP-7 (also known as osteogenic protein-1), another member of the TGF-β superfamily, is perhaps the most well-studied anabolic growth factor in cartilage repair. It is expressed in cartilage and exerts potent anabolic effects by stimulating differentiation and metabolic functions of both osteocytes and chondrocytes (166). In bone, a variety of animal models have clearly demonstrated a therapeutic potential of BMP-7 in bone repair applications, paving the way for BMP-7 to be used as the first commercial BMP to be used for bone repair clinically (149). In articular cartilage, BMP-7 has potent anabolic effects by stimulating matrix biosynthesis in both human adult articular chondrocytes (167) and human IVD cells (168).

In vitro, BMP-7 has several anabolic and anti-catabolic effects on articular cartilage. It promotes cell survival and upregulates chondrocyte metabolism (169) and protein synthesis without creating uncontrolled cell proliferation and formation of osteophytes, unlike other chondrogenic growth factors (149, 151). In a comparison study examining BMP-2, -4, -6, and -7, as well as cartilage-derived morphogenetic protein (CDMP)-1 (also known as GDF-5, growth differentiation factor-5) and CDMP-2, PG synthesis was stimulated to a greater extent by BMP-2 and -4, and the most significant upregulation after stimulation with BMP-7 (150). Importantly, its actions in cartilage are age-independent as BMP-7 induced similar anabolic responses in normal and OA chondrocytes from both young and old donors without inducing chondrocyte hypertrophy or changes in phenotype (151, 170, 171). Chubinskaya and colleagues have revealed that the anabolic effect of BMP-7 extends beyond stimulation of cartilage ECM proteins and their receptors, but also modulates the expression of various anabolic growth factors as well (IGF-1, TGF-β/BMPs) (151). In addition to its anabolic capacity, BMP-7 effectively counteracts chondrocyte catabolism, revealing a potent anti-catabolic effect in human articular cartilage. BMP-7 inhibits the expression of pro-inflammatory cytokines (IL-1 and IL-6), inhibits endogenous expression of cytokines (ie. IL-6, IL-8, IL-11) and their downstream signaling molecules (receptors, transcription factors, and mitogen-activated kinases), and blocks both a baseline and cytokine-induced expression of MMP-1 and MMP-13 (151). BMP-7 has also been shown to enhance the gene expression of the anabolic molecule tissue inhibitor of metalloproteinase (TIMP) in normal and OA chondrocytes (151), and acts synergistically with the anabolic growth actors IGF-1 (169) and TGF-β (172).

Data from animal studies reveal that BMP-7 clearly has therapeutic potential for cartilage repair. In a large chondral defect study in sheep cartilage, BMP-7 was shown to induce significant cartilage repair in a model where no repair takes place in the controls (173). Studies evaluating models of OA, however, are less numerous, but BMP-7 has been shown to prevent development of damage and in some models reverse the damage (151). Finally, although BMP-7 is highly effective at stimulating bone repair, it does not appear to lead to osteophyte formation when administered into a joint, nor does it stimulate uncontrolled fibroblast proliferation (leading to fibrosis) (149). Studies have demonstrated that recombinant BMP-7 use has a relatively safe profile with few side effects in rabbits, dogs, goats and sheep. Overall, the data clearly indicate that BMP-7 has an important role in cartilage, both in normal homeostasis and in repair, but several unknowns continue to exist, such as concentration, dosing, the use of scaffolds, methods of administration, and possibly combinations with other factors.

4.3.3 IGF-1

IGF-1 is a single chain polypeptide that is structurally similar to insulin, a key growth factor that enhances PG synthesis in articular cartilage (174). Much like BMP-7, IGF-1 has a promising future in the field of cartilage repair and regeneration therapy. *In vitro*, IGF-1 induces anabolic and anti-catabolic effects in normal articular cartilage from a variety of species (53, 175). *In vivo* studies support *in vitro* findings, as IGF-1 deficiency in rats leads to the development of articular cartilage lesions (176). In animal models, IGF-1 enhances repair of extensive cartilage defects and protects synovial membrane tissue from chronic inflammation (177, 178). Other studies in spine cartilage demonstrate similar results. Osada *et al* showed that IGF-1 stimulates PG synthesis in bovine NP cells in serum-free conditions in a dose-dependent manner and proposed an autocrine/paracrine mechanism of action (179). Gruber and colleagues found that the addition of IGF-1 increased cell survival upon experimental induction of apoptosis in spine disc annulus fibrosus cells (180), consistent with the anti-catabolic capacity of IGF-1 in both intervertebral disc (IVD) and articular cartilage tissues.

Despite its potent anabolic and anti-catabolic effects on normal cartilage tissue, however, IGF-1 appears to have a diminished ability to stimulate ECM formation and decrease catabolism with both age (181, 182) and OA (68, 149, 181). There appears to be an uncoupling of IGF-1 responsiveness in OA, as IGF-1 is able to stimulate matrix synthesis but is unable to decrease matrix catabolism (183). Nevertheless, combination growth factor therapy with IGF-1 and BMP-7 results in greater repair potential than either factor alone

(169), and the effects of combination factor therapy on aged and old cartilage defects have yet to be determined.

4.3.4 Resveratrol

The phytoestrogen resveratrol (trans-3,4',5-trihydroxystilbene; RSV) is a natural polyphenol compound found in peanuts, cranberries, and the skin of red grapes, and is thought to be one of the compounds responsible for the health benefits of moderate red wine consumption (184, 185). The anti-inflammatory, anti-oxidant, cardioprotective, and antitumor properties of RSV have been well-documented in a variety of tissues (186-194), and recent studies have begun to analyze the effects of RSV on cartilage homeostasis. Elmali *et al* reported a significant protective effect of RSV injections on articular cartilage degradation in rabbit models for OA and RA via histological analysis *in vivo* (195, 196). In human articular chondrocytes, Shakibaei (197) and Czaki (198) have elucidated both anti-apoptotic and anti-inflammatory regulatory mechanisms mediated by RSV. In our laboratory, we have demonstrated potent anabolic and anti-catabolic potential of RSV in bovine spine nucleus pulposus IVD tissue (199) and human adult articular chondrocytes (Im et al., unpublished data) via inhibition of matrix-degrading enzyme expression at the transcriptional and translational level. Further, combination therapy of RSV with BMP-7 induces synergistic effects on PG accumulation, and RSV reverses the catabolic effects of FGF-2 and IL-1 on matrix-degrading enzyme expression, PG accumulation, and the expression of factors (iNOS, IL-1, IL-6) associated with oxidative stress and inflammatory states (199). Future studies are needed to assess the appropriate dose, route of administration, and downstream effects of RSV, as well as elucidate its role in old or degenerative cartilage *in vivo*. Nevertheless, these findings reveal considerable promise for use of RSV as a unique biological therapy for treatment of cartilage degenerative diseases in the future.

4.3.5 Lactoferricin

Bovine lactoferricin (LfcinB) is a 25-amino acid cationic peptide with an amphipatic, anti-parallel β-sheet structure that is obtained by acid-pepsin hydrolysis of the N-terminal region of lactoferrin (Lf) found in cow's milk (200, 201). It exerts more potent biological effects than equimolar amounts of Lf, is cell membrane-permeable, and interacts electrostatically with negatively-charged matrix and cell surface glycosaminoglycans (GAGs), heparin and chondroitin sulfate (200, 201). The anti-inflammatory, anti-viral, anti-bacterial, anti-oxidant, anti-pain, and anti-cancer properties of LfcinB have been reported in a variety of tissues (202, 203). The natural anti-oxidative effect of LfcinB has also been reported, suggesting a possible chondroprotective biological role in articular cartilage (204), and several recent studies have attempted to elucidate the role of LfcinB in musculoskeletal disease. In a mouse collagen-induced and septic arthritis model, periarticular injection of human Lf substantially suppresses local inflammation (205). Further, in a rat adjuvant arthritis model, oral administration of bovine Lf suppresses the development of arthritis and hyperalgesia in the adjuvant-injected paw, suggesting Lf has preventative and therapeutic effects on the adjuvant-induced inflammation and pain (206). Human iron-free Lf delays the apoptosis of neutrophils isolated from synovial fluid of patients with established rheumatoid arthritis (207). Lf was also identified as a novel bone growth factor, as local injection of Lf above the hemicalvaria of adult mice in vivo results in substantial increases in the dynamic histomorphometric indices of bone formation and bone area (208).

Previously in our laboratory, LfcinB was found to exert potent anabolic and anti-catabolic effects in bovine nucleus pulposus matrix homeostasis in the IVD, similar to RSV (209). Similar to the IVD, we also found similar anabolic and anti-catabolic effects of LfcinB in human articular cartilage (Im et al, unpublished data). LfcinB reverses the catabolic effects of FGF-2 and IL-1 on matrix-degrading enzyme production, PG accumulation, and expression of factors associated with oxidative stress and inflammation, suggesting the promise of LfcinB as an anti-catabolic and anti-inflammatory molecule in human articular cartilage. Further, LfcinB abolishes the expression of iNOS, increases the expression of SOD-1, and antagonizes the catabolic effects mediated by bFGF and IL-1 on iNOS and SOD-1 expression, suggesting an anti-oxidative role of LfcinB in cartilage. Taken together, much like RSV, LfcinB may play an important role in prevention and treatment of diseases such as OA. Nevertheless, caution must be advised as further studies are warranted to determine, among other things, possible detrimental effects of its use *in vivo*.

5. Pain modulators in OA

Clinically, pain is the most prominent and disabling symptom of OA, and arthritic pain is associated with inferior functional outcomes and reduced quality of life compared with a range of other chronic conditions (210). Like other chronic pain conditions, OA pain is a complex integration of sensory, affective and cognitive processes that involves a variety of abnormal cellular mechanisms at both peripheral (joints) and central (spinal and supraspinal) levels of the nervous system. For the development of new therapies aimed at pain relief, a thorough understanding of the pathological mechanisms eliciting pain in OA is required. Unfortunately, many of these mechanisms remain elusive because the primary site of pathology (i.e., articular cartilage) does not have neuronal pain receptors that can directly detect tissue injury due to mechanical damage. The process by which painful mechanical stimuli from arthritic joints are converted into electrical signals that propagate along sensory nerves to the central nervous system remains to be fully explored.

Nociceptors are located throughout the joint in tissues peripheral to cartilage, including the joint capsule, ligaments, periosteum and subchondral bone. Joint cartilage and synovial injury influences peripheral afferent and dorsal root ganglion (DRG) neurons and sensitizes symptomatic pain perception through the dynamic interactions between neuropathic pathways and OA tissues. Nociceptive input from the joint is processed via different spinal cord pathways, and inflammation may potentially reduce the threshold for pain. The relative contribution of these processes into peripheral and central pathways appears to be strongly segmented (211), with intra-articular anesthetic studies in hip and knee OA suggesting a peripheral drive to pain in approximately 60% to 80% of patients, depending on the affected joint (212). In some individuals, however, central mechanisms such as dysfunction of descending inhibitory control or altered cortical processing of noxious information, may play a greater role (213). Therefore, research and pharmacotherapy for OA pain may be separated into two broad classes: central sensitization and peripheral sensitization, both leading to one final outcome: pain in a patient with OA.

A detailed overview of the multiple, complex pathways associated with OA pain, particularly relating to central sensitization mechanisms, is outside the scope of this chapter. For example, current targets of pharmacotherapy for OA pain are numerous and include opioids, kinins, cannabinoids, and their respective receptors, in addition to adrenergic receptors, glutamate receptors, specific ion channels, and neurotrophins. The literature is replete with data on the alteration of pain pathways via inhibition of both central and peripheral processes (211). Here, we will focus on select pro-inflammatory cytokines and mediators previously discussed in this chapter, and report their known roles in pain processing. Our laboratory and others have mechanistically linked OA to pathological changes in the metabolism of ECM proteins and inflammatory states that may be controlled by epigenetic, epigenomic, and systemic processes involved in pain processing (5, 9, 89, 93, 94, 199, 214, 215).

5.1 Cytokines

Inflammatory stimuli initiate a cascade of events, including the production of TNF-α, interleukins, chemokines, sympathetic amines, substance P, leukotrienes and prostaglandins, each demonstrating a complex interplay with other mediators to induce pain (211, 216). Cytokines stimulate hyperalgesia by a number of direct and indirect actions. Sensitization of primary afferent fibers for mechanical stimuli is thought to be induced by inflammatory mediators. IL-1β activates nociceptors directly via intracellular kinase activation, but it may also induce indirect nociceptor sensitization via the production of kinins and prostanoids (217).

IL-6, a well-known pro-inflammatory mediator, has been associated with hyperalgesia and hypersensitivity in articular cartilage (218). As previously discussed, IL-6 plays an important role in the pathogenesis of rheumatoid arthritis, and its concentration is elevated in the serum and synovial fluid of arthritic patients (219, 220). Interestingly, primary afferent neurons also respond to IL-6 (221), suggesting an important role of IL-6 in pain propagation in arthritic states.

TNF-α also activates sensory neurons directly via the receptors TNFR1 and TNFR2, and initiates a cascade of inflammatory reactions via the production of IL-1, IL-6 and IL-8 (217, 222). Direct TNF-α application in the periphery induces neuropathic pain, and this pain may be blocked by anti-inflammatory medications such as ibuprofen and celecoxib (223). Anti-TNF-α treatment with a TNF antibody produces a prolonged reduction of pain symptoms in OA (224), and neutralization of TNF-α in mice rescues both mechanical hyperalgesia (testing of withdrawal responses in behavioral experiments) and the inflammatory process (225). Taken together, TNF-α induces an algesic effect, at least in part, via both neuronal and inflammatory stimulation. Antagonists to TNF-α, such as etanercept or infliximab, may indeed serve as a potential therapeutic strategy to decrease OA pain clinically (211). Further controlled studies are needed to substantiate these promising preliminary data on TNF inhibitors in OA.

5.2 Prostanoids and PGE2

During pro-inflammatory states, numerous prostanoid cyclooxygenase (COX) enzyme products are produced and released, including PGE2, PGD2, PGF2a, thromboxane, and PGI2 (211). These factors serve as the premise for blocking the major synthetic enzymes COX-1 and COX-2 with selective or non-selective COX-inhibitor medications (ie. nonsteroidal anti-inflammatory drugs) (226). Of these mediators, PGE2 is considered to be the major contributor to inflammatory pain in arthritic conditions. PGE2 exerts its effects via a variety of E prostanoid (EP) receptors (EP1, EP2, EP3, EP4), which are present in both peripheral sensory neurons and the spinal cord (211). Activation of these receptors produces a variety of effects, ranging from calcium influx to cAMP activation or inhibition.

Peripherally, sensitization of nociceptors by PGE2 is caused by the cAMP-mediated enhancement of sodium currents after ion channel phosphorylation (227). However, in the spinal cord, PGE2 acts via different receptors than peripherally, suggesting further complexity in the prostanoid regulation of pain (228).

In our laboratory, we have assessed the role of PGE2 in human adult articular cartilage homeostasis and its relation to possible pain pathways (58). PGE2 utilizes the EP2 and EP4 receptors downstream to induce its downstream catabolic effects, and PGE2 may mediate pain pathways in articular cartilage via its stimulatory effect on the pain-associated factors IL-6 (218) and iNOS (229). Further, when combined with the catabolic cytokine IL-1, PGE2 synergistically upregulates both IL-6 and iNOS mRNA levels *in vitro* (58). Similar synergistic results were found with iNOS expression as well. Therefore, the EP2/4 receptor may be an important signaling initiator of the PGE2-signaling cascade and a potential target for therapeutic strategies aimed at preventing progression of arthritic disease and pain in the future.

As opposed to PGE2 EP receptor blockade, an alternative route of PGE2 inhibition is via the blockade of PGE synthase (PGES), a major route of conversion of prostaglandin H2 to PGE2 (211). Two isoforms of the enzyme have been identified, membrane or microsomal associated (mPGES-1) and cytosolic (cPGES/p23), which are linked with COX-2 and COX-1 dependent PGE2 production, respectively (230). Both isoforms are upregulated by inflammatory mediators, and gene deletion studies in mice indicate an important role for mPGES in acute and chronic inflammation and inflammatory pain, revealing a potential target for pain treatment in OA (211, 231).

6. Discussion

In summary, the literature reveals important roles of catabolic and anabolic growth factors and cytokines in articular cartilage homeostasis and the development of OA. Each factor discussed plays a critical role in cartilage, both in normal homeostasis and in repair. Currently, many of these specific roles remain unknown, but recent efforts have begun to increase our understanding. Catabolic factors include pro-inflammatory mediators (IL-1, IL-6, IL-17, TNF-α and PGE2), oxidative mediators (iNOS), glycoproteins (fibronectin, osteonectin, and osteopontin), and even growth factors (FGF-2). In contrast, anabolic mediators include select interleukins, TGF-β, IGF-1, BMPs (BMP-2 and BMP-7), RSV and LfcinB. Upregulation of catabolic processes and/or downregulation of anabolic processes leads to disruption of equilibrium with subsequent cartilage degradation and OA, and several of these pathways are known to induce pain in OA as well (ie. IL-1, IL-6, NO, TNF-α, PGE2). The goal of biologic therapy is to retard this process via inhibition of catabolic processes and upregulation of anabolic processes with the hope of clinically preserving joint cartilage, thereby slowing or preventing the process of OA.

Despite a tremendous research effort in recent years to elucidate these processes, however, biologic therapy for OA remains experimental in nature, and several unknowns exist. Given the wide array of interactions of growth factors that are necessary for proper cartilage development and homeostasis *in vivo*, it is unlikely that any single growth factor will lead to complete cartilage repair or affect the arthritic joint clinically, and rather a combination approach will be required (149). Further, appropriate dosing, scaffolds, and routes of administration must be determined before any of these factors plays a role clinically. Nevertheless, this chapter reviews several of the most well-studied biochemical mediators involved in OA and provides a framework for the understanding of potential biologic therapies in the treatment of degenerative joint disease in the future.

7. References

[1] Lewis PB, McCarty LP, 3rd, Kang RW, Cole BJ. Basic science and treatment options for articular cartilage injuries. J Orthop Sports Phys Ther. 2006;36(10):717-27.

[2] Sandell LJ, Aigner T. Articular cartilage and changes in arthritis. An introduction: cell biology of osteoarthritis. Arthritis Res. 2001;3(2):107-13.

[3] Valverde-Franco G, Binette JS, Li W, Wang H, Chai S, Laflamme F, et al. Defects in articular cartilage metabolism and early arthritis in fibroblast growth factor receptor 3 deficient mice. Hum Mol Genet. 2006;15(11):1783-92.

[4] Nakata K, Ono K, Miyazaki J, Olsen BR, Muragaki Y, Adachi E, et al. Osteoarthritis associated with mild chondrodysplasia in transgenic mice expressing alpha 1(IX) collagen chains with a central deletion. Proc Natl Acad Sci U S A. 1993;90(7):2870-4.

[5] Im HJ, Li X, Muddasani P, Kim GH, Davis F, Rangan J, et al. Basic fibroblast growth factor accelerates matrix degradation via a neuro-endocrine pathway in human adult articular chondrocytes. J Cell Physiol. 2008;215(2):452-63.

[6] Bau B, Gebhard PM, Haag J, Knorr T, Bartnik E, Aigner T. Relative messenger RNA expression profiling of collagenases and aggrecanases in human articular chondrocytes in vivo and in vitro. Arthritis Rheum. 2002;46(10):2648-57.

[7] Liu MH, Sun JS, Tsai SW, Sheu SY, Chen MH. Icariin protects murine chondrocytes from lipopolysaccharide-induced inflammatory responses and extracellular matrix degradation. Nutr Res.30(1):57-65.

[8] Iannone F, Lapadula G. The pathophysiology of osteoarthritis. Aging Clin Exp Res. 2003;15(5):364-72.

[9] Ellman MB, An HS, Muddasani P, Im HJ. Biological impact of the fibroblast growth factor family on articular cartilage and intervertebral disc homeostasis. Gene. 2008;420(1):82-9.

[10] Del Carlo M, Schwartz D, Erickson EA, Loeser RF. Endogenous production of reactive oxygen species is required for stimulation of human articular chondrocyte matrix metalloproteinase production by fibronectin fragments. Free Radic Biol Med. 2007;42(9):1350-8.

[11] Goldring MB, Birkhead J, Sandell LJ, Kimura T, Krane SM. Interleukin 1 suppresses expression of cartilage-specific types II and IX collagens and increases types I and III collagens in human chondrocytes. J Clin Invest. 1988;82(6):2026-37.

[12] Lefebvre V, Peeters-Joris C, Vaes G. Modulation by interleukin 1 and tumor necrosis factor alpha of production of collagenase, tissue inhibitor of metalloproteinases and collagen types in differentiated and dedifferentiated articular chondrocytes. Biochim Biophys Acta. 1990;1052(3):366-78.

[13] Richardson DW, Dodge GR. Effects of interleukin-1beta and tumor necrosis factor-alpha on expression of matrix-related genes by cultured equine articular chondrocytes. Am J Vet Res. 2000;61(6):624-30.

[14] Goldring MB. Osteoarthritis and cartilage: the role of cytokines. Curr Rheumatol Rep. 2000;2(6):459-65.

[15] Kapoor M, Martel-Pelletier J, Lajeunesse D, Pelletier JP, Fahmi H. Role of proinflammatory cytokines in the pathophysiology of osteoarthritis. Nat Rev Rheumatol.7(1):33-42.

[16] Benito MJ, Veale DJ, FitzGerald O, van den Berg WB, Bresnihan B. Synovial tissue inflammation in early and late osteoarthritis. Ann Rheum Dis. 2005;64(9):1263-7.

[17] Smith MD, Triantafillou S, Parker A, Youssef PP, Coleman M. Synovial membrane inflammation and cytokine production in patients with early osteoarthritis. J Rheumatol. 1997;24(2):365-71.

[18] Martel-Pelletier J, McCollum R, DiBattista J, Faure MP, Chin JA, Fournier S, et al. The interleukin-1 receptor in normal and osteoarthritic human articular chondrocytes. Identification as the type I receptor and analysis of binding kinetics and biologic function. Arthritis Rheum. 1992;35(5):530-40.

[19] Evans CH, Gouze JN, Gouze E, Robbins PD, Ghivizzani SC. Osteoarthritis gene therapy. Gene Ther. 2004;11(4):379-89.

[20] Guerne PA, Carson DA, Lotz M. IL-6 production by human articular chondrocytes. Modulation of its synthesis by cytokines, growth factors, and hormones in vitro. J Immunol. 1990;144(2):499-505.

[21] Doss F, Menard J, Hauschild M, Kreutzer HJ, Mittlmeier T, Muller-Steinhardt M, et al. Elevated IL-6 levels in the synovial fluid of osteoarthritis patients stem from plasma cells. Scand J Rheumatol. 2007;36(2):136-9.

[22] Moktar NM, Yusof HM, Yahaya NH, Muhamad R, Das S. The transcript level of interleukin-6 in the cartilage of idiopathic osteoarthritis of knee. Clin Ter.161(1):25-8.

[23] Guerne PA, Desgeorges A, Jaspar JM, Relic B, Peter R, Hoffmeyer P, et al. Effects of IL-6 and its soluble receptor on proteoglycan synthesis and NO release by human articular chondrocytes: comparison with IL-1. Modulation by dexamethasone. Matrix Biol. 1999;18(3):253-60.

[24] Jikko A, Wakisaka T, Iwamoto M, Hiranuma H, Kato Y, Maeda T, et al. Effects of interleukin-6 on proliferation and proteoglycan metabolism in articular chondrocyte cultures. Cell Biol Int. 1998;22(9-10):615-21.

[25] Flannery CR, Little CB, Hughes CE, Curtis CL, Caterson B, Jones SA. IL-6 and its soluble receptor augment aggrecanase-mediated proteoglycan catabolism in articular cartilage. Matrix Biol. 2000;19(6):549-53.

[26] Poree B, Kypriotou M, Chadjichristos C, Beauchef G, Renard E, Legendre F, et al. Interleukin-6 (IL-6) and/or soluble IL-6 receptor down-regulation of human type II collagen gene expression in articular chondrocytes requires a decrease of Sp1.Sp3 ratio and of the binding activity of both factors to the COL2A1 promoter. J Biol Chem. 2008;283(8):4850-65.

[27] Mathy-Hartert M, Hogge L, Sanchez C, Deby-Dupont G, Crielaard JM, Henrotin Y. Interleukin-1beta and interleukin-6 disturb the antioxidant enzyme system in bovine chondrocytes: a possible explanation for oxidative stress generation. Osteoarthritis Cartilage. 2008;16(7):756-63.

[28] de Hooge AS, van de Loo FA, Bennink MB, Arntz OJ, de Hooge P, van den Berg WB. Male IL-6 gene knock out mice developed more advanced osteoarthritis upon aging. Osteoarthritis Cartilage. 2005;13(1):66-73.

[29] Ryu JH, Yang S, Shin Y, Rhee J, Chun CH, Chun JS. Interleukin 6 plays an essential role in hypoxia-inducible factor-2alpha-induced experimental osteoarthritic cartilage destruction in mice. Arthritis Rheum.

[30] Distel E, Cadoudal T, Durant S, Poignard A, Chevalier X, Benelli C. The infrapatellar fat pad in knee osteoarthritis: an important source of interleukin-6 and its soluble receptor. Arthritis Rheum. 2009;60(11):3374-7.

[31] Sylvester J, Liacini A, Li WQ, Zafarullah M. Interleukin-17 signal transduction pathways implicated in inducing matrix metalloproteinase-3, -13 and aggrecanase-1 genes in articular chondrocytes. Cell Signal. 2004;16(4):469-76.

[32] Benderdour M, Tardif G, Pelletier JP, Di Battista JA, Reboul P, Ranger P, et al. Interleukin 17 (IL-17) induces collagenase-3 production in human osteoarthritic chondrocytes via AP-1 dependent activation: differential activation of AP-1 members by IL-17 and IL-1beta. J Rheumatol. 2002;29(6):1262-72.

[33] Pacquelet S, Presle N, Boileau C, Dumond H, Netter P, Martel-Pelletier J, et al. Interleukin 17, a nitric oxide-producing cytokine with a peroxynitrite-independent inhibitory effect on proteoglycan synthesis. J Rheumatol. 2002;29(12):2602-10.

[34] Honorati MC, Neri S, Cattini L, Facchini A. Interleukin-17, a regulator of angiogenic factor release by synovial fibroblasts. Osteoarthritis Cartilage. 2006;14(4):345-52.

[35] Attur MG, Patel RN, Abramson SB, Amin AR. Interleukin-17 up-regulation of nitric oxide production in human osteoarthritis cartilage. Arthritis Rheum. 1997;40(6):1050-3.

[36] Koshy PJ, Henderson N, Logan C, Life PF, Cawston TE, Rowan AD. Interleukin 17 induces cartilage collagen breakdown: novel synergistic effects in combination with proinflammatory cytokines. Ann Rheum Dis. 2002;61(8):704-13.

[37] Martel-Pelletier J, Mineau F, Jovanovic D, Di Battista JA, Pelletier JP. Mitogen-activated protein kinase and nuclear factor kappaB together regulate interleukin-17-induced nitric oxide production in human osteoarthritic chondrocytes: possible role of transactivating factor mitogen-activated protein kinase-activated proten kinase (MAPKAPK). Arthritis Rheum. 1999;42(11):2399-409.

[38] LeGrand A, Fermor B, Fink C, Pisetsky DS, Weinberg JB, Vail TP, et al. Interleukin-1, tumor necrosis factor alpha, and interleukin-17 synergistically up-regulate nitric oxide and prostaglandin E2 production in explants of human osteoarthritic knee menisci. Arthritis Rheum. 2001;44(9):2078-83.

[39] Shalom-Barak T, Quach J, Lotz M. Interleukin-17-induced gene expression in articular chondrocytes is associated with activation of mitogen-activated protein kinases and NF-kappaB. J Biol Chem. 1998;273(42):27467-73.

[40] Honorati MC, Bovara M, Cattini L, Piacentini A, Facchini A. Contribution of interleukin 17 to human cartilage degradation and synovial inflammation in osteoarthritis. Osteoarthritis Cartilage. 2002;10(10):799-807.

[41] Jovanovic DV, Di Battista JA, Martel-Pelletier J, Jolicoeur FC, He Y, Zhang M, et al. IL-17 stimulates the production and expression of proinflammatory cytokines, IL-beta and TNF-alpha, by human macrophages. J Immunol. 1998;160(7):3513-21.

[42] Koenders MI, Marijnissen RJ, Devesa I, Lubberts E, Joosten LA, Roth J, et al. TNF / IL-17 interplay induces S100A8, IL-1beta, and MMPs, and drives irreversible cartilage destruction In Vivo: Rationale for combination treatment during arthritis. Arthritis Rheum.

[43] Nakae S, Nambu A, Sudo K, Iwakura Y. Suppression of immune induction of collagen-induced arthritis in IL-17-deficient mice. J Immunol. 2003;171(11):6173-7.

[44] Westacott CI, Atkins RM, Dieppe PA, Elson CJ. Tumor necrosis factor-alpha receptor expression on chondrocytes isolated from human articular cartilage. J Rheumatol. 1994;21(9):1710-5.

[45] Webb GR, Westacott CI, Elson CJ. Osteoarthritic synovial fluid and synovium supernatants up-regulate tumor necrosis factor receptors on human articular chondrocytes. Osteoarthritis Cartilage. 1998;6(3):167-76.

[46] Marks PH, Donaldson ML. Inflammatory cytokine profiles associated with chondral damage in the anterior cruciate ligament-deficient knee. Arthroscopy. 2005;21(11):1342-7.

[47] Shinmei M, Masuda K, Kikuchi T, Shimomura Y, Okada Y. Production of cytokines by chondrocytes and its role in proteoglycan degradation. J Rheumatol Suppl. 1991;27:89-91.

[48] Malfait AM, Verbruggen G, Veys EM, Lambert J, De Ridder L, Cornelissen M. Comparative and combined effects of interleukin 6, interleukin 1 beta, and tumor necrosis factor alpha on proteoglycan metabolism of human articular chondrocytes cultured in agarose. J Rheumatol. 1994;21(2):314-20.

[49] Steenvoorden MM, Bank RA, Ronday HK, Toes RE, Huizinga TW, DeGroot J. Fibroblast-like synoviocyte-chondrocyte interaction in cartilage degradation. Clin Exp Rheumatol. 2007;25(2):239-45.

[50] Muller RD, John T, Kohl B, Oberholzer A, Gust T, Hostmann A, et al. IL-10 overexpression differentially affects cartilage matrix gene expression in response to TNF-alpha in human articular chondrocytes in vitro. Cytokine. 2008;44(3):377-85.

[51] Ray A, Bal BS, Ray BK. Transcriptional induction of matrix metalloproteinase-9 in the chondrocyte and synoviocyte cells is regulated via a novel mechanism: evidence for functional cooperation between serum amyloid A-activating factor-1 and AP-1. J Immunol. 2005;175(6):4039-48.

[52] Shinmei M, Masuda K, Kikuchi T, Shimomura Y. The role of cytokines in chondrocyte mediated cartilage degradation. J Rheumatol Suppl. 1989;18:32-4.

[53] Tyler JA. Insulin-like growth factor 1 can decrease degradation and promote synthesis of proteoglycan in cartilage exposed to cytokines. Biochem J. 1989;260(2):543-8.

[54] Polzer K, Schett G, Zwerina J. The lonely death: chondrocyte apoptosis in TNF-induced arthritis. Autoimmunity. 2007;40(4):333-6.

[55] Lee SW, Song YS, Lee SY, Yoon YG, Lee SH, Park BS, et al. Downregulation of Protein Kinase CK2 Activity Facilitates Tumor Necrosis Factor-alpha-Mediated Chondrocyte Death through Apoptosis and Autophagy. PLoS One.6(4):e19163.

[56] Mitrovic D, Lippiello L, Gruson F, Aprile F, Mankin HJ. Effects of various prostanoids on the in vitro metabolism of bovine articular chondrocytes. Prostaglandins. 1981;22(3):499-511.

[57] Amin AR, Dave M, Attur M, Abramson SB. COX-2, NO, and cartilage damage and repair. Curr Rheumatol Rep. 2000;2(6):447-53.

[58] Li X, Ellman M, Muddasani P, Wang JH, Cs-Szabo G, van Wijnen AJ, et al. Prostaglandin E2 and its cognate EP receptors control human adult articular cartilage homeostasis and are linked to the pathophysiology of osteoarthritis. Arthritis Rheum. 2009;60(2):513-23.

[59] Attur M, Al-Mussawir HE, Patel J, Kitay A, Dave M, Palmer G, et al. Prostaglandin E2 exerts catabolic effects in osteoarthritis cartilage: evidence for signaling via the EP4 receptor. J Immunol. 2008;181(7):5082-8.

[60] Otsuka S, Aoyama T, Furu M, Ito K, Jin Y, Nasu A, et al. PGE2 signal via EP2 receptors evoked by a selective agonist enhances regeneration of injured articular cartilage. Osteoarthritis Cartilage. 2009;17(4):529-38.

[61] Miwa M, Saura R, Hirata S, Hayashi Y, Mizuno K, Itoh H. Induction of apoptosis in bovine articular chondrocyte by prostaglandin E(2) through cAMP-dependent pathway. Osteoarthritis Cartilage. 2000;8(1):17-24.

[62] Notoya K, Jovanovic DV, Reboul P, Martel-Pelletier J, Mineau F, Pelletier JP. The induction of cell death in human osteoarthritis chondrocytes by nitric oxide is related to the production of prostaglandin E2 via the induction of cyclooxygenase-2. J Immunol. 2000;165(6):3402-10.

[63] Campbell IK, Piccoli DS, Hamilton JA. Stimulation of human chondrocyte prostaglandin E2 production by recombinant human interleukin-1 and tumour necrosis factor. Biochim Biophys Acta. 1990;1051(3):310-8.

[64] Tawara T, Shingu M, Nobunaga M, Naono T. Effects of recombinant human IL-1 beta on production of prostaglandin E2, leukotriene B4, NAG, and superoxide by human synovial cells and chondrocytes. Inflammation. 1991;15(2):145-57.

[65] Verbruggen G, Veys EM, Malfait AM, De Clercq L, Van den Bosch F, de Vlam K. Influence of human recombinant interleukin-1 beta on human articular cartilage. Mitotic activity and proteoglycan metabolism. Clin Exp Rheumatol. 1991;9(5):481-8.

[66] Gosset M, Pigenet A, Salvat C, Berenbaum F, Jacques C. Inhibition of matrix metalloproteinase-3 and -13 synthesis induced by IL-1beta in chondrocytes from mice lacking microsomal prostaglandin E synthase-1. J Immunol.185(10):6244-52.

[67] Di Battista JA, Dore S, Martel-Pelletier J, Pelletier JP. Prostaglandin E2 stimulates incorporation of proline into collagenase digestible proteins in human articular chondrocytes: identification of an effector autocrine loop involving insulin-like growth factor I. Mol Cell Endocrinol. 1996;123(1):27-35.

[68] Dore S, Pelletier JP, DiBattista JA, Tardif G, Brazeau P, Martel-Pelletier J. Human osteoarthritic chondrocytes possess an increased number of insulin-like growth factor 1 binding sites but are unresponsive to its stimulation. Possible role of IGF-1-binding proteins. Arthritis Rheum. 1994;37(2):253-63.

Biochemical Mediators Involved in Cartilage Degradation and the Induction of Pain in Osteoarthritis

[69] Taskiran D, Stefanovic-Racic M, Georgescu H, Evans C. Nitric oxide mediates suppression of cartilage proteoglycan synthesis by interleukin-1. Biochem Biophys Res Commun. 1994;200(1):142-8.

[70] Hauselmann HJ, Oppliger L, Michel BA, Stefanovic-Racic M, Evans CH. Nitric oxide and proteoglycan biosynthesis by human articular chondrocytes in alginate culture. FEBS Lett. 1994;352(3):361-4.

[71] Vuolteenaho K, Moilanen T, Knowles RG, Moilanen E. The role of nitric oxide in osteoarthritis. Scand J Rheumatol. 2007;36(4):247-58.

[72] Tamura T, Nakanishi T, Kimura Y, Hattori T, Sasaki K, Norimatsu H, et al. Nitric oxide mediates interleukin-1-induced matrix degradation and basic fibroblast growth factor release in cultured rabbit articular chondrocytes: a possible mechanism of pathological neovascularization in arthritis. Endocrinology. 1996;137(9):3729-37.

[73] Abramson SB. Nitric oxide in inflammation and pain associated with osteoarthritis. Arthritis Res Ther. 2008;10 Suppl 2:S2.

[74] Studer R, Jaffurs D, Stefanovic-Racic M, Robbins PD, Evans CH. Nitric oxide in osteoarthritis. Osteoarthritis Cartilage. 1999;7(4):377-9.

[75] Borderie D, Hilliquin P, Hernvann A, Lemarechal H, Menkes CJ, Ekindjian OG. Apoptosis induced by nitric oxide is associated with nuclear p53 protein expression in cultured osteoarthritic synoviocytes. Osteoarthritis Cartilage. 1999;7(2):203-13.

[76] Del Carlo M, Jr., Loeser RF. Nitric oxide-mediated chondrocyte cell death requires the generation of additional reactive oxygen species. Arthritis Rheum. 2002;46(2):394-403.

[77] Studer RK, Levicoff E, Georgescu H, Miller L, Jaffurs D, Evans CH. Nitric oxide inhibits chondrocyte response to IGF-I: inhibition of IGF-IRbeta tyrosine phosphorylation. Am J Physiol Cell Physiol. 2000;279(4):C961-9.

[78] van der Kraan PM, Vitters EL, van Beuningen HM, van de Loo FA, van den Berg WB. Role of nitric oxide in the inhibition of BMP-2-mediated stimulation of proteoglycan synthesis in articular cartilage. Osteoarthritis Cartilage. 2000;8(2):82-6.

[79] Amin AR, Di Cesare PE, Vyas P, Attur M, Tzeng E, Billiar TR, et al. The expression and regulation of nitric oxide synthase in human osteoarthritis-affected chondrocytes: evidence for up-regulated neuronal nitric oxide synthase. J Exp Med. 1995;182(6):2097-102.

[80] Melchiorri C, Meliconi R, Frizziero L, Silvestri T, Pulsatelli L, Mazzetti I, et al. Enhanced and coordinated in vivo expression of inflammatory cytokines and nitric oxide synthase by chondrocytes from patients with osteoarthritis. Arthritis Rheum. 1998;41(12):2165-74.

[81] Amin AR, Attur M, Abramson SB. Nitric oxide synthase and cyclooxygenases: distribution, regulation, and intervention in arthritis. Curr Opin Rheumatol. 1999;11(3):202-9.

[82] Vuolteenaho K, Moilanen T, Hamalainen M, Moilanen E. Effects of TNFalpha-antagonists on nitric oxide production in human cartilage. Osteoarthritis Cartilage. 2002;10(4):327-32.

[83] Jarvinen K, Vuolteenaho K, Nieminen R, Moilanen T, Knowles RG, Moilanen E. Selective iNOS inhibitor 1400W enhances anti-catabolic IL-10 and reduces

destructive MMP-10 in OA cartilage. Survey of the effects of 1400W on inflammatory mediators produced by OA cartilage as detected by protein antibody array. Clin Exp Rheumatol. 2008;26(2):275-82.

[84] Huang CY, Hung LF, Liang CC, Ho LJ. COX-2 and iNOS are critical in advanced glycation end product-activated chondrocytes in vitro. Eur J Clin Invest. 2009;39(5):417-28.

[85] Vuolteenaho K, Koskinen A, Kukkonen M, Nieminen R, Paivarinta U, Moilanen T, et al. Leptin enhances synthesis of proinflammatory mediators in human osteoarthritic cartilage--mediator role of NO in leptin-induced PGE2, IL-6, and IL-8 production. Mediators Inflamm. 2009;2009:345838.

[86] Pelletier JP, Jovanovic D, Fernandes JC, Manning P, Connor JR, Currie MG, et al. Reduced progression of experimental osteoarthritis in vivo by selective inhibition of inducible nitric oxide synthase. Arthritis Rheum. 1998;41(7):1275-86.

[87] Presle N, Cipolletta C, Jouzeau JY, Abid A, Netter P, Terlain B. Cartilage protection by nitric oxide synthase inhibitors after intraarticular injection of interleukin-1beta in rats. Arthritis Rheum. 1999;42(10):2094-102.

[88] Sah RL, Trippel SB, Grodzinsky AJ. Differential effects of serum, insulin-like growth factor-I, and fibroblast growth factor-2 on the maintenance of cartilage physical properties during long-term culture. J Orthop Res. 1996;14(1):44-52.

[89] Loeser RF, Chubinskaya S, Pacione C, Im HJ. Basic fibroblast growth factor inhibits the anabolic activity of insulin-like growth factor 1 and osteogenic protein 1 in adult human articular chondrocytes. Arthritis Rheum. 2005;52(12):3910-7.

[90] Schmal H, Zwingmann J, Fehrenbach M, Finkenzeller G, Stark GB, Sudkamp NP, et al. bFGF influences human articular chondrocyte differentiation. Cytotherapy. 2007;9(2):184-93.

[91] Stewart K, Pabbruwe M, Dickinson S, Sims T, Hollander AP, Chaudhuri JB. The effect of growth factor treatment on meniscal chondrocyte proliferation and differentiation on polyglycolic acid scaffolds. Tissue Eng. 2007;13(2):271-80.

[92] Sonal D. Prevention of IGF-1 and TGFbeta stimulated type II collagen and decorin expression by bFGF and identification of IGF-1 mRNA transcripts in articular chondrocytes. Matrix Biol. 2001;20(4):233-42.

[93] Muddasani P, Norman JC, Ellman M, van Wijnen AJ, Im HJ. Basic fibroblast growth factor activates the MAPK and NFkappaB pathways that converge on Elk-1 to control production of matrix metalloproteinase-13 by human adult articular chondrocytes. J Biol Chem. 2007;282(43):31409-21.

[94] Im HJ, Muddasani P, Natarajan V, Schmid TM, Block JA, Davis F, et al. Basic fibroblast growth factor stimulates matrix metalloproteinase-13 via the molecular cross-talk between the mitogen-activated protein kinases and protein kinase Cdelta pathways in human adult articular chondrocytes. J Biol Chem. 2007;282(15):11110-21.

[95] Yan D, Muddasani P, Cool SM, van Wijnen AJ, Mikecz K, Murphy G, et al. Fibroblast Growth Factor Receptor 1 Is Principally Responsible For Fibroblast Growth Factor 2-Induced Catabolic Activities In Human Articular Chondrocytes. Arthritis Res Ther. 2011:In press.

[96]   Sawaji Y, Hynes J, Vincent T, Saklatvala J. Fibroblast growth factor 2 inhibits induction of aggrecanase activity in human articular cartilage. Arthritis Rheum. 2008;58(11):3498-509.

[97]   Chia SL, Sawaji Y, Burleigh A, McLean C, Inglis J, Saklatvala J, et al. Fibroblast growth factor 2 is an intrinsic chondroprotective agent that suppresses ADAMTS-5 and delays cartilage degradation in murine osteoarthritis. Arthritis Rheum. 2009;60(7):2019-27.

[98]   Yasuda T. Cartilage destruction by matrix degradation products. Mod Rheumatol. 2006;16(4):197-205.

[99]   Homandberg GA, Wen C, Hui F. Cartilage damaging activities of fibronectin fragments derived from cartilage and synovial fluid. Osteoarthritis Cartilage. 1998;6(4):231-44.

[100] Jones KL, Brown M, Ali SY, Brown RA. An immunohistochemical study of fibronectin in human osteoarthritic and disease free articular cartilage. Ann Rheum Dis. 1987;46(11):809-15.

[101] Zack MD, Malfait AM, Skepner AP, Yates MP, Griggs DW, Hall T, et al. ADAM-8 isolated from human osteoarthritic chondrocytes cleaves fibronectin at Ala(271). Arthritis Rheum. 2009;60(9):2704-13.

[102] Xie DL, Meyers R, Homandberg GA. Fibronectin fragments in osteoarthritic synovial fluid. J Rheumatol. 1992;19(9):1448-52.

[103] Chevalier X, Groult N, Emod I, Planchenault T. Proteoglycan-degrading activity associated with the 40 kDa collagen-binding fragment of fibronectin. Br J Rheumatol. 1996;35(6):506-14.

[104] Yasuda T, Poole AR. A fibronectin fragment induces type II collagen degradation by collagenase through an interleukin-1-mediated pathway. Arthritis Rheum. 2002;46(1):138-48.

[105] Johnson A, Smith R, Saxne T, Hickery M, Heinegard D. Fibronectin fragments cause release and degradation of collagen-binding molecules from equine explant cultures. Osteoarthritis Cartilage. 2004;12(2):149-59.

[106] Kang Y, Koepp H, Cole AA, Kuettner KE, Homandberg GA. Cultured human ankle and knee cartilage differ in susceptibility to damage mediated by fibronectin fragments. J Orthop Res. 1998;16(5):551-6.

[107] Long D, Blake S, Song XY, Lark M, Loeser RF. Human articular chondrocytes produce IL-7 and respond to IL-7 with increased production of matrix metalloproteinase-13. Arthritis Res Ther. 2008;10(1):R23.

[108] Saito S, Yamaji N, Yasunaga K, Saito T, Matsumoto S, Katoh M, et al. The fibronectin extra domain A activates matrix metalloproteinase gene expression by an interleukin-1-dependent mechanism. J Biol Chem. 1999;274(43):30756-63.

[109] Stanton H, Ung L, Fosang AJ. The 45 kDa collagen-binding fragment of fibronectin induces matrix metalloproteinase-13 synthesis by chondrocytes and aggrecan degradation by aggrecanases. Biochem J. 2002;364(Pt 1):181-90.

[110] Dodds RA, Connor JR, James IE, Rykaczewski EL, Appelbaum E, Dul E, et al. Human osteoclasts, not osteoblasts, deposit osteopontin onto resorption surfaces: an in vitro and ex vivo study of remodeling bone. J Bone Miner Res. 1995;10(11):1666-80.

[111] Pullig O, Weseloh G, Gauer S, Swoboda B. Osteopontin is expressed by adult human osteoarthritic chondrocytes: protein and mRNA analysis of normal and osteoarthritic cartilage. Matrix Biol. 2000;19(3):245-55.

[112] Honsawek S, Tanavalee A, Sakdinakiattikoon M, Chayanupatkul M, Yuktanandana P. Correlation of plasma and synovial fluid osteopontin with disease severity in knee osteoarthritis. Clin Biochem. 2009;42(9):808-12.

[113] Gao SG, Li KH, Zeng KB, Tu M, Xu M, Lei GH. Elevated osteopontin level of synovial fluid and articular cartilage is associated with disease severity in knee osteoarthritis patients. Osteoarthritis Cartilage.18(1):82-7.

[114] Rosenthal AK, Gohr CM, Uzuki M, Masuda I. Osteopontin promotes pathologic mineralization in articular cartilage. Matrix Biol. 2007;26(2):96-105.

[115] Gericke A, Qin C, Spevak L, Fujimoto Y, Butler WT, Sorensen ES, et al. Importance of phosphorylation for osteopontin regulation of biomineralization. Calcif Tissue Int. 2005;77(1):45-54.

[116] Attur MG, Dave MN, Stuchin S, Kowalski AJ, Steiner G, Abramson SB, et al. Osteopontin: an intrinsic inhibitor of inflammation in cartilage. Arthritis Rheum. 2001;44(3):578-84.

[117] Matsui Y, Iwasaki N, Kon S, Takahashi D, Morimoto J, Denhardt DT, et al. Accelerated development of aging-associated and instability-induced osteoarthritis in osteopontin-deficient mice. Arthritis Rheum. 2009;60(8):2362-71.

[118] Jundt G, Berghauser KH, Termine JD, Schulz A. Osteonectin--a differentiation marker of bone cells. Cell Tissue Res. 1987;248(2):409-15.

[119] Chandrasekhar S, Harvey AK, Johnson MG, Becker GW. Osteonectin/SPARC is a product of articular chondrocytes/cartilage and is regulated by cytokines and growth factors. Biochim Biophys Acta. 1994;1221(1):7-14.

[120] Nakamura S, Kamihagi K, Satakeda H, Katayama M, Pan H, Okamoto H, et al. Enhancement of SPARC (osteonectin) synthesis in arthritic cartilage. Increased levels in synovial fluids from patients with rheumatoid arthritis and regulation by growth factors and cytokines in chondrocyte cultures. Arthritis Rheum. 1996;39(4):539-51.

[121] Nanba Y, Nishida K, Yoshikawa T, Sato T, Inoue H, Kuboki Y. Expression of osteonectin in articular cartilage of osteoarthritic knees. Acta Med Okayama. 1997;51(5):239-43.

[122] Tremble PM, Lane TF, Sage EH, Werb Z. SPARC, a secreted protein associated with morphogenesis and tissue remodeling, induces expression of metalloproteinases in fibroblasts through a novel extracellular matrix-dependent pathway. J Cell Biol. 1993;121(6):1433-44.

[123] Arend WP, Welgus HG, Thompson RC, Eisenberg SP. Biological properties of recombinant human monocyte-derived interleukin 1 receptor antagonist. J Clin Invest. 1990;85(5):1694-7.

[124] Smith RJ, Chin JE, Sam LM, Justen JM. Biologic effects of an interleukin-1 receptor antagonist protein on interleukin-1-stimulated cartilage erosion and chondrocyte responsiveness. Arthritis Rheum. 1991;34(1):78-83.

[125] Woodell-May J, Matuska A, Oyster M, Welch Z, O'Shaughnessey K, Hoeppner J. Autologous protein solution inhibits MMP-13 production by IL-1beta and TNFalpha-stimulated human articular chondrocytes. J Orthop Res.

[126] Pelletier JP, Mineau F, Ranger P, Tardif G, Martel-Pelletier J. The increased synthesis of inducible nitric oxide inhibits IL-1ra synthesis by human articular chondrocytes: possible role in osteoarthritic cartilage degradation. Osteoarthritis Cartilage. 1996;4(1):77-84.

[127] Baragi VM, Renkiewicz RR, Jordan H, Bonadio J, Hartman JW, Roessler BJ. Transplantation of transduced chondrocytes protects articular cartilage from interleukin 1-induced extracellular matrix degradation. J Clin Invest. 1995;96(5):2454-60.

[128] Muller-Ladner U, Roberts CR, Franklin BN, Gay RE, Robbins PD, Evans CH, et al. Human IL-1Ra gene transfer into human synovial fibroblasts is chondroprotective. J Immunol. 1997;158(7):3492-8.

[129] Caron JP, Fernandes JC, Martel-Pelletier J, Tardif G, Mineau F, Geng C, et al. Chondroprotective effect of intraarticular injections of interleukin-1 receptor antagonist in experimental osteoarthritis. Suppression of collagenase-1 expression. Arthritis Rheum. 1996;39(9):1535-44.

[130] Doi H, Nishida K, Yorimitsu M, Komiyama T, Kadota Y, Tetsunaga T, et al. Interleukin-4 downregulates the cyclic tensile stress-induced matrix metalloproteinases-13 and cathepsin B expression by rat normal chondrocytes. Acta Med Okayama. 2008;62(2):119-26.

[131] Yorimitsu M, Nishida K, Shimizu A, Doi H, Miyazawa S, Komiyama T, et al. Intra-articular injection of interleukin-4 decreases nitric oxide production by chondrocytes and ameliorates subsequent destruction of cartilage in instability-induced osteoarthritis in rat knee joints. Osteoarthritis Cartilage. 2008;16(7):764-71.

[132] Yeh LA, Augustine AJ, Lee P, Riviere LR, Sheldon A. Interleukin-4, an inhibitor of cartilage breakdown in bovine articular cartilage explants. J Rheumatol. 1995;22(9):1740-6.

[133] Relic B, Guicheux J, Mezin F, Lubberts E, Togninalli D, Garcia I, et al. Il-4 and IL-13, but not IL-10, protect human synoviocytes from apoptosis. J Immunol. 2001;166(4):2775-82.

[134] Manning K, Rachakonda PS, Rai MF, Schmidt MF. Co-expression of insulin-like growth factor-1 and interleukin-4 in an in vitro inflammatory model. Cytokine.50(3):297-305.

[135] Iannone F, De Bari C, Dell'Accio F, Covelli M, Cantatore FP, Patella V, et al. Interleukin-10 and interleukin-10 receptor in human osteoarthritic and healthy chondrocytes. Clin Exp Rheumatol. 2001;19(2):139-45.

[136] Fernandes JC, Martel-Pelletier J, Pelletier JP. The role of cytokines in osteoarthritis pathophysiology. Biorheology. 2002;39(1-2):237-46.

[137] Zhang X, Mao Z, Yu C. Suppression of early experimental osteoarthritis by gene transfer of interleukin-1 receptor antagonist and interleukin-10. J Orthop Res. 2004;22(4):742-50.

[138] Maier R, Ganu V, Lotz M. Interleukin-11, an inducible cytokine in human articular chondrocytes and synoviocytes, stimulates the production of the tissue inhibitor of metalloproteinases. J Biol Chem. 1993;268(29):21527-32.

[139] Trepicchio WL, Dorner AJ. The therapeutic utility of Interleukin-11 in the treatment of inflammatory disease. Expert Opin Investig Drugs. 1998;7(9):1501-4.

[140] Alaaeddine N, Di Battista JA, Pelletier JP, Kiansa K, Cloutier JM, Martel-Pelletier J. Differential effects of IL-8, LIF (pro-inflammatory) and IL-11 (anti-inflammatory) on TNF-alpha-induced PGE(2)release and on signalling pathways in human OA synovial fibroblasts. Cytokine. 1999;11(12):1020-30.

[141] Hermann JA, Hall MA, Maini RN, Feldmann M, Brennan FM. Important immunoregulatory role of interleukin-11 in the inflammatory process in rheumatoid arthritis. Arthritis Rheum. 1998;41(8):1388-97.

[142] Walmsley M, Butler DM, Marinova-Mutafchieva L, Feldmann M. An anti-inflammatory role for interleukin-11 in established murine collagen-induced arthritis. Immunology. 1998;95(1):31-7.

[143] Trontzas P, Kamper EF, Potamianou A, Kyriazis NC, Kritikos H, Stavridis J. Comparative study of serum and synovial fluid interleukin-11 levels in patients with various arthritides. Clin Biochem. 1998;31(8):673-9.

[144] Tardif G, Pelletier JP, Dupuis M, Geng C, Cloutier JM, Martel-Pelletier J. Collagenase 3 production by human osteoarthritic chondrocytes in response to growth factors and cytokines is a function of the physiologic state of the cells. Arthritis Rheum. 1999;42(6):1147-58.

[145] Chabaud M, Durand JM, Buchs N, Fossiez F, Page G, Frappart L, et al. Human interleukin-17: A T cell-derived proinflammatory cytokine produced by the rheumatoid synovium. Arthritis Rheum. 1999;42(5):963-70.

[146] Jovanovic D, Pelletier JP, Alaaeddine N, Mineau F, Geng C, Ranger P, et al. Effect of IL-13 on cytokines, cytokine receptors and inhibitors on human osteoarthritis synovium and synovial fibroblasts. Osteoarthritis Cartilage. 1998;6(1):40-9.

[147] Alaaeddine N, Di Battista JA, Pelletier JP, Kiansa K, Cloutier JM, Martel-Pelletier J. Inhibition of tumor necrosis factor alpha-induced prostaglandin E2 production by the antiinflammatory cytokines interleukin-4, interleukin-10, and interleukin-13 in osteoarthritic synovial fibroblasts: distinct targeting in the signaling pathways. Arthritis Rheum. 1999;42(4):710-8.

[148] Woods JM, Haines GK, Shah MR, Rayan G, Koch AE. Low-level production of interleukin-13 in synovial fluid and tissue from patients with arthritis. Clin Immunol Immunopathol. 1997;85(2):210-20.

[149] Fortier LA, Barker JU, Strauss EJ, McCarrel TM, Cole BJ. The Role of Growth Factors in Cartilage Repair. Clin Orthop Relat Res.

[150] Chubinskaya S, Segalite D, Pikovsky D, Hakimiyan AA, Rueger DC. Effects induced by BMPS in cultures of human articular chondrocytes: comparative studies. Growth Factors. 2008;26(5):275-83.

[151] Chubinskaya S, Hurtig M, Rueger DC. OP-1/BMP-7 in cartilage repair. Int Orthop. 2007;31(6):773-81.

[152] van der Kraan PM, Blaney Davidson EN, van den Berg WB. A role for age-related changes in TGFbeta signaling in aberrant chondrocyte differentiation and osteoarthritis. Arthritis Res Ther.12(1):201.

[153] Blaney Davidson EN, van der Kraan PM, van den Berg WB. TGF-beta and osteoarthritis. Osteoarthritis Cartilage. 2007;15(6):597-604.

[154] Fan J, Gong Y, Ren L, Varshney RR, Cai D, Wang DA. In vitro engineered cartilage using synovium-derived mesenchymal stem cells with injectable gellan hydrogels. Acta Biomater.6(3):1178-85.

[155] Kizawa H, Kou I, Iida A, Sudo A, Miyamoto Y, Fukuda A, et al. An aspartic acid repeat polymorphism in asporin inhibits chondrogenesis and increases susceptibility to osteoarthritis. Nat Genet. 2005;37(2):138-44.

[156] Jiang Q, Shi D, Yi L, Ikegawa S, Wang Y, Nakamura T, et al. Replication of the association of the aspartic acid repeat polymorphism in the asporin gene with knee-osteoarthritis susceptibility in Han Chinese. J Hum Genet. 2006;51(12):1068-72.

[157] Yang X, Chen L, Xu X, Li C, Huang C, Deng CX. TGF-beta/Smad3 signals repress chondrocyte hypertrophic differentiation and are required for maintaining articular cartilage. J Cell Biol. 2001;153(1):35-46.

[158] Serra R, Johnson M, Filvaroff EH, LaBorde J, Sheehan DM, Derynck R, et al. Expression of a truncated, kinase-defective TGF-beta type II receptor in mouse skeletal tissue promotes terminal chondrocyte differentiation and osteoarthritis. J Cell Biol. 1997;139(2):541-52.

[159] Blaney Davidson EN, Scharstuhl A, Vitters EL, van der Kraan PM, van den Berg WB. Reduced transforming growth factor-beta signaling in cartilage of old mice: role in impaired repair capacity. Arthritis Res Ther. 2005;7(6):R1338-47.

[160] Morales TI. Transforming growth factor-beta 1 stimulates synthesis of proteoglycan aggregates in calf articular cartilage organ cultures. Arch Biochem Biophys. 1991;286(1):99-106.

[161] Bakker AC, van de Loo FA, van Beuningen HM, Sime P, van Lent PL, van der Kraan PM, et al. Overexpression of active TGF-beta-1 in the murine knee joint: evidence for synovial-layer-dependent chondro-osteophyte formation. Osteoarthritis Cartilage. 2001;9(2):128-36.

[162] Livne E, Laufer D, Blumenfeld I. Differential response of articular cartilage from young growing and mature old mice to IL-1 and TGF-beta. Arch Gerontol Geriatr. 1997;24(2):211-21.

[163] Gouttenoire J, Valcourt U, Ronziere MC, Aubert-Foucher E, Mallein-Gerin F, Herbage D. Modulation of collagen synthesis in normal and osteoarthritic cartilage. Biorheology. 2004;41(3-4):535-42.

[164] Arai Y, Kubo T, Kobayashi K, Takeshita K, Takahashi K, Ikeda T, et al. Adenovirus vector-mediated gene transduction to chondrocytes: in vitro evaluation of therapeutic efficacy of transforming growth factor-beta 1 and heat shock protein 70 gene transduction. J Rheumatol. 1997;24(9):1787-95.

[165] Blaney Davidson EN, Vitters EL, van Lent PL, van de Loo FA, van den Berg WB, van der Kraan PM. Elevated extracellular matrix production and degradation upon

bone morphogenetic protein-2 (BMP-2) stimulation point toward a role for BMP-2 in cartilage repair and remodeling. Arthritis Res Ther. 2007;9(5):R102.

[166] Im HJ, Pacione C, Chubinskaya S, Van Wijnen AJ, Sun Y, Loeser RF. Inhibitory effects of insulin-like growth factor-1 and osteogenic protein-1 on fibronectin fragment- and interleukin-1beta-stimulated matrix metalloproteinase-13 expression in human chondrocytes. J Biol Chem. 2003;278(28):25386-94.

[167] Flechtenmacher J, Huch K, Thonar EJ, Mollenhauer JA, Davies SR, Schmid TM, et al. Recombinant human osteogenic protein 1 is a potent stimulator of the synthesis of cartilage proteoglycans and collagens by human articular chondrocytes. Arthritis Rheum. 1996;39(11):1896-904.

[168] Imai Y, Okuma M, An HS, Nakagawa K, Yamada M, Muehleman C, et al. Restoration of disc height loss by recombinant human osteogenic protein-1 injection into intervertebral discs undergoing degeneration induced by an intradiscal injection of chondroitinase ABC. Spine (Phila Pa 1976). 2007;32(11):1197-205.

[169] Loeser RF, Pacione CA, Chubinskaya S. The combination of insulin-like growth factor 1 and osteogenic protein 1 promotes increased survival of and matrix synthesis by normal and osteoarthritic human articular chondrocytes. Arthritis Rheum. 2003;48(8):2188-96.

[170] Merrihew C, Kumar B, Heretis K, Rueger DC, Kuettner KE, Chubinskaya S. Alterations in endogenous osteogenic protein-1 with degeneration of human articular cartilage. J Orthop Res. 2003;21(5):899-907.

[171] Chubinskaya S, Kumar B, Merrihew C, Heretis K, Rueger DC, Kuettner KE. Age-related changes in cartilage endogenous osteogenic protein-1 (OP-1). Biochim Biophys Acta. 2002;1588(2):126-34.

[172] Miyamoto C, Matsumoto T, Sakimura K, Shindo H. Osteogenic protein-1 with transforming growth factor-beta1: potent inducer of chondrogenesis of synovial mesenchymal stem cells in vitro. J Orthop Sci. 2007;12(6):555-61.

[173] Jelic M, Pecina M, Haspl M, Kos J, Taylor K, Maticic D, et al. Regeneration of articular cartilage chondral defects by osteogenic protein-1 (bone morphogenetic protein-7) in sheep. Growth Factors. 2001;19(2):101-13.

[174] Luyten FP, Hascall VC, Nissley SP, Morales TI, Reddi AH. Insulin-like growth factors maintain steady-state metabolism of proteoglycans in bovine articular cartilage explants. Arch Biochem Biophys. 1988;267(2):416-25.

[175] Sah RL, Chen AC, Grodzinsky AJ, Trippel SB. Differential effects of bFGF and IGF-I on matrix metabolism in calf and adult bovine cartilage explants. Arch Biochem Biophys. 1994;308(1):137-47.

[176] Ekenstedt KJ, Sonntag WE, Loeser RF, Lindgren BR, Carlson CS. Effects of chronic growth hormone and insulin-like growth factor 1 deficiency on osteoarthritis severity in rat knee joints. Arthritis Rheum. 2006;54(12):3850-8.

[177] Goodrich LR, Hidaka C, Robbins PD, Evans CH, Nixon AJ. Genetic modification of chondrocytes with insulin-like growth factor-1 enhances cartilage healing in an equine model. J Bone Joint Surg Br. 2007;89(5):672-85.

[178] Fortier LA, Mohammed HO, Lust G, Nixon AJ. Insulin-like growth factor-I enhances cell-based repair of articular cartilage. J Bone Joint Surg Br. 2002;84(2):276-88.

[179] Osada R, Ohshima H, Ishihara H, Yudoh K, Sakai K, Matsui H, et al. Autocrine/paracrine mechanism of insulin-like growth factor-1 secretion, and the effect of insulin-like growth factor-1 on proteoglycan synthesis in bovine intervertebral discs. J Orthop Res. 1996;14(5):690-9.

[180] Gruber HE, Norton HJ, Hanley EN, Jr. Anti-apoptotic effects of IGF-1 and PDGF on human intervertebral disc cells in vitro. Spine (Phila Pa 1976). 2000;25(17):2153-7.

[181] Loeser RF, Shanker G, Carlson CS, Gardin JF, Shelton BJ, Sonntag WE. Reduction in the chondrocyte response to insulin-like growth factor 1 in aging and osteoarthritis: studies in a non-human primate model of naturally occurring disease. Arthritis Rheum. 2000;43(9):2110-20.

[182] Boehm AK, Seth M, Mayr KG, Fortier LA. Hsp90 mediates insulin-like growth factor 1 and interleukin-1beta signaling in an age-dependent manner in equine articular chondrocytes. Arthritis Rheum. 2007;56(7):2335-43.

[183] Morales TI. The quantitative and functional relation between insulin-like growth factor-I (IGF) and IGF-binding proteins during human osteoarthritis. J Orthop Res. 2008;26(4):465-74.

[184] Wang Z, Huang Y, Zou J, Cao K, Xu Y, Wu JM. Effects of red wine and wine polyphenol resveratrol on platelet aggregation in vivo and in vitro. Int J Mol Med. 2002;9(1):77-9.

[185] Orallo F, Alvarez E, Camina M, Leiro JM, Gomez E, Fernandez P. The possible implication of trans-Resveratrol in the cardioprotective effects of long-term moderate wine consumption. Mol Pharmacol. 2002;61(2):294-302.

[186] Haider UG, Sorescu D, Griendling KK, Vollmar AM, Dirsch VM. Resveratrol suppresses angiotensin II-induced Akt/protein kinase B and p70 S6 kinase phosphorylation and subsequent hypertrophy in rat aortic smooth muscle cells. Mol Pharmacol. 2002;62(4):772-7.

[187] Bhat KPL, Kosmeder JW, 2nd, Pezzuto JM. Biological effects of resveratrol. Antioxid Redox Signal. 2001;3(6):1041-64.

[188] Bertelli AA, Ferrara F, Diana G, Fulgenzi A, Corsi M, Ponti W, et al. Resveratrol, a natural stilbene in grapes and wine, enhances intraphagocytosis in human promonocytes: a co-factor in antiinflammatory and anticancer chemopreventive activity. Int J Tissue React. 1999;21(4):93-104.

[189] Fremont L. Biological effects of resveratrol. Life Sci. 2000;66(8):663-73.

[190] Huang KS, Lin M, Cheng GF. Anti-inflammatory tetramers of resveratrol from the roots of Vitis amurensis and the conformations of the seven-membered ring in some oligostilbenes. Phytochemistry. 2001;58(2):357-62.

[191] Jang M, Cai L, Udeani GO, Slowing KV, Thomas CF, Beecher CW, et al. Cancer chemopreventive activity of resveratrol, a natural product derived from grapes. Science. 1997;275(5297):218-20.

[192] Martinez J, Moreno JJ. Effect of resveratrol, a natural polyphenolic compound, on reactive oxygen species and prostaglandin production. Biochem Pharmacol. 2000;59(7):865-70.

[193] Ignatowicz E, Baer-Dubowska W. Resveratrol, a natural chemopreventive agent against degenerative diseases. Pol J Pharmacol. 2001;53(6):557-69.

[194] Leiro J, Alvarez E, Arranz JA, Laguna R, Uriarte E, Orallo F. Effects of cis-resveratrol on inflammatory murine macrophages: antioxidant activity and down-regulation of inflammatory genes. J Leukoc Biol. 2004;75(6):1156-65.

[195] Elmali N, Esenkaya I, Harma A, Ertem K, Turkoz Y, Mizrak B. Effect of resveratrol in experimental osteoarthritis in rabbits. Inflamm Res. 2005;54(4):158-62.

[196] Elmali N, Baysal O, Harma A, Esenkaya I, Mizrak B. Effects of resveratrol in inflammatory arthritis. Inflammation. 2007;30(1-2):1-6.

[197] Shakibaei M, John T, Seifarth C, Mobasheri A. Resveratrol inhibits IL-1 beta-induced stimulation of caspase-3 and cleavage of PARP in human articular chondrocytes in vitro. Ann N Y Acad Sci. 2007;1095:554-63.

[198] Csaki C, Keshishzadeh N, Fischer K, Shakibaei M. Regulation of inflammation signalling by resveratrol in human chondrocytes in vitro. Biochem Pharmacol. 2008;75(3):677-87.

[199] Li X, Phillips FM, An HS, Ellman M, Thonar EJ, Wu W, et al. The action of resveratrol, a phytoestrogen found in grapes, on the intervertebral disc. Spine (Phila Pa 1976). 2008;33(24):2586-95.

[200] Gitay-Goren H, Soker S, Vlodavsky I, Neufeld G. The binding of vascular endothelial growth factor to its receptors is dependent on cell surface-associated heparin-like molecules. J Biol Chem. 1992;267(9):6093-8.

[201] Baker EN, Baker HM. A structural framework for understanding the multifunctional character of lactoferrin. Biochimie. 2009;91(1):3-10.

[202] Mader JS, Richardson A, Salsman J, Top D, de Antueno R, Duncan R, et al. Bovine lactoferricin causes apoptosis in Jurkat T-leukemia cells by sequential permeabilization of the cell membrane and targeting of mitochondria. Exp Cell Res. 2007;313(12):2634-50.

[203] Gifford JL, Hunter HN, Vogel HJ. Lactoferricin: a lactoferrin-derived peptide with antimicrobial, antiviral, antitumor and immunological properties. Cell Mol Life Sci. 2005;62(22):2588-98.

[204] Henrotin YE, Bruckner P, Pujol JP. The role of reactive oxygen species in homeostasis and degradation of cartilage. Osteoarthritis Cartilage. 2003;11(10):747-55.

[205] Guillen C, McInnes IB, Vaughan D, Speekenbrink AB, Brock JH. The effects of local administration of lactoferrin on inflammation in murine autoimmune and infectious arthritis. Arthritis Rheum. 2000;43(9):2073-80.

[206] Hayashida K, Kaneko T, Takeuchi T, Shimizu H, Ando K, Harada E. Oral administration of lactoferrin inhibits inflammation and nociception in rat adjuvant-induced arthritis. J Vet Med Sci. 2004;66(2):149-54.

[207] Wong SH, Francis N, Chahal H, Raza K, Salmon M, Scheel-Toellner D, et al. Lactoferrin is a survival factor for neutrophils in rheumatoid synovial fluid. Rheumatology (Oxford). 2009;48(1):39-44.

[208] Cornish J, Callon KE, Naot D, Palmano KP, Banovic T, Bava U, et al. Lactoferrin is a potent regulator of bone cell activity and increases bone formation in vivo. Endocrinology. 2004;145(9):4366-74.

[209] Kim JS, Ellman MB, An HS, Yan D, van Wijnen AJ, Murphy G, et al. Lactoferricin mediates anabolic and anti-catabolic effects in the intervertebral disc. J Cell Physiol.

[210] Sprangers MA, de Regt EB, Andries F, van Agt HM, Bijl RV, de Boer JB, et al. Which chronic conditions are associated with better or poorer quality of life? J Clin Epidemiol. 2000;53(9):895-907.

[211] Dray A, Read SJ. Arthritis and pain. Future targets to control osteoarthritis pain. Arthritis Res Ther. 2007;9(3):212.

[212] Creamer P, Hunt M, Dieppe P. Pain mechanisms in osteoarthritis of the knee: effect of intraarticular anesthetic. J Rheumatol. 1996;23(6):1031-6.

[213] Kosek E, Ordeberg G. Lack of pressure pain modulation by heterotopic noxious conditioning stimulation in patients with painful osteoarthritis before, but not following, surgical pain relief. Pain. 2000;88(1):69-78.

[214] Loeser RF, Yammani RR, Carlson CS, Chen H, Cole A, Im HJ, et al. Articular chondrocytes express the receptor for advanced glycation end products: Potential role in osteoarthritis. Arthritis Rheum. 2005;52(8):2376-85.

[215] Li X, An HS, Ellman M, Phillips F, Thonar EJ, Park DK, et al. Action of fibroblast growth factor-2 on the intervertebral disc. Arthritis Res Ther. 2008;10(2):R48.

[216] Schaible HG, Richter F, Ebersberger A, Boettger MK, Vanegas H, Natura G, et al. Joint pain. Exp Brain Res. 2009;196(1):153-62.

[217] Sommer C, Kress M. Recent findings on how proinflammatory cytokines cause pain: peripheral mechanisms in inflammatory and neuropathic hyperalgesia. Neurosci Lett. 2004;361(1-3):184-7.

[218] Brenn D, Richter F, Schaible HG. Sensitization of unmyelinated sensory fibers of the joint nerve to mechanical stimuli by interleukin-6 in the rat: an inflammatory mechanism of joint pain. Arthritis Rheum. 2007;56(1):351-9.

[219] Arvidson NG, Gudbjornsson B, Elfman L, Ryden AC, Totterman TH, Hallgren R. Circadian rhythm of serum interleukin-6 in rheumatoid arthritis. Ann Rheum Dis. 1994;53(8):521-4.

[220] Desgeorges A, Gabay C, Silacci P, Novick D, Roux-Lombard P, Grau G, et al. Concentrations and origins of soluble interleukin 6 receptor-alpha in serum and synovial fluid. J Rheumatol. 1997;24(8):1510-6.

[221] Obreja O, Biasio W, Andratsch M, Lips KS, Rathee PK, Ludwig A, et al. Fast modulation of heat-activated ionic current by proinflammatory interleukin 6 in rat sensory neurons. Brain. 2005;128(Pt 7):1634-41.

[222] Ohtori S, Takahashi K, Moriya H, Myers RR. TNF-alpha and TNF-alpha receptor type 1 upregulation in glia and neurons after peripheral nerve injury: studies in murine DRG and spinal cord. Spine (Phila Pa 1976). 2004;29(10):1082-8.

[223] Schafers M, Marziniak M, Sorkin LS, Yaksh TL, Sommer C. Cyclooxygenase inhibition in nerve-injury- and TNF-induced hyperalgesia in the rat. Exp Neurol. 2004;185(1):160-8.

[224] Grunke M, Schulze-Koops H. Successful treatment of inflammatory knee osteoarthritis with tumour necrosis factor blockade. Ann Rheum Dis. 2006;65(4):555-6.

[225] Inglis JJ, Notley CA, Essex D, Wilson AW, Feldmann M, Anand P, et al. Collagen-induced arthritis as a model of hyperalgesia: functional and cellular analysis of the analgesic actions of tumor necrosis factor blockade. Arthritis Rheum. 2007;56(12):4015-23.

[226] Yaksh TL, Dirig DM, Conway CM, Svensson C, Luo ZD, Isakson PC. The acute antihyperalgesic action of nonsteroidal, anti-inflammatory drugs and release of spinal prostaglandin E2 is mediated by the inhibition of constitutive spinal cyclooxygenase-2 (COX-2) but not COX-1. J Neurosci. 2001;21(16):5847-53.

[227] England S, Bevan S, Docherty RJ. PGE2 modulates the tetrodotoxin-resistant sodium current in neonatal rat dorsal root ganglion neurones via the cyclic AMP-protein kinase A cascade. J Physiol. 1996;495 (Pt 2):429-40.

[228] Bar KJ, Natura G, Telleria-Diaz A, Teschner P, Vogel R, Vasquez E, et al. Changes in the effect of spinal prostaglandin E2 during inflammation: prostaglandin E (EP1-EP4) receptors in spinal nociceptive processing of input from the normal or inflamed knee joint. J Neurosci. 2004;24(3):642-51.

[229] Castro RR, Cunha FQ, Silva FS, Jr., Rocha FA. A quantitative approach to measure joint pain in experimental osteoarthritis--evidence of a role for nitric oxide. Osteoarthritis Cartilage. 2006;14(8):769-76.

[230] Claveau D, Sirinyan M, Guay J, Gordon R, Chan CC, Bureau Y, et al. Microsomal prostaglandin E synthase-1 is a major terminal synthase that is selectively up-regulated during cyclooxygenase-2-dependent prostaglandin E2 production in the rat adjuvant-induced arthritis model. J Immunol. 2003;170(9):4738-44.

[231] Trebino CE, Stock JL, Gibbons CP, Naiman BM, Wachtmann TS, Umland JP, et al. Impaired inflammatory and pain responses in mice lacking an inducible prostaglandin E synthase. Proc Natl Acad Sci U S A. 2003;100(15):9044-9.

5

Toll-Like Receptors: At the Intersection of Osteoarthritis Pathology and Pain

Qi Wu and James L. Henry

*Department of Psychiatry and Behavioural Neurosciences,
McMaster University, Hamilton,
Canada*

1. Introduction

Osteoarthritis (OA) is a common chronic joint disease projected to affect an astounding 18% of the population in the western world by the year 2020 (Lawrence et al., 1998). In addition, it has a cost of $15.5 billion per year in the US alone, taking into account the accompanying disability and social consequences (Yelin and Callahan, 1995). Current hypotheses of OA pathology and OA pain tend to be exclusive to either. Here we present a hypothesis that is an attempt to identify a common aetiology for both.

2. OA pathology

The features of OA constitute a group of conditions that are diagnosed upon common pathological and radiological characteristics (Felson et al., 1997) and are believed to be caused by material failure of the cartilage network leading to tissue breakdown (Poole, 1999) or by injury of chondrocytes with increased degradative responses (Aigner and Kim, 2002).

3. OA pain

Pain has been defined as the primary symptom of OA (Creamer, 2000). Physicians typically rely on scores of pain and measures of joint function to make treatment decisions for OA (Swagerty, Jr. and Hellinger, 2001), as pain rather than joint pathology is more pronounced in this disorder.

4. Immunologic mechanisms in OA

OA has been considered to primarily affect cartilage and bone. However, there is increasing awareness that all tissues of the synovial joint, including synovium, ligaments and nerve terminals, are likely affected by this complex disease. Moreover, OA has been described as a non-inflammatory degenerative condition that is characterized by the imbalance of articular cartilage degradation and repair. Traumatic injury of the joint, either acute sport injuries or chronic aging accumulation is the leading cause of this imbalance. But genetic factors also play a role in some OA. Surprisingly, C-reactive protein (CRP), a systemic marker of inflammation, is increased in serum in OA patients at early phases (Saxne et al.,

2003b;Sowers et al., 2002) although it has been suggested that inflammation is actually related to complication by crystalline arthritis (Rothschild and Martin, 2006). This suggests the presence of low-grade inflammation at early stages of the disease process.

Recently, the research of the genetic linkages and the innate immune activation in OA further supports a possible pathogenic role of inflammation and a "chronic wound repair" type of immunologic mechanisms in OA (Kato et al., 2004;Scanzello et al., 2008). There have been reports about linkages between HLA haplotypes and OA, including the linkages of HLA-Cw1, 4, 10 (Wakitani et al., 2001), HLA B35-DQ1, B40-DQ1, DR2-DQ1 (Merlotti et al., 2003), HLA DR2, DR4 (Riyazi et al., 2003). These HLAs are polymorphologic molecules presenting antigens to T cells, which supports a role of immune activation at the onset of OA.

Synovial inflammation is milder than in rheumatoid arthritis (RA). Despite this, cellular infiltration of activated lymphocytes and neo-vascularisation are documented in many advanced OA, as well as patients at early stages (Walsh et al., 2007;Pearle et al., 2007;Saito et al., 2002;Saxne et al., 2003a). The severity of synovial inflammation defined by MRI is correlated with pain intensities in OA patients (Hill et al., 2007). Synovitis seen under arthroscopy is associated with cartilage degradation (Ayral et al., 2005).

Increased levels of immunoglobulins have been reported in OA. Jasin reported IgM and IgG levels in OA cartilage tissue are three times more than in normal cartilage tissue (Jasin, 1985). This suggests that antibodies are synthesized within the affected joint by infiltrating immune cells or that the cartilage is more permeable to immunoglobulins.

5. Toll-like receptors (TLRs)

TLRs are a group of pattern recognition receptors (Barton and Medzhitov, 2002), which gate the immune response. Up to now, a total of 13 TLRs have been identified -TLR1 to TLR10 in human; TLR1 to TLR13 (except TLR10) in murine (Beutler, 2005). A highly specific pattern governs the TLR recognition of various microbial ligands. Each of these TLRs responds only to a limited number of microbial ligands summarized in Table 1 of Akira and Takeda (2004).

TLRs adopt either the myeloid differentiation primary response gene 88 (MyD88)-dependent or MyD88-independent pathway following activation. TLR signalling pathways lead to the production of several critical transcription factors, including NF-κB, interferon regulatory factor (IRF) and activator protein-1 (AP-1). Three most common TLR-mediated signalling pathways are the MyD88-dependent and MyD88-independent release of NF-κB, and the MyD88-independent production of IRF. Each of TLRs seems to recruit different subsequent signalling pathways (Akira and Takeda, 2004). But detailed information remains unclear to us. Mollen et al. (2006) proposed the theory of "TLRs and danger signalling": During tissue stress or injury, a variety of damage-associated molecules are actively secreted by stressed cells, passively released from necrotic cells, or originally from the degradation of the extracellular matrix. These damage-associated molecular patterns are recognized by TLRs in a similar manner as that of exogenous pathogen-associated molecular patterns.

A long list of damage-associated molecules have been proposed as putative endogenous TLR ligands (Beg, 2002), including hyaluronan, heparin sulphate, fibrinogen, high-mobility group protein (HMGB1), HSP 60, host mRNA, host chromatin and small ribonucleoprotein particles as well. Therefore, TLRs seem to be critical players in determining the nature of tissue injure, and initiating corresponding signalling pathways that result in distinct forms of pain.

Increasing evidence supports TLR4 as the main TLR sensing tissue damage in that it responds to a couple of endogenous ligands, such as HSP 60, fibrinogen, heparin sulphate and hyaluronan (Johnson et al., 2002;Ohashi et al., 2000;Smiley et al., 2001;Taylor et al., 2004a;Termeer et al., 2002). TLR4-dependent signalling pathway has been linked to sterile inflammation resulted from various neural and non-neural tissue injuries. Studies reveal that the production of inflammatory cytokines is compromised during tissue injuries in C3H/HeJ strain mice featured with TLR4 mutation - reduced TNF level in would incision (Bettinger et al., 1994); low circulating IL-6 in hemorrhagic shock (Prince et al., 2006); and decreased IL-1β expression at the nerve stump in sciatic nerve lesion (Boivin et al., 2007). As a consequence, the overall inflammatory response in TLR4-deficient animals is attenuated. Evidence includes reduced accumulation and activation of macrophages in injured nerve tissue (Boivin et al., 2007); less severe systemic inflammatory response (e.g. lower hepatic IL-6 level, less liver injury) after bilateral femur fracture with soft tissue crush injury (Levy et al., 2006).

TLR2 was implicated in the pathogenesis of arthritis (Cho et al., 2007). TLR2, IL-8, and vascular endothelial growth factor (VEGF) were upregulated in arthritic joints in human synovial tissue culture, which was block by anti-TLR2 antibodies. Interestingly, HMGB1 was up-regulated at the same time frame in arthritic joints in human (Kokkola et al., 2002;Taniguchi et al., 2003). HMGB1 has been proposed as the primary putative endogenous TLR2 ligand (Park et al., 2004;van Beijnum et al., 2008;Yu et al., 2006). Although there is no direct evidence for the involvement of HMGB1-TLR2-mediated pathway in arthritis, some results favour the notion. Park et al. (2006) showed the protein-protein interaction between HMGB1 and TLR2 was functional in term of initiating intracellular signal transductions. Yu et al. (2006) demonstrated that anti-TLR2 antibody blocked HMGB1-induced TLR2-dependent IL-8 release in HEK cells.

TLR3 and TLR9 are known to recognize microbial nucleic acids. However, host nucleic acids are also capable of initiating immune response via TLR activation - chromatin can induce the production of anti-DNA antibodies via a TLR9-dependent mechanism (Leadbetter et al., 2002). In Alzheimer's patients, TLR3 expression was identified in brains without previous viral infection (Jackson et al., 2006). The up-regulation of TLR3 expression might partly be explained by the finding that RNA is a constituent in senile plaques (Marcinkiewicz, 2002). The inflammatory nature of the disease may result from TLR3 activation by host RNA. Necrotic cells resulted from various processes including tissue injuries release host nucleic acids. Kariko et al. (2004) demonstrated that it was RNA released from necrotic cells that led to TLR3-dependent release of TNF-α. Necrotic cell lysates lost the capability to stimulate TNF-α release once they were pretreated with Benzonase, a potent and nonspecific nuclease that degrades all RNA into oligomers of 2–5 nucleotides in length.

6. TLR pathways in OA pathology

Age and joint trauma are two risk factors for the development and progression of OA. Endogenous damage-associated molecules, including hyaluronan, fibronectin, have been identified in OA in response to initial tissue injury. Hyaluronan is highly viscous polysaccharide found in the extracellular matrix, and is a major component of synovial fluid and cartilage, which plays an important role in the lubrication and shock absorption for the joint tissue. Its molecular weight/length is reduced in exercise and joint injury (Brown et al., 2007). In OA, both of the concentration and molecular weight of hyaluronan are reduced (Dahl et al., 1985). Hyaluronan fragments of specific sizes have been shown to promote angiogenesis and have immune regulatory effects mediated by the TLR-4 receptor (Taylor et al., 2004b). However, TLR-4 responses initiated by bacterial product lipopolysaccharide (LPS) and endogenous product hyaluronan are different, due to the recruitment of different accessory molecules, CD14 for the LPS-TLR-4 response and CD44 for the hyaluronan-TLR-4 response (Taylor et al., 2007). Fibronectin is another extracellular matrix component affected by both age and tissue injury, and the presence of fibronectin and a specific isoform containing the B sequence, Ed-B fibronectin, in osteoarthritic cartilage but not in normal cartilage has led to the suggestion that the isoform might play a role in extracellular matrix remodelling (Chevalier et al., 1996). In addition to the traditional integrin-mediated pathways, certain splice variants of fibronectin are also capable of activating a TLR-4 dependant pathway (Lasarte et al., 2007;Gondokaryono et al., 2007;Okamura et al., 2001).

Although TLRs are constitutively expressed on immune cells, the expression of TLR can be induced on other cell types as a result of IL-1 stimulation or TLR-4 activation (Matsumura et al., 2003;Kim et al., 2006;Ojaniemi et al., 2006). Radstake et al. (2004) reported the expression of TLR-2 and TLR-4 in osteoarthritic synovial membrane. Moreover, cultured synovial cells and chondrocytes from OA subjects show responsiveness to TLR-4 agonist LPS and TLR-2 agonist peptidoglycan (Kim et al., 2006;Kyburz et al., 2003;Ozawa et al., 2007). TLR-4 deficiency rescues cartilage and bone erosion in arthritis, while TLR-2 deficiency promotes the disease severity (Abdollahi-Roodsaz et al., 2008).

Activation of TLR-2 and TLR-4 recruits downstream adaptors such as MyD88 and Toll-interleukin 1 receptor domain containing adaptor protein (TIRAP), and ultimately leads to the activation of various transcription factors including IRFs, AP-1, and NF-κB. All TLR pathways are capable of activating NF-κB, and recent evidence suggests a role of NF-κB in OA. The activation of NF-κB requires the degradation of IκB bounding to it. Amos et al. (2006) showed that inhibiting NF-κB via over-expressing IκBα inhibited the production of many inflammatory and destructive mediators in OA, including TNF-α, IL-6, IL-8, oncostatin M, and metaloproteinase (MMP)-1, 3, 9, 13. The Bondeson group further showed that several MMPs and aggrecanases such as a disintegrin and metalloprotease with thrombospondin motifs 4 and 5 (ADAMTS 4, 5) are NF-κB dependent (Bondeson et al., 2007). MMP-1 and MMP-13 are capable of cleaving collagen type II, and MMP-3 cleaves other components of extracellular matrix, such as fibronectin and laminin (Yoshihara et al., 2000). ADAMTS4 and ADAMTS5 work together to cleave aggregating proteoglycan aggrecan in cartilage (Song et al., 2007;Lohmander et al., 1993). Chen et al. (2008) reported the suppression of early surgically induced OA, such as minimized synovitis and articular cartilage damage, by intra-articular delivery of NF-κBp65 specific siRNA NF-kB.

Several autoantibodies against degradative products of cartilage tissues have been identified in OA, in both humans and other animal species. These include antibodies against collagen 2 (Jasin, 1985;Niebauer et al., 1987;Osborne et al., 1995), cartilage link protein (Guerassimov et al., 1998), G1 domain proteoglycan aggrecan (Niebauer et al., 1987), cartilage intermediate layer protein (Tsuruha et al., 2001), human chondrocyte gp-39 homologous, YKL-39 (Tsuruha et al., 2002), and osteopontin (Sakata et al., 2001). Collagen II has been indentified as one of the major autoantigens in human and other animal models of RA, but much remains to be known about the autoantigen(s) driving the synovitis in OA. MyD88 dependent TLR signalling is critical for the induction of adaptive immune responses, including B-cell activation and antibody production (for review see Pasare and Medzhitov, 2005). Stimulating TLRs on B cells can result in polyclonal activation and production of low-affinity immunoglobulin M (IgM) antibodies, which may be one of mechanisms producing autoreactive antibodies (Iwasaki and Medzhitov, 2004).

7. TLR bridges traumatic injury and OA pain

Chronic pain can arise from a wide variety of causes - arthritis pain, low back pain, migraine, cancer pain, post-herpetic neuralgia, diabetic neuropathy, and others. Currently, chronic pain is explained more or less on the basis of structural abnormalities, such as osteoarthritis or herniated disk (Omoigui, 2007a). Chronic pain has not been able to be classified into well mechanism-based entities. To distinguish inflammatory pain from neuropathic pain is the best attempt so far. Hawker et al. (2008) revealed two distinct types of OA pain: an early predictable dull, aching, throbbing "background" pain and an unpredictable short episode of intense pain that develops later (Hawker et al., 2008). During the progression of OA, pain evolves from the "background" pain that is use-related in early OA (Kidd, 2006), to unpredictable short episodes of intense pain on top of the "background" pain in advanced OA (Hawker et al., 2008). However, the nature of the pain in OA still remains unclear (Hunter et al., 2008;Kidd, 2006;McDougall, 2006;Wu and Henry, 2010). Our poor understanding of chronic pain results in poor mechanism-based treatments, particularly for neuropathic pain (Gordon and Dahl, 2004;Colombo et al., 2006;Jackson, 2006;Rice and Hill, 2006;Dworkin et al., 2007).

One critical fact about chronic pain is that its nature is determined shortly after the initial insult. For example, nerve section induces neuropathic pain only, but never inflammatory pain, no matter how complicated the subsequent cytokine cascade is. Different types of tissue injury are associated with distinct forms of chronic pain. TLRs likely play an important role in the "judgment of pain" in various tissue injuries, as they are the most important interface initiating the release of cytokines following cellular response to distinct pathogen- or damage-associated molecular patterns, and they have limited yet highly specific subtypes associated with distinct intracellular signalling pathways.

The notion that inflammatory mechanisms are underlying all pain syndromes was recently proposed in two review papers (Moalem et al., 2005;Omoigui, 2007b). Alteration of the chemical environment surrounding sensory neurons changes nociception (Clatworthy et al., 1995) demonstrated that the development of the thermal hyperalgesia was tightly governed by peri-axonal inflammation. These findings lead to a re-examination of the significance of the accumulation of immune cells and inflammatory factors in nerve injuries. Cytokines likely play critical roles in the above processes. TNF-α, IL-1 and IL-6 have been shown to induced hyperalgesia if injected peripherally into the paw (Cunha et al., 1992;Ferreira et al., 1988), which can be blocked by the application of antibodies against each of these cytokines (Cunha et al., 1992;Schafers et al., 2001;Sommer et al., 1999). A second line of evidence is from inflammatory models of neuropathic pain. Those models are able to mimic neuropathic type of pain by means that are unlikely to injure sensory axons. Neuropathic pain can be induced by placing chromic gut thread next to sciatic nerve (Maves et al., 1993), by cutting ventral roots of spinal nerves which are motor efferents (Li et al., 2002;Sheth et al., 2002), by applying complete Freund's adjuvant (CFA) (Eliav et al., 1999) or zymosan (Chacur et al., 2001) around the intact sciatic nerve. Third line of evidence is from neurology clinics. Neurologists surprisingly found that pain is a common comorbidity in autoimmune diseases of nervous system: 65% of multiple sclerosis patients reported pain during the course of their disease (Kerns et al., 2002); 70-90% of Guillain-Barre syndrome patients complained pain (Pentland and Donald, 1994;Moulin et al., 1997).

A sundry of signalling pathways – such as PKA, PKC, PKG, ERK, P38 MAPK, NF-κB and JAK/STAT have been implicated to be involved in the development of chronic pain (Hanada and Yoshimura, 2002;Ji and Woolf, 2001;Obata and Noguchi, 2004). Among them, NF-κB, JAK/STAT and MAPK pathways are of particular importance in chronic pain: NF-κB pathway is the most important cellular pathway responsible for the production of inflammatory cytokines (Nguyen et al., 2002); JAK/STAT pathway is the primary pathway responsible for cytokine receptor signalling (Ihle, 1995); and MAPKs play a pivotal role in transducing extracellular stimuli into intracellular posttranslational and transcriptional responses, and are hot topics in recent pain mechanism studies, particularly ERK and P38 (Ji and Suter, 2007;Ma and Quirion, 2005;Obata and Noguchi, 2004). TLR signalling pathways have intensive crosstalk with the above mentioned pain-related pathways.

TLR and NF-κB pathway - Different adaptor molecules recruited by different TLRs result in differences in NF-κB activation. TLR signalling via the MyD88-dependent pathway leads to the early phase release of NF-κB. During TLR2 or TLR4 signalling, TIRAP/MAL is recruited to TIR domain, and then MyD88, whereas during TLR5, TLR7 or TLR9 signalling, MyD88 is recruited to TIR domain. Activation of MyD88-independent pathway downstream of TLR3 or TLR4 accounts for the late phase release of NF-κB, where TRIF is the key adaptor recruited.

TLR and IFN-JAK-STAT pathway – Type I IFNs previously were found mainly due to the activation of the MyD88-independent pathway which triggers the expression of IFN-β and chemokine genes (Sakaguchi et al., 2003). Recruitment of MyD88 by TLR7, TLR8 or TLR9 also results in the release of different set of type I IFNs, including both IFN-α and IFN-β species. (Honda et al., 2004;Takaoka and Yanai, 2006). The activation of IFN-receptors by Type I IFNs is an important mechanism linking TLR pathway and the JAK-STAT pathway (Akira and Takeda, 2004;Kawai and Akira, 2005), as the JAK-STAT pathway is one of the best characterized IFN-signalling pathways (Stark et al., 1998).

TLR and MAPK pathway - TGF-β–activated protein kinase 1 (TAK1) is a member of the MAP3K family, which is a key regulator of MAP kinase activity (Yamaguchi et al., 1995). TAK1 can be activated by TLR3 or TLR4 signalling via the MyD88-independent pathway. Moreover, another MAP3K, MEKK3 could be activated via the MyD88-dependent pathway. TLR4 but not TLR9 signalling via MEKK3 induced the activation of JNK/P38 but not ERK, suggesting differential activation of MAPKs during TLR signalling (Huang et al., 2004).

Accumulating evidence shows that TLRs are involved in chronic pain determination, likely at the level of primary sensory neurons. Dorsal root ganglion (DRG) neurons are located at the first stop of the sensory pathway. Different types of pain seem to affect different subgroups of DRG neurons. TLRs are constitutively expressed in immune cells. However, TLR expression is also found in CNS and PNS - in microglia, astrocytes (Bsibsi et al., 2002) and sensory ganglia neurons (Wadachi and Hargreaves, 2006). In polyarthritis models induced by CFA injection (Djouhri and Lawson, 1999;Xu et al., 2000), only A δ neurons and C neurons were significantly altered in electrophysiological properties, with C neurons the more severely altered. In complete sciatic nerve transection model (Abdulla and Smith, 2001), partial sciatic nerve transection model (Liu and Eisenach, 2005), or lumbar spinal nerve transection models (Kim et al., 1998;Liu et al., 2000;Ma et al., 2003;Sapunar et al., 2005;Stebbing et al., 1999), changes in A type neurons were common, even in the large size neurons. In some studies (Abdulla and Smith, 2001;Kim et al., 1998;Ma et al., 2003), changes in C neurons were also reported, but are less prominent than those in A neurons. Therefore, it seems that there are distinct changes in subgroups of DRG neurons in various chronic pain models resulted from different mechanisms, which can be regarded as pain manifestation at the neuronal level. Several TLRs have clearly established their correlation with hyperalgesia or allodynia. Compared with wild type mice, TLR2 knock-out mice showed reduced mechanical allodynia and thermal hyperalgesia after spinal nerve axotomy (Kim et al., 2007). Intrathecal administration of TLR3 antisense oligodeoxynucleotide (ODN) suppressed the spinal nerve ligation-induced tactile allodynia, whereas intrathecal injection of TLR3 agonist induced behavioural changes similar to the nerve-injury induced sensory hypersensitivity (Obata et al., 2008). TLR4 knock-out mice and the rats treated with TLR4 antisense ODN both showed significantly attenuated mechanical allodynia and thermal hyperalgesia in L5 spinal nerve transection (Tanga et al., 2005). TLR activation in microglia in spinal cord was proven to play a critical role in spinal nerve axotomy-induced sensory hypersensitivity (Kim et al., 2007;Tanga et al., 2005;Obata et al., 2008).

8. Conclusion

We propose a novel concept regarding the mechanism underlying the pain in OA induced by traumatic injuries. Following an initial trauma to the joint, two distinct yet interacting processes are initiated. One is neural injury of joint afferents and ensuing maladaptive changes of the nervous system, which results in pain in OA. The other is the cartilage degradation and bony changes in the joint, which generates characteristic pathology in OA. These two processes are likely initiated by damage-associated molecules produced during the initial joint injury, such as hyaluronan, fibronectin and proteoglycan aggrecan, mediated by pattern-recognition receptors like the TLRs. The TLR-dependent pathways lead to the activation of NF-$_\kappa$B and downstream transcription factors to produce various inflammatory and destructive mediators and autoantibodies. Thus, various downstream pathways, such as the MMP-mediated, ADAMITS-mediated, MAPK-mediated, are activated to generate a spectrum of osteoarthritic changes, both functional (pain) and structural (deficit in cartilage and bone deformity). TLRs, maybe other pattern-recognition receptors, are at the intersection of OA pathology and pain.

9. Acknowledgement

This work was supported by an operating grant from the Canadian Arthritis Network and the Canadian Institutes of Health Research as well as funds from McMaster University. QW was supported by the Canadian Pain Society, the Canadian Arthritis Network and the Canadian Institutes of Health Research.

10. List of abbreviations

AP-1, Activator Protein-1; **CFA,** Complete Freund's Adjuvant; **CRP,** C-Reactive Protein; **DRG,** Dorsal Root Ganglion; **HMGB,** High-Mobility Group Protein; **IRF,** Interferon Regulatory Factor; **LPS,** Lipopolysaccharide; **MyD88,** Myeloid Differentiation Primary Response Gene 88; **OA,** Osteoarthritis; **ODN,** Oligodeoxynucleotide; **RA,** Rheumatoid Arthritis; **TAK1,** Transforming Growth Factor (TGF)-β–Activated Protein Kinase 1; **TIRAP,**

Toll-Interleukin 1 Receptor (TIR) Domain Containing Adaptor Protein; **TLR**, Toll-like Receptor ; **VEGF**, Vascular Endothelial Growth Factor

11. References

[1] Abdollahi-Roodsaz S, Joosten LA, Koenders MI, Devesa I, Roelofs MF, Radstake TR, Heuvelmans-Jacobs M, Akira S, Nicklin MJ, Ribeiro-Dias F, van den Berg WB (2008) Stimulation of TLR2 and TLR4 differentially skews the balance of T cells in a mouse model of arthritis. J Clin Invest 118:205-216.

[2] Abdulla FA, Smith PA (2001) Axotomy- and autotomy-induced changes in the excitability of rat dorsal root ganglion neurons. J Neurophysiol 85:630-643.

[3] Aigner T, Kim HA (2002) Apoptosis and cellular vitality: issues in osteoarthritic cartilage degeneration. Arthritis Rheum 46:1986-1996.

[4] Akira S, Takeda K (2004) Toll-like receptor signalling. Nat Rev Immunol 4:499-511.

[5] Amos N, Lauder S, Evans A, Feldmann M, Bondeson J (2006) Adenoviral gene transfer into osteoarthritis synovial cells using the endogenous inhibitor IkappaBalpha reveals that most, but not all, inflammatory and destructive mediators are NFkappaB dependent. Rheumatology (Oxford) 45:1201-1209.

[6] Ayral X, Pickering EH, Woodworth TG, Mackillop N, Dougados M (2005) Synovitis: a potential predictive factor of structural progression of medial tibiofemoral knee osteoarthritis -- results of a 1 year longitudinal arthroscopic study in 422 patients. Osteoarthritis Cartilage 13:361-367.

[7] Barton GM, Medzhitov R (2002) Toll-like receptors and their ligands. Curr Top Microbiol Immunol 270:81-92.

[8] Beg AA (2002) Endogenous ligands of Toll-like receptors: implications for regulating inflammatory and immune responses. Trends Immunol 23:509-512.

[9] Bettinger DA, Pellicane JV, Tarry WC, Yager DR, Diegelmann RF, Lee R, Cohen IK, DeMaria EJ (1994) The role of inflammatory cytokines in wound healing: accelerated healing in endotoxin-resistant mice. J Trauma 36:810-813.

[10] Beutler B (2005) The Toll-like receptors: analysis by forward genetic methods. Immunogenetics 57:385-392.

[11] Boivin A, Pineau I, Barrette B, Filali M, Vallieres N, Rivest S, Lacroix S (2007) Toll-like receptor signaling is critical for Wallerian degeneration and functional recovery after peripheral nerve injury. J Neurosci 27:12565-12576.

[12] Bondeson J, Lauder S, Wainwright S, Amos N, Evans A, Hughes C, Feldmann M, Caterson B (2007) Adenoviral gene transfer of the endogenous inhibitor IkappaBalpha into human osteoarthritis synovial fibroblasts demonstrates that several matrix metalloproteinases and aggrecanases are nuclear factor-kappaB-dependent. J Rheumatol 34:523-533.

[13] Brown MP, Trumble TN, Plaas AH, Sandy JD, Romano M, Hernandez J, Merritt KA (2007) Exercise and injury increase chondroitin sulfate chain length and decrease hyaluronan chain length in synovial fluid. Osteoarthritis Cartilage 15:1318-1325.

[14] Bsibsi M, Ravid R, Gveric D, van Noort JM (2002) Broad expression of Toll-like receptors in the human central nervous system. J Neuropathol Exp Neurol 61:1013-1021.

[15] Chacur M, Milligan ED, Gazda LS, Armstrong C, Wang H, Tracey KJ, Maier SF, Watkins LR (2001) A new model of sciatic inflammatory neuritis (SIN): induction of unilateral and bilateral mechanical allodynia following acute unilateral peri-sciatic immune activation in rats. Pain 94:231-244.

[16] Chen LX, Lin L, Wang HJ, Wei XL, Fu X, Zhang JY, Yu CL (2008) Suppression of early experimental osteoarthritis by in vivo delivery of the adenoviral vector-mediated NF-kappaBp65-specific siRNA. Osteoarthritis Cartilage 16:174-184.

[17] Chevalier X, Groult N, Hornebeck W (1996) Increased expression of the Ed-B-containing fibronectin (an embryonic isoform of fibronectin) in human osteoarthritic cartilage. Br J Rheumatol 35:407-415.

[18] Cho ML, Ju JH, Kim HR, Oh HJ, Kang CM, Jhun JY, Lee SY, Park MK, Min JK, Park SH, Lee SH, Kim HY (2007) Toll-like receptor 2 ligand mediates the upregulation of angiogenic factor, vascular endothelial growth factor and interleukin-8/CXCL8 in human rheumatoid synovial fibroblasts. Immunol Lett 108:121-128.

[19] Clatworthy AL, Illich PA, Castro GA, Walters ET (1995) Role of peri-axonal inflammation in the development of thermal hyperalgesia and guarding behavior in a rat model of neuropathic pain. Neurosci Lett 184:5-8.

[20] Colombo B, Annovazzi PO, Comi G (2006) Medications for neuropathic pain: current trends. Neurol Sci 27 Suppl 2:S183-S189.

[21] Creamer P (2000) Osteoarthritis pain and its treatment. Curr Opin Rheumatol 12:450-455.

[22] Cunha FQ, Poole S, Lorenzetti BB, Ferreira SH (1992) The pivotal role of tumour necrosis factor alpha in the development of inflammatory hyperalgesia. Br J Pharmacol 107:660-664.

[23] Dahl LB, Dahl IM, Engstrom-Laurent A, Granath K (1985) Concentration and molecular weight of sodium hyaluronate in synovial fluid from patients with rheumatoid arthritis and other arthropathies. Ann Rheum Dis 44:817-822.

[24] Djouhri L, Lawson SN (1999) Changes in somatic action potential shape in guinea-pig nociceptive primary afferent neurones during inflammation in vivo. J Physiol 520:565-576.

[25] Dworkin RH, O'connor AB, Backonja M, Farrar JT, Finnerup NB, Jensen TS, Kalso EA, Loeser JD, Miaskowski C, Nurmikko TJ, Portenoy RK, Rice AS, Stacey BR, Treede RD, Turk DC, Wallace MS (2007) Pharmacologic management of neuropathic pain: evidence-based recommendations. Pain 132:237-251.

[26] Eliav E, Herzberg U, Ruda MA, Bennett GJ (1999) Neuropathic pain from an experimental neuritis of the rat sciatic nerve. Pain 83:169-182.

[27] Felson DT, McAlindon TE, Anderson JJ, Naimark A, Weissman BW, Aliabadi P, Evans S, Levy D, LaValley MP (1997) Defining radiographic osteoarthritis for the whole knee. Osteoarthritis Cartilage 5:241-250.

[28] Ferreira SH, Lorenzetti BB, Bristow AF, Poole S (1988) Interleukin-1 beta as a potent hyperalgesic agent antagonized by a tripeptide analogue. Nature 334:698-700.

[29] Gondokaryono SP, Ushio H, Niyonsaba F, Hara M, Takenaka H, Jayawardana ST, Ikeda S, Okumura K, Ogawa H (2007) The extra domain A of fibronectin stimulates murine mast cells via toll-like receptor 4. J Leukoc Biol 82:657-665.

[30] Gordon DB, Dahl JL (2004) Quality improvement challenges in pain management. Pain 107:1-4.

[31] Guerassimov A, Zhang Y, Banerjee S, Cartman A, Webber C, Esdaile J, Fitzcharles MA, Poole AR (1998) Autoimmunity to cartilage link protein in patients with rheumatoid arthritis and ankylosing spondylitis. J Rheumatol 25:1480-1484.

[32] Hanada T, Yoshimura A (2002) Regulation of cytokine signaling and inflammation. Cytokine Growth Factor Rev 13:413-421.

[33] Hawker GA, Stewart L, French MR, Cibere J, Jordan JM, March L, Suarez-Almazor M, Gooberman-Hill R (2008) Understanding the pain experience in hip and knee osteoarthritis--an OARSI/OMERACT initiative. Osteoarthritis Cartilage 16:415-422.

[34] Hill CL, Hunter DJ, Niu J, Clancy M, Guermazi A, Genant H, Gale D, Grainger A, Conaghan P, Felson DT (2007) Synovitis detected on magnetic resonance imaging and its relation to pain and cartilage loss in knee osteoarthritis. Ann Rheum Dis 66:1599-1603.

[35] Honda K, Yanai H, Mizutani T, Negishi H, Shimada N, Suzuki N, Ohba Y, Takaoka A, Yeh WC, Taniguchi T (2004) Role of a transductional-transcriptional processor complex involving MyD88 and IRF-7 in Toll-like receptor signaling. Proc Natl Acad Sci U S A 101:15416-15421.

[36] Huang Q, Yang J, Lin Y, Walker C, Cheng J, Liu ZG, Su B (2004) Differential regulation of interleukin 1 receptor and Toll-like receptor signaling by MEKK3. Nat Immunol 5:98-103.

[37] Hunter DJ, McDougall JJ, Keefe FJ (2008) The symptoms of osteoarthritis and the genesis of pain. Rheum Dis Clin North Am 34:623-643.

[38] Ihle JN (1995) Cytokine receptor signalling. Nature 377:591-594.

[39] Iwasaki A, Medzhitov R (2004) Toll-like receptor control of the adaptive immune responses. Nat Immunol 5:987-995.

[40] Jackson AC, Rossiter JP, Lafon M (2006) Expression of Toll-like receptor 3 in the human cerebellar cortex in rabies, herpes simplex encephalitis, and other neurological diseases. J Neurovirol 12:229-234.

[41] Jackson KC (2006) Pharmacotherapy for neuropathic pain. Pain Pract 6:27-33.

[42] Jasin HE (1985) Autoantibody specificities of immune complexes sequestered in articular cartilage of patients with rheumatoid arthritis and osteoarthritis. Arthritis Rheum 28:241-248.

[43] Ji RR, Suter MR (2007) p38 MAPK, microglial signaling, and neuropathic pain. Mol Pain 3:33.

[44] Ji RR, Woolf CJ (2001) Neuronal plasticity and signal transduction in nociceptive neurons: implications for the initiation and maintenance of pathological pain. Neurobiol Dis 8:1-10.

[45] Johnson GB, Brunn GJ, Kodaira Y, Platt JL (2002) Receptor-mediated monitoring of tissue well-being via detection of soluble heparan sulfate by Toll-like receptor 4. J Immunol 168:5233-5239.

[46] Kariko K, Ni H, Capodici J, Lamphier M, Weissman D (2004) mRNA is an endogenous ligand for Toll-like receptor 3. J Biol Chem 279:12542-12550.

[47] Kato T, Xiang Y, Nakamura H, Nishioka K (2004) Neoantigens in osteoarthritic cartilage. Curr Opin Rheumatol 16:604-608.

[48] Kawai T, Akira S (2005) Toll-like receptor downstream signaling. Arthritis Res Ther 7:12-19.

[49] Kerns RD, Kassirer M, Otis J (2002) Pain in multiple sclerosis: a biopsychosocial perspective. J Rehabil Res Dev 39:225-232.

[50] Kidd BL (2006) Osteoarthritis and joint pain. Pain 123:6-9.

[51] Kim D, Kim MA, Cho IH, Kim MS, Lee S, Jo EK, Choi SY, Park K, Kim JS, Akira S, Na HS, Oh SB, Lee SJ (2007) A critical role of toll-like receptor 2 in nerve injury-induced spinal cord glial cell activation and pain hypersensitivity. J Biol Chem 282:14975-14983.

[52] Kim HA, Cho ML, Choi HY, Yoon CS, Jhun JY, Oh HJ, Kim HY (2006) The catabolic pathway mediated by Toll-like receptors in human osteoarthritic chondrocytes. Arthritis Rheum 54:2152-2163.

[53] Kim YI, Na HS, Kim SH, Han HC, Yoon YW, Sung B, Nam HJ, Shin SL, Hong SK (1998) Cell type-specific changes of the membrane properties of peripherally-axotomized dorsal root ganglion neurons in a rat model of neuropathic pain. Neuroscience 86:301-309.

[54] Kokkola R, Sundberg E, Ulfgren AK, Palmblad K, Li J, Wang H, Ulloa L, Yang H, Yan XJ, Furie R, Chiorazzi N, Tracey KJ, Andersson U, Harris HE (2002) High mobility group box chromosomal protein 1: a novel proinflammatory mediator in synovitis. Arthritis Rheum 46:2598-2603.

[55] Kyburz D, Rethage J, Seibl R, Lauener R, Gay RE, Carson DA, Gay S (2003) Bacterial peptidoglycans but not CpG oligodeoxynucleotides activate synovial fibroblasts by toll-like receptor signaling. Arthritis Rheum 48:642-650.

[56] Lasarte JJ, Casares N, Gorraiz M, Hervas-Stubbs S, Arribillaga L, Mansilla C, Durantez M, Llopiz D, Sarobe P, Borras-Cuesta F, Prieto J, Leclerc C (2007) The extra domain A from fibronectin targets antigens to TLR4-expressing cells and induces cytotoxic T cell responses in vivo. J Immunol 178:748-756.

[57] Lawrence RC, Helmick CG, Arnett FC, Deyo RA, Felson DT, Giannini EH, Heyse SP, Hirsch R, Hochberg MC, Hunder GG, Liang MH, Pillemer SR, Steen VD, Wolfe F (1998) Estimates of the prevalence of arthritis and selected musculoskeletal disorders in the United States. Arthritis Rheum 41:778-799.

[58] Leadbetter EA, Rifkin IR, Hohlbaum AM, Beaudette BC, Shlomchik MJ, Marshak-Rothstein A (2002) Chromatin-IgG complexes activate B cells by dual engagement of IgM and Toll-like receptors. Nature 416:603-607.

[59] Levy RM, Prince JM, Yang R, Mollen KP, Liao H, Watson GA, Fink MP, Vodovotz Y, Billiar TR (2006) Systemic inflammation and remote organ damage following bilateral femur fracture requires Toll-like receptor 4. Am J Physiol Regul Integr Comp Physiol 291:R970-R976.

[60] Li L, Xian CJ, Zhong JH, Zhou XF (2002) Effect of lumbar 5 ventral root transection on pain behaviors: a novel rat model for neuropathic pain without axotomy of primary sensory neurons. Exp Neurol 175:23-34.

[61] Liu B, Eisenach JC (2005) Hyperexcitability of axotomized and neighboring unaxotomized sensory neurons is reduced days after perineural clonidine at the site of injury. J Neurophysiol 94:3159-3167.

[62] Liu CN, Wall PD, Ben-Dor E, Michaelis M, Amir R, Devor M (2000) Tactile allodynia in the absence of C-fiber activation: altered firing properties of DRG neurons following spinal nerve injury. Pain 85:503-521.

[63] Lohmander LS, Neame PJ, Sandy JD (1993) The structure of aggrecan fragments in human synovial fluid. Evidence that aggrecanase mediates cartilage degradation in inflammatory joint disease, joint injury, and osteoarthritis. Arthritis Rheum 36:1214-1222.

[64] Ma C, Shu Y, Zheng Z, Chen Y, Yao H, Greenquist KW, White FA, LaMotte RH (2003) Similar electrophysiological changes in axotomized and neighboring intact dorsal root ganglion neurons. J Neurophysiol 89:1588-1602.

[65] Ma W, Quirion R (2005) The ERK/MAPK pathway, as a target for the treatment of neuropathic pain. Expert Opin Ther Targets 9:699-713.

[66] Marcinkiewicz M (2002) BetaAPP and furin mRNA concentrates in immature senile plaques in the brain of Alzheimer patients. J Neuropathol Exp Neurol 61:815-829.

[67] Matsumura T, Degawa T, Takii T, Hayashi H, Okamoto T, Inoue J, Onozaki K (2003) TRAF6-NF-kappaB pathway is essential for interleukin-1-induced TLR2 expression and its functional response to TLR2 ligand in murine hepatocytes. Immunology 109:127-136.

[68] Maves TJ, Pechman PS, Gebhart GF, Meller ST (1993) Possible chemical contribution from chromic gut sutures produces disorders of pain sensation like those seen in man. Pain 54:57-69.

[69] McDougall JJ (2006) Pain and OA. J Musculoskelet Neuronal Interact 6:385-386.

[70] Merlotti D, Santacroce C, Gennari L, Geraci S, Acquafredda V, Conti T, Bargagli G, Canto ND, Biagi F, Gennari C, Giordano N (2003) HLA antigens and primary osteoarthritis of the hand. J Rheumatol 30:1298-1304.

[71] Moalem G, Grafe P, Tracey DJ (2005) Chemical mediators enhance the excitability of unmyelinated sensory axons in normal and injured peripheral nerve of the rat. Neuroscience 134:1399-1411.

[72] Mollen KP, Anand RJ, Tsung A, Prince JM, Levy RM, Billiar TR (2006) Emerging paradigm: toll-like receptor 4-sentinel for the detection of tissue damage. Shock 26:430-437.

[73] Moulin DE, Hagen N, Feasby TE, Amireh R, Hahn A (1997) Pain in Guillain-Barre syndrome. Neurology 48:328-331.

[74] Nguyen MD, Julien JP, Rivest S (2002) Innate immunity: the missing link in neuroprotection and neurodegeneration? Nat Rev Neurosci 3:216-227.

[75] Niebauer GW, Wolf B, Bashey RI, Newton CD (1987) Antibodies to canine collagen types I and II in dogs with spontaneous cruciate ligament rupture and osteoarthritis. Arthritis Rheum 30:319-327.

[76] Obata K, Katsura H, Miyoshi K, Kondo T, Yamanaka H, Kobayashi K, Dai Y, Fukuoka T, Akira S, Noguchi K (2008) Toll-like receptor 3 contributes to spinal glial activation and tactile allodynia after nerve injury. J Neurochem.

[77] Obata K, Noguchi K (2004) MAPK activation in nociceptive neurons and pain hypersensitivity. Life Sci 74:2643-2653.

[78] Ohashi K, Burkart V, Flohe S, Kolb H (2000) Cutting edge: heat shock protein 60 is a putative endogenous ligand of the toll-like receptor-4 complex. J Immunol 164:558-561.

[79] Ojaniemi M, Liljeroos M, Harju K, Sormunen R, Vuolteenaho R, Hallman M (2006) TLR-2 is upregulated and mobilized to the hepatocyte plasma membrane in the space of

Disse and to the Kupffer cells TLR-4 dependently during acute endotoxemia in mice. Immunol Lett 102:158-168.

[80] Okamura Y, Watari M, Jerud ES, Young DW, Ishizaka ST, Rose J, Chow JC, Strauss JF, III (2001) The extra domain A of fibronectin activates Toll-like receptor 4. J Biol Chem 276:10229-10233.

[81] Omoigui S (2007b) The biochemical origin of pain: the origin of all pain is inflammation and the inflammatory response. Part 2 of 3 - inflammatory profile of pain syndromes. Med Hypotheses 69:1169-1178.

[82] Omoigui S (2007a) The biochemical origin of pain--proposing a new law of pain: the origin of all pain is inflammation and the inflammatory response. Part 1 of 3--a unifying law of pain. Med Hypotheses 69:70-82.

[83] Osborne AC, Carter SD, May SA, Bennett D (1995) Anti-collagen antibodies and immune complexes in equine joint diseases. Vet Immunol Immunopathol 45:19-30.

[84] Ozawa T, Koyama K, Ando T, Ohnuma Y, Hatsushika K, Ohba T, Sugiyama H, Hamada Y, Ogawa H, Okumura K, Nakao A (2007) Thymic stromal lymphopoietin secretion of synovial fibroblasts is positively and negatively regulated by Toll-like receptors/nuclear factor-kappaB pathway and interferon-gamma/dexamethasone. Mod Rheumatol 17:459-463.

[86] Park JS, Svetkauskaite D, He Q, Kim JY, Strassheim D, Ishizaka A, Abraham E (2004) Involvement of toll-like receptors 2 and 4 in cellular activation by high mobility group box 1 protein. J Biol Chem 279:7370-7377.

[87] Pasare C, Medzhitov R (2005) Control of B-cell responses by Toll-like receptors. Nature 438:364-368.

[88] Pearle AD, Scanzello CR, George S, Mandl LA, DiCarlo EF, Peterson M, Sculco TP, Crow MK (2007) Elevated high-sensitivity C-reactive protein levels are associated with local inflammatory findings in patients with osteoarthritis. Osteoarthritis Cartilage 15:516-523.

[89] Pentland B, Donald SM (1994) Pain in the Guillain-Barre syndrome: a clinical review. Pain 59:159-164.

[90] Poole AR (1999) An introduction to the pathophysiology of osteoarthritis. Front Biosci 4:D662-D670.

[91] Prince JM, Levy RM, Yang R, Mollen KP, Fink MP, Vodovotz Y, Billiar TR (2006) Toll-like receptor-4 signaling mediates hepatic injury and systemic inflammation in hemorrhagic shock. J Am Coll Surg 202:407-417.

[92] Radstake TR, Roelofs MF, Jenniskens YM, Oppers-Walgreen B, van Riel PL, Barrera P, Joosten LA, van den Berg WB (2004) Expression of toll-like receptors 2 and 4 in rheumatoid synovial tissue and regulation by proinflammatory cytokines interleukin-12 and interleukin-18 via interferon-gamma. Arthritis Rheum 50:3856-3865.

[93] Rice AS, Hill RG (2006) New treatments for neuropathic pain. Annu Rev Med 57:535-551.

[94] Riyazi N, Spee J, Huizinga TW, Schreuder GM, de Vries RR, Dekker FW, Kloppenburg M (2003) HLA class II is associated with distal interphalangeal osteoarthritis. Ann Rheum Dis 62:227-230.

[95] Rothschild BM, Martin LD. Skeletal Impact of Disease. Albuquerque: New Mexico Museum of Natural History Press, 2006.

[96] Saito I, Koshino T, Nakashima K, Uesugi M, Saito T (2002) Increased cellular infiltrate in inflammatory synovia of osteoarthritic knees. Osteoarthritis Cartilage 10:156-162.

[97] Sakaguchi S, Negishi H, Asagiri M, Nakajima C, Mizutani T, Takaoka A, Honda K, Taniguchi T (2003) Essential role of IRF-3 in lipopolysaccharide-induced interferon-beta gene expression and endotoxin shock. Biochem Biophys Res Commun 306:860-866.

[98] Sakata M, Tsuruha JI, Masuko-Hongo K, Nakamura H, Matsui T, Sudo A, Nishioka K, Kato T (2001) Autoantibodies to osteopontin in patients with osteoarthritis and rheumatoid arthritis. J Rheumatol 28:1492-1495.

[99] Sapunar D, Ljubkovic M, Lirk P, McCallum JB, Hogan QH (2005) Distinct membrane effects of spinal nerve ligation on injured and adjacent dorsal root ganglion neurons in rats. Anesthesiology 103:360-376.

[100] Saxne T, Lindell M, Mansson B, Petersson IF, Heinegard D (2003a) Inflammation is a feature of the disease process in early knee joint osteoarthritis. Rheumatology (Oxford) 42:903-904.

[101] Saxne T, Lindell M, Mansson B, Petersson IF, Heinegard D (2003b) Inflammation is a feature of the disease process in early knee joint osteoarthritis. Rheumatology (Oxford) 42:903-904.

[102] Scanzello CR, Plaas A, Crow MK (2008) Innate immune system activation in osteoarthritis: is osteoarthritis a chronic wound? Curr Opin Rheumatol 20:565-572.

[103] Schafers M, Brinkhoff J, Neukirchen S, Marziniak M, Sommer C (2001) Combined epineurial therapy with neutralizing antibodies to tumor necrosis factor-alpha and interleukin-1 receptor has an additive effect in reducing neuropathic pain in mice. Neurosci Lett 310:113-116.

[104] Sheth RN, Dorsi MJ, Li Y, Murinson BB, Belzberg AJ, Griffin JW, Meyer RA (2002) Mechanical hyperalgesia after an L5 ventral rhizotomy or an L5 ganglionectomy in the rat. Pain 96:63-72.

[105] Smiley ST, King JA, Hancock WW (2001) Fibrinogen stimulates macrophage chemokine secretion through toll-like receptor 4. J Immunol 167:2887-2894.

[106] Sommer C, Petrausch S, Lindenlaub T, Toyka KV (1999) Neutralizing antibodies to interleukin 1-receptor reduce pain associated behavior in mice with experimental neuropathy. Neurosci Lett 270:25-28.

[107] Song RH, Tortorella MD, Malfait AM, Alston JT, Yang Z, Arner EC, Griggs DW (2007) Aggrecan degradation in human articular cartilage explants is mediated by both ADAMTS-4 and ADAMTS-5. Arthritis Rheum 56:575-585.

[108] Sowers M, Jannausch M, Stein E, Jamadar D, Hochberg M, Lachance L (2002) C-reactive protein as a biomarker of emergent osteoarthritis. Osteoarthritis Cartilage 10:595-601.

[109] Stark GR, Kerr IM, Williams BR, Silverman RH, Schreiber RD (1998) How cells respond to interferons. Annu Rev Biochem 67:227-264.

[110] Stebbing MJ, Eschenfelder S, Habler HJ, Acosta MC, Janig W, McLachlan EM (1999) Changes in the action potential in sensory neurones after peripheral axotomy in vivo. Neuroreport 10:201-206.

[111] Swagerty DL, Jr., Hellinger D (2001) Radiographic assessment of osteoarthritis. Am Fam Physician 64:279-286.

[112] Takaoka A, Yanai H (2006) Interferon signalling network in innate defence. Cell Microbiol 8:907-922.

[113] Tanga FY, Nutile-McMenemy N, DeLeo JA (2005) The CNS role of Toll-like receptor 4 in innate neuroimmunity and painful neuropathy. Proc Natl Acad Sci U S A 102:5856-5861.

[114] Taniguchi N, Kawahara K, Yone K, Hashiguchi T, Yamakuchi M, Goto M, Inoue K, Yamada S, Ijiri K, Matsunaga S, Nakajima T, Komiya S, Maruyama I (2003) High mobility group box chromosomal protein 1 plays a role in the pathogenesis of rheumatoid arthritis as a novel cytokine. Arthritis Rheum 48:971-981.

[115] Taylor KR, Trowbridge JM, Rudisill JA, Termeer CC, Simon JC, Gallo RL (2004a) Hyaluronan fragments stimulate endothelial recognition of injury through TLR4. J Biol Chem 279:17079-17084.

[116] Taylor KR, Trowbridge JM, Rudisill JA, Termeer CC, Simon JC, Gallo RL (2004b) Hyaluronan fragments stimulate endothelial recognition of injury through TLR4. J Biol Chem 279:17079-17084.

[117] Taylor KR, Yamasaki K, Radek KA, Di NA, Goodarzi H, Golenbock D, Beutler B, Gallo RL (2007) Recognition of hyaluronan released in sterile injury involves a unique receptor complex dependent on Toll-like receptor 4, CD44, and MD-2. J Biol Chem 282:18265-18275.

[118] Termeer C, Benedix F, Sleeman J, Fieber C, Voith U, Ahrens T, Miyake K, Freudenberg M, Galanos C, Simon JC (2002) Oligosaccharides of Hyaluronan activate dendritic cells via toll-like receptor 4. J Exp Med 195:99-111.

[119] Tsuruha J, Masuko-Hongo K, Kato T, Sakata M, Nakamura H, Nishioka K (2001) Implication of cartilage intermediate layer protein in cartilage destruction in subsets of patients with osteoarthritis and rheumatoid arthritis. Arthritis Rheum 44:838-845.

[120] Tsuruha J, Masuko-Hongo K, Kato T, Sakata M, Nakamura H, Sekine T, Takigawa M, Nishioka K (2002) Autoimmunity against YKL-39, a human cartilage derived protein, in patients with osteoarthritis. J Rheumatol 29:1459-1466.

[121] van Beijnum JR, Buurman WA, Griffioen AW (2008) Convergence and amplification of toll-like receptor (TLR) and receptor for advanced glycation end products (RAGE) signaling pathways via high mobility group B1 (HMGB1). Angiogenesis 11:91-99.

[122] Wadachi R, Hargreaves KM (2006) Trigeminal nociceptors express TLR-4 and CD14: a mechanism for pain due to infection. J Dent Res 85:49-53.

[123] Wakitani S, Imoto K, Mazuka T, Kim S, Murata N, Yoneda M (2001) Japanese generalised osteoarthritis was associated with HLA class I--a study of HLA-A, B, Cw, DQ, DR in 72 patients. Clin Rheumatol 20:417-419.

[124] Walsh DA, Bonnet CS, Turner EL, Wilson D, Situ M, McWilliams DF (2007) Angiogenesis in the synovium and at the osteochondral junction in osteoarthritis. Osteoarthritis Cartilage 15:743-751.

[125] Wu Q, Henry JL (2010) Changes in Aβ non-nociceptive primary sensory neurons in a rat model of osteoarthritis pain. Mol Pain 6:37.

[126] Xu GY, Huang LY, Zhao ZQ (2000) Activation of silent mechanoreceptive cat C and Adelta sensory neurons and their substance P expression following peripheral inflammation. J Physiol 528:339-348.

[127] Yamaguchi K, Shirakabe K, Shibuya H, Irie K, Oishi I, Ueno N, Taniguchi T, Nishida E, Matsumoto K (1995) Identification of a member of the MAPKKK family as a potential mediator of TGF-beta signal transduction. Science 270:2008-2011.

[128] Yelin E, Callahan LF (1995) The economic cost and social and psychological impact of musculoskeletal conditions. National Arthritis Data Work Groups. Arthritis Rheum 38:1351-1362.

[129] Yoshihara Y, Nakamura H, Obata K, Yamada H, Hayakawa T, Fujikawa K, Okada Y (2000) Matrix metalloproteinases and tissue inhibitors of metalloproteinases in synovial fluids from patients with rheumatoid arthritis or osteoarthritis. Ann Rheum Dis 59:455-461.

[130] Yu M, Wang H, Ding A, Golenbock DT, Latz E, Czura CJ, Fenton MJ, Tracey KJ, Yang H (2006) HMGB1 signals through toll-like receptor (TLR) 4 and TLR2. Shock 26:174-179.

6

Anion Channels in Osteoarthritic Chondrocytes

Elizabeth Perez-Hernandez[1], Nury Perez-Hernandez[2],
Fidel de la C. Hernandez-Hernandez[3] and Juan B. Kouri-Flores[3]
[1]Hospital de Ortopedia Dr. Victorio de la Fuente Narváez –IMSS,
[2]Departamento de Biomedicina Molecular, Escuela Nacional de
Medicina y Homeopatía- IPN,
[3]Departamento de Infectómica y Patogénesis Molecular, CINVESTAV-IPN,
México

1. Introduction

Osteoarthritis (OA) is the most common form of arthritis and represents a global health problem. OA is estimated to affect 40% of the population over 70 years of age and is a major cause of pain and physical disability (Lawrence, 2008). This is a condition that predominantly involves hip, knee, spine, foot and hands. Several risk factors have been associated with the initiation and progression of OA, increasing age, sex, obesity, occupational loading, malalignment, articular trauma and crystal deposition.

OA is a chronic degenerative joint disorder characterized primarily by destruction of articular cartilage, formation of reparative fibrocartilage and subchondral bone remodelling. However, not only the cartilage and bone are affected, also the synovium and the joint-stabilizing structures such as ligaments and meniscus (Baker-LePain, 2010). Apparently, all the tissues of the joint respond to mechanical stress with the consequent loss of function and clinical deterioration.

The application of mechanical forces under physiological conditions is a preponderant factor in cartilage homeostasis. It is now well know, that environmental factors, such as compressive and tensile forces, load and shear stress have a significant influence on the chondrocyte metabolism. Also, conditions that alter the load distribution on the articular surface can induce the development of OA (Roos, 2005).

This degradative process of the cartilage in OA is a consequence of an imbalance between anabolism and catabolism of chondrocytes. Generally, chondrocytes respond with increased expression of inflammatory mediators and matrix-degrading proteinases (Kurz, 2005).

Other effect observed in chondrocytes under mechanical stimulation is the change in membrane and osmotic potential (Wright, 1992, Bush, 2001). In OA, chondrocytes undergo depolarization instead of hyperpolarization (Millward-Sadler, 2000), and the decrease of the osmotic potential has been associated with loss of volume control in early stages of OA (Stockwell, 1991, Bush, 2003). However, the sequence of mechanobiological events necessary for the maintenance of extracellular matrix (ECM) homeostasis and its involvement in the pathogenesis of OA is still poorly understood.

2. Articular cartilage structure

Articular cartilage is a specialized connective tissue that contains a single cell type, the chondrocytes, embedded in an ECM which is composed of water and macromolecules. Collagens, proteoglycans and noncollagenous proteins are the main components of matrix. The chondrocytes are highly differentiated cells and constitute 1% of the total cartilage volume (Stockwell, 1967). These cells are responsible of the production and organization of ECM. Cartilage is divided into four horizontal zones: superficial, transitional o middle, radial o deep, and calcified zones. Each of these layers has specific morphological and functional characteristics related to the metabolic activity.

In the superficial zone, chondrocytes are flattened and oriented parallel to the surface. This layer consists of a low proportion of proteoglycans, thin collagen fibers and higher water content (Weiss, 1968). Functionally, this zone is responsible of the highest resistance to compressive forces during joint movement.

The transitional or middle zone consist of rounded chondrocytes, a network of collagen fibers arranged radially and an increased proteoglycan content.

In the deep zone, the chondrocytes are grouped in perpendicular columns to the articular surface. This layer contains the highest proportion of aggrecan and long collagen fibers, approximately of 55 µm across (Minns, 1977).

The calcified zone links and anchors the articular cartilage to subchondral bone through collagen fibers arranged perpendicularly. The hypertrophic chondrocytes are scarce and located in uncalcified lacunae.

Also, the matrix is subdivided into the pericellular, territorial and interterritorial regions which are arranged around the chondrocytes. The pericellular matrix is composed for sulfated proteoglycans and glycoproteins. They provide protection to chondrocytes when exposed to chondrocyte load and maintain water homeostasis. Together, the chondrocyte and pericellular matrix constitute the chondron (Poole, 1997). Adjacent to this region, the territorial matrix contains a dense meshwork of collagen fibers that provide mechanical protection to the chondrocytes. The concentration of proteoglycans rich in chondroitin sulfate is higher in this region. In the interterritorial region predominates proteoglycans rich in keratan sulfate and the collagen fibers of largest diameter (Stockwell, 1990).

The biochemical properties of cartilage are dependent of the integrity of the matrix. In the ECM of mature mammalian articular cartilage, the collagen represents 50-60% dry weight. The network consists of collagen IX (1%), collagen XI (3%) and collagen II (≥90%) (Eyre, 1987). Type II collagen, a fibrillar protein, is composed of three identical α-1 chains in form triple helix and constitutes the basic structure of cartilage. Type XI collagen is probably copolymerized and type IX collagen is covalently linked to the type II collagen fibrils (Mendler, 1989). Among other types of collagen found in cartilage, type X collagen is described in the calcified zone (Gannon, 1991), type VI collagen promotes the chondrocyte-matrix attachment (Wu, 1987) and type III collagen is copolymerized and linked to collagen II (Wu, 1996). Generally, these collagen fibers provided to the cartilage the tensile stiffness and strength.

The second largest component of the ECM are the proteoglycans, which constitute 5 to 10% of the tissue wet weight. These are molecules consisting of glycosaminglycans (GAGs) chains bound to a protein core. Also, the aggrecan are composed of proteoglycan aggregates in association with hyaluronic acid (HA) and link protein (Hardingham, 1974). The keratan sulfate and chondroitin sulfate are the main types of GAGs. The anionic groups of aggrecan attract cations such as Na+, this allows an osmotic imbalance and the accumulation of fluid in the ECM, which is critical for the biomechanical properties of cartilage. Collagen fibrils interact with aggrecan monomers in the keratan sulfate-rich regions (Hedlund, 1999). Other proteoglycans include decorin, biglycan, lumican and fibromodulin, consisting of small leucine-rich repeat. They bind to fibrillar collagen via its core protein regulating the fibril diameter and fibril-fibril interaction in the ECM.

In addition, there are nocollagenous proteins such as fibronectin and tenascin favoring chondrocyte-matrix interaction.

3. Chondrocytes mechanotransduction

The articular cartilage is continuously exposed to mechanical stress which significantly affects the response of chondrocytes to their environment (Grodzinsky, 2000). Under conditions of continuous compression, the chondrocytes undergo changes in potential membrane (Wright, 1992), matrix water content, ion concentrations and pH (Mobasheri, 1998; Mow, 1999). The process of converting physical forces into biochemical signals and the subsequent transduction into cellular responses is referred to as mechanotransduction (Huang, 2004).

Miscellaneous "mechanoreceptors" including ion channels and cell adhesion molecules, such as integrins have been described in chondrocytes. Thus far, $\alpha 1\beta 1$ integrin, a receptor for collagen, $\alpha 5\beta 1$ integrin, a receptor for fibronectin and $\alpha V\beta 5$ integrin, a receptor for vitronectin have been implicated in the regulation of chondrocyte behaviour (Ostergaard, 1998; Loeser, 1995). Voltage-gated Na+ and K+ channels (Sugimoto, 1996), epithelial sodium channels (ENaC) (Mobasheri, 1999) and N-/L-type voltage-gated Ca^{2+} channels (Wang, 2000) have been considered as potential mechanosensitive ion channels.

3.1 Membrane potential

The negative resting membrane potential (RMP) in most cells, is the result from activity of K+ (Wilson, 2004) and Cl⁻ channels (ClC) (Tsuga, 2002; Funabashi, 2010). In chondrocytes, the RMP ranging from -10.6 mV to -46 mV (Wright, 1992; Clark, 2010; Lewis 2011), and those values are determined by the influx and efflux of cations and anions in the cell membrane. Consequently, the stability of the ECM is linked to the ionic changes and the RMP in chondrocytes. Several studies related the use of ionic blockers such as lidocaine and verapamil, showed a decrease in the synthesis of GAGs (Wu, 2000; Mouw, 2007), inhibition of chondrocytes proliferation (Wohlrab, 2002) and induction of apoptosis (Wohlrab, 2005). The permeability of ion channels is regulated by chondrocyte channelome (Barret-Jolley, 2010).

The ion channels so far identified in chondrocytes are summarized in Table 1.

The membrane potential in articular chondrocytes is primarily related to the Cl⁻ conductance greater than K+ conductance (Tsuga, 2002; Funabashi, 2010). More recently, it was showed the involvement of TRPV5 (gadolinium-sensitive cation channels) in the relatively positive RMP of the chondrocytes. Furthermore, has been suggested that the positive membrane potential is due to TRVP5 higher than that generated by potassium ions, which would allow efflux of potassium ions into the cell limiting the increase in cell volume in situations of reduced osmolarity (Lewis, 2011).

Ion channels	Reference
Voltage-gated K$^+$ channels	Walsh, 1992
	Sugimoto, 1996
	Wilson, 2004
	Mobasheri, 2005
	Ponce, 2006
	Clark, 2010
Voltage-gated Na$^+$ channels	Sugimoto, 1996
	Ramage, 2008
Voltage-gated Ca^{2+} channels	Shakibaei, 2003
	Sanchez, 2004
	Mancilla, 2007
	Xu, 2009
Voltage-activated H$^+$ channels	Sanchez, 2006
Cl$^-$ channels (ClC)	Sugimoto, 1996
	Tsuga, 2002
	Isoya, 2009
	Okumura, 2009
	Funabashi, 2010
	Perez, 2010
ATP-dependent K$^+$ channels	Mobasheri, 2007
Ca^{2+}-dependent K$^+$ channels	Grandolfo, 1992
	Long, 1994
	Martina, 1997
	Mozrzymas, 1997
	Mobasheri, 2010
Transient receptor potential (TRP) channel	Sanchez, 2003
	Phan, 2009
	Lewis, 2010
Epithelial sodium channels (ENaC)	Trujillo, 1999
	Shakibaei, 2003
	Lewis, 2008

Table 1. Ion channels described in chondrocytes

Therefore, it has been proposed that the ClCs functions in chondrocytes could be involved in setting of the membrane potential or anionic osmolyte channels (Barret-Jolley, 2010).

3.2 Mechanotransduction in osteoarthritic chondrocytes

In vivo, the extracellular environment surrounding the chondrocytes is negatively charged and provides a high osmolarity, from 480 mOsm to 55 0mOsm under load (Urban, 1993; 1994; Xu, 2010). Under physiological conditions, chondrocytes are able to regulate their volume through osmotic pressure cycles (Bush, 2001). However, in OA, the chondrocytes have decreased osmotic potential and increased water content (Stockwell, 1991). Furthermore, in osteoarthritic chondrocytes described a high recovery of the increased volume, which promotes the progression of the disease (Jones, 1999; Bush, 2005).

In this matter, in the superficial and middle zones of normal cartilage and the zone of fibrillated osteoarthritic cartilage has been demonstrated the expression of ATP-dependent K+ channels (Mobasheri, 2007). Under normal conditions, mechanical stimulation produces hyperpolarization of the membrane of chondrocytes, but in OA the depolarization is induced. According to studies preformed with sodium channel blockers, this response could be due to the involvement of Ca^{2+}-dependent K+ channels (stretch-activated channels) in the process of chondrocyte mechanotransduction (Wright, 1996).

In osteoarthritic chondrocytes has been suggested that the response of membrane depolarization is due to the autocrine / paracrine activity of soluble factors. *In vitro*, mechanical stimulation of chondrocytes at 0.33 Hz induces membrane hyperpolarization due to IL-4 (Millward-Sadler, 1999) with the consequent increase in aggrecan mRNA levels. Interestingly, in osteoarthritic condrocytes, membrane depolarization is induced by proinflammatory cytokine IL-1 (Salter, 2002). Altered mechanotransduction in OA may contribute to the response of the chondrocyte favoring ECM degradation and disease progression.

Moreover, osmotic fluctuations, in addition to the volume change in chondrocytes (Bush, 2005; Kerrigan, 2006; Lewis, 2011) involve the filamentous actin restructuring (Chao, 2006; Erickson, 2003). Similarly, the osmotic stimulation of chondrocytes increases cytosolic calcium concentrations with the consequent regulation of metabolism, cell volume, and gene expression (Liu, 2006; Hardingham, 1999). In this case, a possible candidate in the chondrocyte mechanotransduction is the transient receptor potential vanilloid 4 channel (TRPV4), a Ca^{2+}-permeable, nonspecific cation channel (Liedtke, 2000; Phan, 2009).

4. Anion channels

The anion channels are a membranal class of porin ion channel that allow the passive diffusion of negatively charged ions along their electrochemical gradient. These channels allow the flow of monovalent anions such as I$^-$, NO$_3^-$, Br$^-$, and Cl, however, these are known as ClC (Fahlke, 2001). The ClC constitute a large family of Cl$^-$ selective channels (Jentsch, 2002). In humans, have been described nine isoforms of ClCs. The first branch of this gene family encodes plasma membrane channels (ClC-1, -2, -Ka and -Kb) and others two branches (ClC-3, -4 and -5; ClC-6/-7) which encode for proteins found on intracellular vesicles (Jentsch, 2005).

In the plasma membrane, the main functions of ClCs are regulation cell volume and ionic homeostasis, transepithelial transport and excitability. Channels in intracellular organelles facilitate the exchange of anionic substrates between the biosynthetic compartments involved in acidification of vesicles in the endosomal pathway (Jentsch, 2002; 2007).

Different diseases have been associated with anionic channels. The loss of ClC-5 is related to Dent's disease (Lloyd, 1996), while the disruption of ClC-3, -6, or -7 in mice promotes the development of neurodegenerative disorders in the central nervous system (Kasper, 2005; Poët, 2006), and ClC-7 mutations have been related with osteopetrosis and lysosomal storage disease (Kasper, 2005; Poët, 2006).

4.1 ClC and chondrocytes proliferation

OA is a complex morphology reflect the severity of damage to articular structures. The histopathological parameters in OA include cartilage degradation with formation of fibrocartilage, fissures, denudation with exposure, repair and remodeling of subchondral bone. In addition, chondrocytes suffer proliferation and apoptosis (Pritzker, 2006) (Fig. 1).

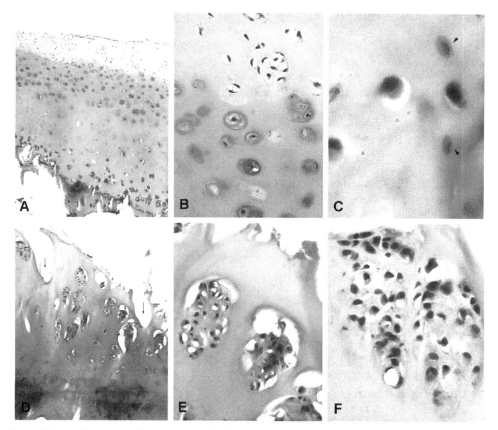

Fig. 1. OA cartilage morphology. A-B fibrillation zone, C apoptotic chondrocytes, D vertical fissures, E-F "clones" or chondrocytes aggregates. Hematoxylin and eosin staining. 10x, 20x and 40x.

This is a condition in which it was reported that the proliferative activity of chondrocytes is low compared with its absence in normal cartilage (Rothwell, 1973; Hulth, 1972). Apparently, the osteoarthritic chondrocytes have a greater access to proliferation factors due to alterations in the ECM (Lee, 1993). It is also possible that aggregates of chondrocytes or clones are a manifestation of the proliferative activity (Horton, 2005).

Moreover, apoptotic cell death is a mechanism widely described in association with OA (Blanco, 1998; Hashimoto, 1998a, 1998b; Kim, 2000; Kouri, 2000). The classic morphologic appearance of this process is characterized by fragmentation and nuclear condensation, and formation of apoptotic bodies (Aigner, 2002). In general, the response of osteoarthritic chondrocytes to the metabolic imbalance (Sandell, 2001), phenotypic modulation (Aigner, 1997) and cell death induces proliferation that compensate the cell loss and the demand of synthetic activity (Aigner, 2001; Rothwell, 1973; Hulth, 1972).

Processes such as proliferation and cell death have been linked to the involvement of ion channels. In this regard, it has been described the association between the activity of K+ channels and the proliferation of Schwann cells and B lymphocytes (Deutsch, 1990), keratinocytes (Harmon, 1993), melanoma (Nilius, 1994), neuroblastoma and astrocytoma cells (Lee YS, 1993). It also has been associated intracellular free Ca^{2+} concentration and cell proliferation (Wohlrab, 1998).

In chondrocytes, there are changes in the membrane potential of human chondrocytes in response to modulators of ion channels such as tetraethylammonium (TEA), 4-aminopyridine (4-AP), 4',4'diisothiocyanato-stilbene-2,2'-disulfonic acid (DIDS), 4-acetamido-4'-isothiocyano-2,2'-disulfonic acid (SITS), verapamil and lidocaine. About this, it was reported an increase in DNA synthesis with lidocaine and 4-AP after 12 days in chondrocytes culture (Wohlrab, 2002). Moreover, the exposure of chondrocytes to high concentrations of SITS induced necrosis while that the use of 4-AP caused cytotoxic effects and suppression of proliferation on the same system (Wohlrab, 2004).

4.2 CLIC proteins

The chloride intracellular channel (CLIC) proteins belong to the glutathione S-transferase (GST) superfamiliy and these are group of proteins with possible role of anion channels. However, they differ from classical GSTs because they contain an active site with cysteine residue, reactive for the protein itself and not through a thiol group (Littler, 2010). The CLICs are proteins highly conserved in vertebrates and these are referred to as CLIC1–CLIC6.

These proteins are present in soluble and membrane-inserted form. CLICs have been reported in membranous organelles, cytoplasmic and vesicular compartments and the nucleus (Valenzuela, 1997; Duncan, 1997; Chuang, 1999). The functions of CLICs include pH-dependent ion channel activity (Tulk, 2002; Littler, 2005) and enzymatic which likely to involve a glutathione (GSH) related cofactor (Littler, 2010). They could also be involved in maintaining the structure of intracellular organelles and their interaction with cytoskeleton proteins (Singh, 2007).

Functions of CLICs reported in the musculoskeletal system involve these proteins in the acidification processes in bone resorption (Edwards, 2006; Schlesinger, 1997). Despite their involvement in different systems with activities of ClC, has not been possible to attribute the channel protein function permanently.

CLICs proteins are implicated in cell cycle regulation, cell differentiation, and apoptosis. Specifically, CLIC4 has been linked to apoptosis and differentiation of fibroblasts into myofibroblasts (Fernandez-Salas, 2002; Ronnov-Jessen, 2002). In addition, it was reported that CLIC3 interacts with ERK7, a mitogen-activated protein kinase, allowing the regulation of the phosphatases or kinases (Qian, 1999).

4.3 CLIC6 protein

CLIC6 consist of 704 aminoacids with decapeptide repeats (Friedli, 2003) and and reportedly bind to the dopamine D(2)-like receptors (Griffon, 2003). It is also suggested that CLIC6 could be involved in the regulation of water and secretion of hormones (Nishizawa, 2000).

In chondrocytes, recently, we reported the identification of CLIC6 protein from proteomic analysis of rat normal articular cartilage (Perez, 2010). In human cartilage obtained from total knee arthroplasty, we found immunoreactivity for CLIC6 protein largely restricted to the aggregates of chondrocytes (clones or clusters) in the superficial zone (Fig. 2).

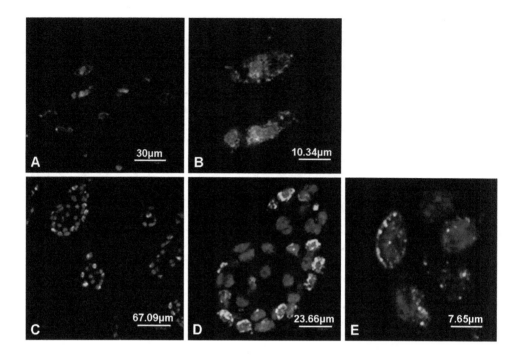

Fig. 2. CLIC6 immunostaining of NoAC and OAC. A-B Surface zone (NoAC), C-E
Chondrocytes clusters (OAC). The anti-CLIC6 antibody was coupled to FITC (fluorescein-5-
isothiocyanate) and the nucleus were counterstained with propidium iodide.

Immunolabelling was arranged in a coarse granular pattern located in the cytoplasm of
most chondrocytes. Comparatively, chondrocytes of non osteoarthritic human articular
cartilage (NoAC) showed scarse immunoreactivity predominantly in cells of superficial
zones (unpublished data).

Although controversial, the formation of cell clusters in osteoarthritic cartilage (OAC) has
been considered an event of repair and regeneration (Horton, 2005). However,
electrophysiological and molecular investigations are required to define role of the CLIC6
protein on healthy and osteoarthritic chondrocytes.

5. Conclusion

The pathogenesis of OA includes homeostatic alterations that induce imbalance in the
anabolic and catabolic processes. These have been associated with changes in the viability
and chondrocytes proliferation. Previous studies have showed a low proliferative activity of
OAC. However, the arrangement of the chondrocytes in groups (clones), a hallmark of OA,
could possibly be considered a sign of proliferation.

CLIC6 protein expression in normal articular cartilage of rat, and immunolocalization in
chondrocytes clusters removed from patients with OA, could suggest the involvement of
this anion channel in the pathophysiologic processes of disease.

6. Acknowledgment

We wish to thank Jose C. Luna Muñoz, PhD, for image capture support at the Departamento de Fisiología y Unidad de Microscopia Confocal, CINVESTAV-IPN, México.

7. References

Aigner, T.; Dudhia, J. (1997). Phenotypic modulation of chondrocytes as a potential therapeutic target in osteoarthritis: a hypothesis. *Ann Rheum Dis.* Vol. 56, pp. 287-291.

Aigner, T.; Hemmel, M.; Neureiter, D.; Gebhard, P.M.; Zeiler, G.; Kirchner, T.; McKenna, L. (2001). Apoptotic cell death is not a widespread phenomenon in normal aging and osteoarthritis human articular knee cartilage: a study of proliferation, programmed cell death (apoptosis), and viability of chondrocytes in normal and osteoarthritic human knee cartilage. *Arthritis Rheum.* Vol. 44, pp. 1304-1312.

Aigner, T.; Kim, H.A. (2002). Apoptosis and cellular vitality: issues in osteoarthritic cartilage degeneration. *Arthritis Rheum.* Vol. 46, pp. 1986-1996.

Baker-LePain, J.C.; Lane, N.E. (2010). Relationship between joint shape and the development of osteoarthritis. *Curr Opin Rheumatol* Vol. 22, pp. 538–543.

Barrett-Jolley, R.; Lewis, R.; Fallman, R.; Mobasheri, A. (2010). The emerging chondrocyte channelome. *Front Physiol.* Vol. 1, pp. 135.

Blanco, F.J.; Guitian, R.; Vazquez-Martul, E.; de Toro, F.J.; Galdo, F. (1998). Osteoarthritis chondrocytes die by apoptosis. A possible pathway for osteoarthritis pathology. *Arthritis Rheum* Vol. 41, pp. 284–289.

Bush, P.G.; Hall, A.C. (2001). The osmotic sensitivity of isolated and in situ bovine articular chondrocytes. *J Orthop Res* Vol. 19, pp. 768-778.

Bush, P.G.; Hall, A.C. (2003). The volume and morphology of chondrocytes within non-degenerate and degenerate human articular cartilage. *Osteoarthritis Cartilage* Vol. 11, pp. 242-251.

Bush, P.G.; Hodkinson, P.D.; Hamilton, G.L.; Hall, A.C. (2005). Viability and volume of in situ bovine articular chondrocytes--changes following a single impact and effects of medium osmolarity. *Osteoarthritis Cartilage* Vol. 13, pp. 54-65.

Chao, P.H.; West, A.C.; Hung, C.T. (2006). Chondrocyte intracellular calcium, cytoskeletal organization, and gene expression responses to dynamic osmotic loading. *Am J Physiol Cell Physiol* Vol. 291, pp. C718–725.

Chuang, J.Z.; Milner, T.A.; Zhu, M.; Sung, C.H. (1999). A 29 kDa intracellular chloride channel p64H1 is associated with large dense-core vesicles in rat hippocampal neurons. *J Neurosci* Vol. 19, pp. 2919–2928.

Clark, R.B.; Hatano, N.; Kondo, C.; Belke, D.D.; Brown, B.S.; Kumar, S.; Votta, B.J.; Giles, W.R. (2010). Voltage-gated k+ currents in mouse articular chondrocytes regulate membrane potential. *Channels* Vol. 4, pp. 179-191.

Deutsch, C. (1990). K+ channels and mitogenesis, *Prog Clin Biol Res.* Vol. 334, pp. 251-271.

Duncan, R.R.; Westwood, P.K.; Boyd, A.; Ashley, R.H. (1997). Rat brain p64H1, expression of a new member of the p64 chloride channel protein family in endoplasmic reticulum. *J Biol Chem* Vol. 272, pp. 23880–23886.

Edwards, J.C.; Cohen, C.; Xu, W.; Schlesinger, P.H. (2006). c-Src control of chloride channel support for osteoclast HCl transport and bone resorption. *J Biol Chem* Vol. 281, pp. 28011-28022.

Erickson, G.R.; Northrup, D.L.; Guilak, F. (2003). Hypo-osmotic stress induces calcium-dependent actin reorganization in articular chondrocytes. *Osteoarthritis Cartilage* Vol. 11, pp. 187-197.

Eyre, D.R.; Wu, J.J. (1987). Type XI or 1α2α3α collagen. In *Structure and Function of Collagen Types*. R. Mayne, R.E. Burgeson (Ed), New York: Academic Press, pp. 261-281.

Fahlke, C. (2001) Ion permeation and selectivity in ClC-type chloride channels. *Am J Physiol Renal Physiol*. Vol. 280, pp. F748-F757.

Fernández-Salas, E.; Suh, K.S.; Speransky, V.V.; Bowers, W.L.; Levy, J.M.; Adams, T.; Pathak, K.R.; Edwards, L.E.; Hayes, D.D.; Cheng, C.; Steven, A.C.; Weinberg, W.C.; Yuspa, S.H. (2002). mtCLIC/CLIC4, an organellular chloride channel protein, is increased by DNA damage and participates in the apoptotic response to p53. *Mol Cell Biol* Vol. 22, pp. 3610-3620.

Friedli, M.; Guipponi, M.; Bertrand, S.; Bertrand, D.; Neerman-Arbez, M.; Scott, H.S.; Antonarakis, S.E.; Reymond, A. (2003). Identification of a novel member of the CLIC family, CLIC6, mapping to 21q22.12. *Gene*. Vol. 320, pp. 31-40.

Funabashi, K.; Fujii, M.; Yamamura, H.; Ohya, S.; Imaizumi, Y. (2010). Contribution of chloride channel conductance to the regulation of resting membrane potential in chondrocytes. *J Pharmacol Sci*. Vol. 113, pp. 94-99.

Gannon, J.M.; Walker, G.; Fischer, M.; Carpenter, R.; Thompson, R.C. Jr.; Oegema, T.R. Jr. (1991). Localization of type X collagen in canine growth plate and adult canine articular cartilage. *J Orthop Res* Vol. 9, pp. 485-494.

Grandolfo, M.; D'Andrea, P.; Martina, M.; Ruzzier, F.; Vittur, F. (1992). Calcium-activated potassium channels in chondrocytes. *Biochem Biophys Res Commun*. Vol. 182, pp. 1429-1434.

Griffon, N., Jeanneteau, F., Prieur, F., Diaz, J. and Sokoloff, P. (2003) CLIC6, a member of the intracellular chloride channel family, interacts with dopamine D(2)-like receptors. *Brain Res Mol Brain Res*. Vol. 117, pp. 47-57.

Grodzinsky AJ, Levenston ME, Jin M, Frank EH. (2000). Cartilage tissue remodeling in response to mechanical forces. *Annu Rev Biomed Eng*. Vol. 2, pp. 691-713.

Hardingham, T.E.; Muir, H. (1974). Hyaluronic acid in cartilage and proteoglycan aggregation. *Biochem J*. Vol. 139, pp. 565-581.

Hardingham, G.E.; Bading, H. (1999). Calcium as a versatile second messenger in the control of gene expression. *Microsc Res Tech* Vol. 46, pp. 348-355.

Harmon SC, Lutz D, Ducote J. (1993). Potassium channel openers stimulate DNA synthesis in mouse epidermal keratinocyte and whole hair follicle cultures. *Skin Pharmacol*. Vol. 6, pp. 170-178.

Hashimoto, S.; Ochs, R.L.; Komiya, S.; Lotz, M. (1998a). Linkage of chondrocyte apoptosis and cartilage degradation in human osteoarthritis. *Arthritis Rheum* Vol. 41, pp. 1632-1638.

Hashimoto, S.; Takahashi, K.; Amiel, D.; Coutts, R.D.; Lotz, M. (1998b). Chondrocyte apoptosis and nitric oxide production during experimentally induced osteoarthritis. *Arthritis Rheum* Vol. 41, pp. 1266-1274.

Hedlund, H.; Hedbom, E.; Heineg rd, D.; Mengarelli-Widholm, S.; Reinholt, F.P.; Svensson, O. (1999). Association of the aggrecan keratan sulfate-rich region with collagen in bovine articular cartilage. *J Biol Chem* Vol. 274, pp. 5777-5781.

Horton, W.E. Jr.; Yagi, R.; Laverty, D.; Weiner, S. (2005). Overview of studies comparing human normal cartilage with minimal and advanced osteoarthritic cartilage. *Clin Exp Rheumatol* Vol. 23, pp. 103-112.

Huang, H.; Kamm, R.D.; Lee, R.T. (2004). Cell mechanics and mechanotransduction: pathways, probes, and physiology. *Am J Physiol Cell Physiol*. Vol. 287, pp. C1-11.

Hulth, A.; Lindberg, L.; Telhag, H. (1972). Mitosis in human osteoarthritic cartilage. *Clin Orthop Rel Res* Vol. 84, pp. 197-199.

Isoya, E.; Toyoda, F.; Imai, S.; Okumura, N.; Kumagai, K.; Omatsu-Kanbe, M.; Kubo, M.; Matsuura, H.; Matsusue, Y. (2009). Swelling-activated Cl(-) current in isolated rabbit articular chondrocytes: inhibition by arachidonic acid. *J Pharmacol Sci*. Vol. 109, pp. 293-304.

Jentsch, T.J.; Stein, V.; Weinreich, F.; Zdebik, A.A. (2002). Molecular structure and physiological function of chloride channels. *Physiol Rev*. Vol. 82, pp. 503-568.

Jentsch, T.J.; Poët, M.; Fuhrmann, J.C.; Zdebik, A.A. (2005). Physiological functions of CLC Cl--channels gleaned from human genetic disease and mouse models. *Annu Rev Physiol*. Vol. 67, pp. 779-807.

Jentsch, T.J. (2007) Chloride and the endosomal-lysosomal pathway: emerging roles of CLC chloride transporters. *J Physiol*. Vol. 578, pp. 633-40.

Jones, W.R.; Ting-Beall, H.P.; Lee, G.M.; Kelley, S.S.; Hochmuth, R.M.; Guilak, F. (1999). Alterations in the young's modulus and volumetric properties of chondrocytes isolated from normal and osteoarthritic human cartilage. *J Biomech* Vol. 32, pp. 119-127.

Kasper, D.; Planells-Cases, R.; Fuhrmann, J.C.; Scheel, O.; Zeitz, O.; Ruether, K.; Schmitt, A.; Poët, M.; Steinfeld, R.; Schweizer, M.; Kornak, U.; Jentsch, T.J. (2005). Loss of the chloride channel ClC-7 leads to lysosomal storage disease and neurodegeneration. *EMBO J*. Vol. 24, pp. 1079-1091.

Kerrigan, M.J.; Hook, C.S.; Qusous, A.; Hall, A.C. (2006). Regulatory volume increase (RVI) by in situ and isolated bovine articular chondrocytes. *J Cell Physiol* Vol. 209, pp. 481-492.

Kim, H.A.; Lee, Y.J.; Seong, S.C.; Choe, K.W.; Song, Y.W. (2000). Apoptotic chondrocyte death in human osteoarthritis. *J Rheum* Vol. 27, pp. 455-462.

Kouri, J.B.; Aguilera, J.M.; Reyes, J.; Lozoya, K.A.; Gonzalez S. (2000). Apoptotic chondrocytes from osteoarthrotic human articular cartilage and abnormal calcification of subchondral bone. *J Rheum* Vol. 27, pp. 1005-1019.

Kurz, B.; Lemke, A.K.; Fay, J.; Pufe, T.; Grodzinsky, A.J.; Schünke, M. (2005). Pathomechanisms of cartilage destruction by mechanical injury. *Ann Anat* Vol. 187, pp. 473-485.

Lawrence, R.C.; Felson, D.T.; Helmick, C.G.; Arnold, L.M.; Choi, H.; Deyo, R.A.; Gabriel, S.; Hirsch, R.; Hochberg, M.C.; Hunder, G.G.; Jordan, J.M.; Katz, J.N.; Kremers, H.M.; Wolfe, F. (2008). Estimates of the prevalence of arthritis and other rheumatic conditions in the United States. Part II. *Arthritis Rheum*. Vol. 58, pp. 26-35.

Lee, D.A.; Bentley, G.; Archer, C.W. (1993). The control of cell division in articular chondrocytes. *Osteoarthritis Cartilage* Vol. 1, pp. 137-146.

Lee, Y.S.; Sayeed, M.M.; Wurster, R.D. (1993). Inhibition of cell growth by K1 channel modulators is due to interference with agonist induced Ca2+ release. *Cell Signal* Vol. 5, pp. 803–809.

Lewis, R., Mobasheri, A., and Barrett-Jolley, R. (2008). Electrophysiological identification of epithelial sodium channels in canine articular chondrocytes. *Proc Physiol Soc*. Vol. 11, pp. C47.

Lewis, R.; Purves, G.; Crossley, J.; Barrett-Jolley, R. (2010). Modelling the membrane potential dependence on non-specific cation channels in canine articular chondrocytes. *Biophys J*. Vol. 98. (Suppl. 1), pp. 340A.

Lewis, R.; Asplin, K.E.; Bruce. G.; Dart, C.; Mobasheri, A.; Barrett-Jolley R. (2011). The role of the membrane potential in chondrocyte volume regulation. *J Cell Physiol*. Feb 15.

Liedtke W, Choe Y, Martí-Renom MA, Bell AM, Denis CS, Sali A, Hudspeth AJ, Friedman JM, Heller S. (2000). Vanilloid receptor-related osmotically activated channel (VR-OAC), a candidate vertebrate osmoreceptor. *Cell* Vol. 103, pp. 525–535.

Littler, D.R.; Assaad, N.N.; Harrop, S.J.; Brown, L.J.; Pankhurst, G.J.; Luciani, P.; Aguilar, M.I.; Mazzanti, M.; Berryman, M.A.; Breit, S.N.; Curmi, P.M. (2005). Crystal structure of the soluble form of the redox-regulated chloride ion channel protein CLIC4. *FEBS J*. Vol. 272, pp. 4996–5007.

Littler, D.R.; Harrop, S.J.; Goodchild, S.C.; Phang, J.M.; Mynott, A.V.; Jiang, L.; Valenzuela, S.M.; Mazzanti, M.; Brown, L.J.; Breit, S.N.; Curmi, P.M. (2010). The enigma of the CLIC proteins: Ion channels, redox proteins, enzymes, scaffolding proteins? *FEBS Lett*. Vol. 584, pp. 2093–2101

Liu, X.; Bandyopadhyay, B.C.; Nakamoto, T.; Singh, B.; Liedtke, W.; Melvin, J.E.; Ambudkar I. (2006). A role for AQP5 in activation of TRPV4 by hypotonicity: concerted involvement of AQP5 and TRPV4 in regulation of cell volume recovery. *J Biol Chem* Vol. 281, pp. 15485–15495.

Lloyd, S.E.; Pearce, S.H.; Fisher, S.E.; Steinmeyer, K.; Schwappach, B.; Scheinman, S.J.; Harding, B.; Bolino, A.; Devoto, M.; Goodyer, P.; Rigden, S.P.; Wrong, O.; Jentsch, T.J.; Craig, I.W.; Thakker, R.V. (1996). A common molecular basis for three inherited kidney stone diseases. *Nature* Vol. 379, pp. 445–449.

Loeser, R.F.; Carlson, C.S.; McGee, M.P. (1995). Expression of beta 1 integrins by cultured articular chondrocytes and in osteoarthritic cartilage. *Exp Cell Res* Vol. 217, pp. 248-257.

Long, K.J.; Walsh, K.B. (1994). Calcium-activated potassium channel in growth-plate chondrocytes: regulation by protein-kinase A. *Biochem Biophys Res Commun*. Vol. 201, pp. 776–781.

Mancilla, E.E.; Galindo, M.; Fertilio, B.; Herrera, M.; Salas, K.; Gatica, H.; Goecke, A. (2007). L-type calcium channels in growth plate chondrocytes participate in endochondral ossification. *J Cell Biochem*. Vol. 101, pp. 389–398.

Martina, M.; Mozrzymas, J.W.; Vittur, F. (1997). Membrane stretch activates a potassium channel in pig articular chondrocytes. *Biochim Biophys Acta*. Vol. 1329, pp. 205–210.

Mendler, M.; Eich-Bender, S.V.; Vaughan, L.; Winterhalter, K.M.; Bruckner P. (1989). Cartilage contains mixed fibrils of collagen types II, IX, and XI. *J Cell Biol* Vol. 108, pp. 191–197.

Millward-Sadler, S.J.; Wright, M.O.; Lee, H.S.; Nishida, K.; Caldwell, H.; Nuki, G.; Salter, D.M. (1999). Integrin-regulated secretion of interleukin 4: a novel pathway of mechanotransduction in human articular chondrocytes. *J Cell Biol* Vol. 145, pp. 183-189.

Millward-Sadler, S.J.; Wright, M.O.; Lee, H.S.; Caldwell, H.; Nuki, G.; Salter, D.M. (2000). Altered electrophysiological responses to mechanical stimulation and abnormal signaling through alpha5beta1 integrin in chondrocytes from osteoarthritic cartilage. *Osteoarthritis Cartilage* Vol. 8, pp. 272-278.

Minns, R.J.; Steven, F.S. (1977). The collagen fibril organization in human articular cartilage. *J Anat* Vol. 123, pp. 437- 457.

Mobasheri, A.; Mobasheri, R.; Francis, M.J.; Trujillo, E.; Alvarez de la Rosa, D.; Martín-Vasallo, P. (1998). Ion transport in chondrocytes: membrane transporters involved in intracellular ion homeostasis and the regulation of cell volume, free $[Ca^{2+}]$ and pH. *Histol Histopathol.* Vol. 13, pp. 893-910.

Mobasheri, A.; Martín-Vasallo, P. (1999). Epithelial sodium channels in skeletal cells; a role in mechanotransduction? *Cell Biol Int.* Vol. 23, pp. 237-240.

Mobasheri, A.; Gent, T.C.; Womack, M.D.; Carter, S.D.; Clegg, P.D.; Barrett-Jolley, R. (2005). Quantitative analysis of voltage-gated potassium currents from primary equine (Equus caballus) and elephant (Loxodonta africana) articular chondrocytes. *Am J Physiol Regul Integr Comp Physiol.* Vol. 289, pp. R172-R180.

Mobasheri, A.; Gent, T.C.; Nash, A.I.; Womack, M.D.; Moskaluk, C.A.; Barrett-Jolley, R. (2007). Evidence for functional ATP-sensitive (K(ATP)) potassium channels in human and equine articular chondrocytes. *Osteoarthritis Cartilage.* Vol. 15, pp. 1-8.

Mobasheri, A.; Lewis, R.; Maxwell, J.E.; Hill, C.; Womack, M.; Barrett-Jolley, R. (2010). Characterization of a stretch-activated potassium channel in chondrocytes. *J Cell Physiol.* Vol. 223, pp. 511-518.

Mouw, J.K.; Imler, S.M.; Levenston, M.E. (2007). Ion-channel regulation of chondrocyte matrix synthesis in 3D culture under static and dynamic compression. *Biomech Model Mechanobiol* Vol. 6, pp. 33-41.

Mow, V.C.; Wang, C.C.; Hung, C.T. (1999). The extracellular matrix, interstitial fluid and ions as a mechanical signal transducer in articular cartilage. *Osteoarthritis Cartilage.* Vol. 7, pp. 41-58.

Mozrzymas, J.W.; Martina, M.; Ruzzier, F. (1997). A large-conductance voltage-dependent potassium channel in cultured pig articular chondrocytes. *Pflugers Arch.* Vol. 433, pp. 413-427.

Nilius, B.; Droogmans, G. (1994). A role for potassium channels in cell proliferation?. *News Physiol Sci.* Vol. 16:1-12.

Nishizawa, T., Nagao, T., Iwatsubo, T., Forte, J.G. and Urushidani, T. (2000) Molecular cloning and characterization of a novel chloride intracellular channel-related protein, parchorin, expressed in water-secreting cells. *J Biol Chem.* Vol. 275, pp. 11164-11173.

Okumura, N.; Imai, S.; Toyoda, F.; Isoya, E.; Kumagai, K.; Matsuura, H.; Matsusue, Y. (2009). Regulatory role of tyrosine phosphorylation in the swelling-activated chloride current in isolated rabbit articular chondrocytes. *J Physiol* Vol. 587, pp. 3761-3776.

Ostergaard, K.; Salter, D.M.; Petersen, J.; Bendtzen, K.; Hvolris, J.; Andersen, C.B. (1998). Expression of alpha and beta subunits of the integrin superfamily in articular cartilage from macroscopically normal and osteoarthritic human femoral heads. *Ann Rheum Dis* Vol. 57, pp. 303-308.

Pérez, E.; Gallegos, J.L.; Cortés, L.; Calderón, K.G.; Luna, J.C.; Cázares, F.E.; Velasquillo, M.C,; Kouri, J.B.; Hernández, F.C. (2010). Identification of latexin by a proteomic analysis in rat normal articular cartilage. *Proteome Sci.* Vol. 5, pp. 27.

Phan, M.N.; Leddy, H.A.; Votta, B.J.; Kumar, S.; Levy, D.S.; Lipshutz, D.B.; Lee, S.H.; Liedtke, W.; Guilak, F. (2009). Functional characterization of TRPV4 as an osmotically sensitive ion channel in porcine articular chondrocytes. *Arthritis Rheum.* Vol. 60, pp. 3028-3037.

Poët, M.; Kornak, U.; Schweizer, M.; Zdebik, A.A.; Scheel, O.; Hoelter, S.;Wurst, W.; Schmitt, A.; Fuhrmann, J.C.; Planells-Cases, R.; Mole, S.E.; Hübner, C.A.; Jentsch, T.J. (2006). Lysosomal storage disease upon disruption of the neuronal chloride transport protein ClC-6. *Proc Natl Acad Sci USA* Vol. 103, pp. 13854-13859.

Ponce, A. (2006). Expression of voltage dependent potassium currents in freshly dissociated rat articular chondrocytes. *Cell Physiol Biochem.* Vol. 18, pp. 35-46.

Poole, C.A. (1997). Articular cartilage chondrons: form, function and failure. *J Anat* Vol. 191, pp. 1-13.

Pritzker, K.P.; Gay, S.; Jimenez, S.A.; Ostergaard, K.; Pelletier, J.P.; Revell, P.A.; Salter, D.; van den Berg WB. (2006). Osteoarthritis cartilage histopathology: grading and staging. *Osteoarthritis Cartilage.* Vol. 14, pp. 13-29.

Qian, Z.; Okuhara, D.; Abe, M.K.; Rosner, M.R. (1999). Molecular cloning and characterization of a mitogen activated protein kinase-associated intracellular chloride channel. *J Biol Chem.* Vol. 274, pp. 1621-1627.

Ramage, L.; Martel, M.A.; Hardingham, G.E.; Salter, D.M. (2008). NMDA receptor expression and activity in osteoarthritic human articular chondrocytes. *Osteoarthritis Cartilage.* Vol. 16, pp. 1576-1584.

Ronnov-Jessen, L.; Villadsen, R.; Edwards, J.C.; Petersen, O.W. (2002). Differential expression of a chloride intracellular channel gene, CLIC4, in transforming growth factor-beta1-mediated conversion of fibroblasts to myofibroblasts. *Am J Pathol* Vol. 161, pp. 471-480.

Roos, E.M. (2005). Joint injury causes knee osteoarthritis in young adults. *Curr Opin Rheumatol* Vol. 17, pp. 195-200.

Rothwell, A.G.; Bentley, G. Chondrocyte multiplication in osteoarthritic articular cartilage. (1973). *J Bone Joint Surg Br.* Vol. 55, pp. 588-594.

Salter, D.M.; Millward-Sadler, S.J.; Nuki, G.; Wright, M.O. (2002). Differential responses of chondrocytes from normal and osteoarthritic human articular cartilage to mechanical stimulation. *Biorheology* Vol. 39, pp. 97-108.

Sanchez, J.C.; Danks, T.A.; Wilkins, R.J. (2003). Mechanisms involved in the increase in intracellular calcium following hypotonic shock in bovine articular chondrocytes. *Gen Physiol Biophys.* Vol. 22, pp. 487-500.

Sanchez, J. C., and Wilkins, R. J. (2004). Changes in intracellular calcium concentration in response to hypertonicity in bovine articular chondrocytes. *Comp Biochem Physiol A Mol Integr Physiol.* Vol. 137, pp. 173-182.

Sanchez, J.C.; Powell, T.; Staines, H.M.; Wilkins, R.J. (2006). Electrophysiological demonstration of voltage-activated H+ channels in bovine articular chondrocytes. *Cell Physiol Biochem.* Vol. 18, pp. 85-90.

Sandell, L.J.; Aigner, T. (2001). Articular cartilage and changes in arthritis. An introduction: cell biology of osteoarthritis. *Arthritis Res.* Vol. 3, pp. 107-113.

Schlesinger, P.H.; Blair, H.C.; Teitelbaum, S.L.; Edwards, J.C. (1997). Characterization of the osteoclast ruffled border chloride channel and its role in bone resorption. *J Biol Chem* Vol. 272, pp. 18636–18643.

Shakibaei, M.; Mobasheri, A. (2003). Beta1-integrins co-localize with Na, K-ATPase, epithelial sodium channels (ENaC) and voltage activated calcium channels (VACC) in mechanoreceptor complexes of mouse limb-bud chondrocytes. *Histol Histopathol.* Vol. 18, pp. 343–351.

Singh, H.; Cousin, M.A.; Ashley, R.H. (2007). Functional reconstitution of mammalian 'chloride intracellular channels' CLIC1, CLIC4 and CLIC5 reveals differential regulation by cytoskeletal actin. *FEBS J* Vo.l 274, pp. 6306–6316.

Stockwell, R.A. (1967). The cell density of human articular and costal cartilage. *J Anat* Vol. 101, pp. 753–763.

Stockwell, R.A. (1990). Morphology of cartilage. In *Maroudas A & Keuttner K* (eds.). Methods in cartilage research. San Diego: Academic Press, pp. 61–63.

Stockwell, R.A. (1991). Cartilage failure in osteoarthritis: Relevance of normal structure and function. *Clinical Anatomy* Vol. 4, pp. 161–191.

Sugimoto, T.; Yoshino, M.; Nagao, M.; Ishii, S.; Yabu, H. (1996). Voltage-gated ionic channels in cultured rabbit articular chondrocytes. *Comp Biochem Physiol C Pharmacol Toxicol Endocrinol.* Vol. 115, pp. 223–232.

Trujillo, E., Alvarez de la Rosa, D., Mobasheri, A., Gonzalez, T., Canessa, C. M., and Martin-Vasallo, P. (1999). Sodium transport systems in human chondrocytes. II. Expression of ENaC, Na+/K+/2Cl- cotransporter and Na+/H+ exchangers in healthy and arthritic chondrocytes. *Histol Histopathol.* Vol. 14, pp. 1023–1031.

Tsuga, K.; Tohse, N.; Yoshino, M.; Sugimoto, T.; Yamashita, T.; Ishii, S; Yabu, H. (2002). Chloride conductance determining membrane potential of rabbit articular chondrocytes. *J Membr Biol.* Vol. 185, pp. 75–81.

Tulk, B.M.; Kapadia, S.; Edwards, J.C. (2002). CLIC1 inserts from the aqueous phase into phospholipid membranes, where it functions as an anion channel. *Am J Physiol Cell Physiol.* Vol. 282, pp. C1103-1112.

Urban, J.P.; Hall, A.C.; Gehl, K.A. (1993). Regulation of matrix synthesis rates by the ionic and osmotic environment of articular chondrocytes. *J Cell Physiol.* Vol. 154, pp. 262–270.

Urban, J.P. (1994). The chondrocyte: a cell under pressure. *Br J Rheumatol.* Vol. 33, pp. 901–908.

Valenzuela SM, Martin DK, Por SB, Robbins JM, Warton K, Bootcov MR, Schofield PR, Campbell TJ, Breit SN. (1997). Molecular cloning and expression of a chloride ion channel of cell nuclei. *J Biol Chem* Vol. 272, pp. 12575–12582.

Walsh, K.B.; Cannon, S.D.; Wuthier, R.E. (1992). Characterization of a delayed rectifier potassium current in chicken growth plate chondrocytes. *Am J Physiol.* Vol. 262, pp. C1335–C1340.

Wang, X.T,; Nagaba, S.; Nagaba, Y.; Leung, S.W.; Wang, J.; Qiu, W.; Zhao, P.L.; Guggino, S.E. (2000). Cardiac L-type calcium channel alpha 1-subunit is increased by cyclic adenosine monophosphate: messenger RNA and protein expression in intact bone. *J Bone Miner Res.* Vol. 15, pp. 1275–1285.

Weiss, C.; Rosenberg, L.; Helfet, A.J. (1968). An ultrastructural study of normal young adult human articular cartilage. *J Bone Joint Surg Am* Vol. 50, pp. 663– 674.

Wilson, J.R.; Duncan, N.A.; Giles, W.R.; Clark, R.B. (2004). A voltage dependent K+ current contributes to membrane potential of acutely isolated canine articular chondrocytes. *J Physiol.* Vol. 557, pp. 93–104.

Wohlrab, D. (1998). Der Einfluß elektrophysiologischer Membraneigenschaften auf die Proliferation humaner Keratinozyten. Tectum, Marburg, pp. 1-89

Wohlrab, D.; Lebek, S.; Krüger, T.; Reichel, H. (2002). Influence of ion channels on the proliferation of human chondrocytes. *Biorheology* Vol. 39, pp. 55-61.

Wohlrab, D.; Vocke, M.; Klapperstuck, T.; Hein, W. (2004). Effects of potassium and anion channel blockers on the cellular response of human osteoarthritic chondrocytes. *J Orthop Sci.* Vol. 9, pp. 364–371.

Wohlrab, D.; Vocke, M.; Klapperstück, T.; Hein, W. (2005). The influence of lidocaine and verapamil on the proliferation, CD44 expression and apoptosis behavior of human chondrocytes. *Int J Mol Med.* Vol. 16, pp. 149-57.

Wright, M.O.; Stockwell, R.A.; Nuki, G. (1992). Response of the plasma membrane to applied hydrostatic pressure in chondrocytes and fibroblasts. *Connect Tissue Res* Vol. 28, pp. 49-70.

Wright, M.O.; Jobanputra, P.; Bavington, C.; Salter, D.M.; Nuki, G. (1996). The effects of intermittent pressurisation on the electrophysiology of cultured human articular chondrocytes: evidence for the presence of stretch activated membrane ion channels. *Clin Sci (Lond).* Vol. 90, pp. 61-71.

Wu, J.J.; Eyre, D.R.; Slayter, H.S. (1987). Type VI collagen of the intervertebral disc. Biochemical and electron microscopic characterization of the native protein. *Biochem J* Vol. 248, pp. 373-381.

Wu, J.J.; Murray, J.; Eyre, D.R. (1996). Evidence for copolymeric crosslinking between types II and III collagens in human articular cartilage. *Trans Orthop Res Soc* Vol. 21, pp. 42.

Wu, Q. Q., and Chen, Q. (2000). Mechanoregulation of chondrocyte proliferation, maturation, and hypertrophy: ion-channel dependent transduction of matrix deformation signals. *Exp Cell Res* Vol. 256, pp. 383–391.

Xu, J.; Wang, W.; Clark, C.C.; Brighton, C.T. (2009). Signal transduction in electrically stimulated articular chondrocytes involves translocation of extracellular calcium through voltage-gated channels. *Osteoarthritis Cartilage.* Vol. 17, pp. 397–405.

Xu, X.; Urban, J.P.; Tirlapur, U.K.; Cui, Z. (2010). Osmolarity effects on bovine articular chondrocytes during three-dimensional culture in alginate beads. *Osteoarthritis Cartilage* Vol. 18, pp. 433-439.

7

Transcriptional Regulation of Articular Chondrocyte Function and Its Implication in Osteoarthritis

Jinxi Wang[1,2], William C. Kramer[1] and John P. Schroeppel[1]
[1]Department of Orthopaedic Surgery,
[2]Department of Biochemistry and Molecular Biology,
University of Kansas Medical Center, Kansas City,
USA

1. Introduction

Osteoarthritis (OA) is characterized by joint pain and stiffness with radiographic evidence of joint space narrowing, osteophytes, and subchondral bone sclerosis. Current treatments primarily target symptomatic control of OA, including pharmacologic therapy, local joint injection, and surgical interventions. Pharmaceuticals such as nonsteroidal anti-inflammatory drugs (NSAIDs) and Acetaminophen are aimed to control inflammation and pain by blocking potent inflammatory cytokine pathways. Joint injections including glucocorticoids and hyaluranan-based formulations attempt to control inflammatory mediators locally and improve the glucosaminoglycan concentration within the joint space. Surgical procedures such as debridement, microfracture, osteochondral autografting, and autologous chondrocyte transplantation are currently employed to stimulate articular cartilage repair and delay the need for joint replacement. However, all these therapies are aimed at symptomatic control and have limited impact on impeding or reversing the progression to advanced OA. Therefore, interest has been high in development of structure or disease-modifying OA drugs (DMOADs) aimed at slowing, halting, or reversing the progression of structural damage of articular cartilage. A large number of candidate DMOADs have been tested but none have been approved by American or European regulatory agencies (Hellio Le Graverand-Gastineau, 2009; Lotz & Kraus, 2010).

A critical barrier in drug development for OA is that molecular and cellular mechanisms for the development of OA, especially the mechanisms that control the activity of adult articular chondrocytes, remain unclear. Overexpression of proinflammatory cytokines such as Interleukin-1β (IL-1β) and tumor necrosis factor-α (TNF-α) (Goldring, 2001; Fernandes et al., 2002), matrix-degrading proteinases such as matrix metalloproteinases (MMPs) (Burrage et al., 2006) and a disintegrin and metalloproteinase with thrombospondin motifs (ADAMTS) (Glasson et al., 2005; Karsenty, 2005; Stanton et al., 2005), and nitric oxide (Pelletier et al., 2000; Haudenschild et al., 2008; Lotz, 1999) may cause cartilage degradation. However, no single cytokine or proteinase can stimulate all the metabolic reactions observed in OA. Due to the involvement of multiple proteinases and proinflammatory cytokines in the pathogenesis of OA, a candidate DMOAD that inhibits a single proteinase or inflammatory cytokine is unlikely to produce long-term benefit if other catabolic factors are not blocked. Therefore, it is critical to identify which upstream factors regulate the expression of these catabolic molecules in articular cartilage and other joint tissues (e.g., synovium).

This chapter summarizes the recent advances in identification of potential upstream regulators such as transcription factors and specific growth factors that may control the expression of anabolic and/or catabolic molecules in articular cartilage and their functional implications in the pathogenesis and treatment of OA.

2. Dysfunction of adult articular chondrocytes and its significance in OA

It has been recognized that OA may develop as a result of: 1) abnormal loading on normal joint tissues (articular cartilage and subchondral bone); 2) normal/physiologic loading on abnormal/defective joint tissues; or 3) a combination of the two (Piscoya et al., 2005; Brandt et al., 2008; Segal et al., 2009; Buckwalter et al., 2004; Block & Shakoor, 2009; Drewniak et al., 2009; June & Fyhrie, 2008; Borrelli et al., 2009; van der Meulen & Huiskes, 2002; Rothschild & Panza, 2007). Dysfunction of articular chondrocytes may be the initial change in OA with normal loading on abnormal articular cartilage. For OA associated with abnormal loading on normal joint tissues, dysfunction of articular chondrocytes is not the initial cause. However, mechanical disruption of the extracellular matrix and abnormal mechanotransduction in articular chondrocytes during and after joint injury or malalignment may activate specific signaling pathways, leading to changes in gene expression and cartilage metabolism as a result of dysfunction of articular chondrocytes. In order to develop effective strategies for prevention and treatment of OA, it is critical to understand the regulatory mechanisms of articular chondrocyte function.

Mature cartilage exists in three main types: hyaline cartilage, fibrocartilage, and elastic cartilage. Hyaline cartilage is characterized by matrix containing type-II collagen (collagen-2) fibers, glycosaminoglycans, proteoglycans, and multiadhesive glycoproteins. Fibrocartilage is characterized by abundant type-I collagen (collagen-1) fibers in addition to the matrix material of hyaline cartilage. Elastic cartilage is characterized by elastic fibers and elastic lamellae in addition to the matrix material of hyaline cartilage. Elastic cartilage is found in the external ear, the wall of the external acoustic meatus, the eustacchium, and the epiglottis of the larynx (Ross & Pawlina, 2006). Hyaline cartilage is of particular focus here because it is the innate component of diarthrodial joint surface involved in OA. Normal articular cartilage is composed of hyaline cartilage, which is divided into four zones: 1) the superficial tangential zone, composed of thin tangential collagen fibrils and low aggrecan content, 2) the middle or transitional zone, composed of thick radial collagen bundles, 3) the deep zone, composed of even thicker radial bundles of collagen fibrils, and 4) the calcified cartilage zone located between the tidemark and the subchondral bone (Goldring & Marcu, 2009). The calcified zone persists after growth plate closure and serves as an important mechanical buffer between the uncalcified articular cartilage and the subchondral bone. Generally, cell density decreases and cell volume and relative proteoglycan content increase as the cartilage transitions from superficial to deep. Unlike those chondrocytes involved in endochondral ossification, the chondrocytes within normal articular cartilage do not undergo terminal differentiation, but persist and function to produce extracellular matrix and maintain cartilage homeostasis.

The extracellular matrix is produced and maintained by the chondrocyte. Articular cartilage is characterized by the absence of blood vessels or nerves. Due to the avascularity of articular cartilage, some nutrients are provided by diffusion of the synovial fluid. Articular chondrocytes have adapted to the very low oxygen tension (in the range of 1-7%) and low glucose levels with facilitated glucose transport via upregulation of hypoxia inducible factor-1 (HIF-1), expression of glucose transporter-1 and -3 (GLUT1 and GLUT3), and enhanced anaerobic glycolysis (Wilkins et al., 2000; Mobasheri et al., 2005; Clouet et al., 2009). Much like bone, the physiologic properties of articular cartilage are primarily related to the extracellular matrix, but homeostasis in adult articular cartilage relies on the function of articular chondrocytes. In healthy articular cartilage, chondrocytes maintain a very low turnover rate of its constituents with a good balance of anabolism vs. catabolism.

Articular cartilage undergoes changes in its material properties related to aging which are different from the disease process of OA, but may eventually predispose cartilage to OA or contribute to its progression. One such factor is the development of advanced glycation end products (AGEs), which enhance collagen cross-linking and make the tissue more brittle (Verzijl et al., 2002). Additionally, the ability of chondrocytes to respond to growth factor stimulation appears to decline with age, leading to decreased anabolism (Loeser & Shakoor, 2003). Chondrocytes also demonstrate increasing senescence with age due to erosion of telomere length related to oxidative stress.

OA is a disease process characterized radiographically by narrowing of joint space due to loss of articular cartilage, subchondral bone sclerosis, osteophyte formation, and subchondral cyst formation. In addition to bony changes evident on radiographs, OA also affects the synovium and surrounding connective tissue, indicating it is not simply a disease of articular cartilage (Brandt et al., 2006; Brandt et al., 2008). At the cellular and molecular level, OA is a disruption of normal cartilage homeostasis, generally leading to excessive catabolism relative to anabolism. Risk factors that contribute to development of OA include advanced age, joint trauma, irregular joint mechanics and malalignment, obesity, muscle weakness, and genetic predisposition. Although OA is not commonly referred to as an inflammatory arthropathy due to the lack of neutrophils in the synovial fluid and the absence of a systemic inflammatory response, inflammatory mediators clearly play a role in the progression of OA.

In early OA, global gene expression within the chondrocyte is activated following mechanical injury or biological abnormalities causing increased expression of inflammatory mediators, cartilage-degrading proteinases, and stress-response factors (Fitzgerald et al., 2004; Kurz et al., 2005). Loss of proteoglycans and cleavage of collagen-2 occurs initially at the surface of articular cartilage, causing an increase in water content and reduced tensile strength of the matrix (Goldring & Goldring, 2007). Chondrocyte clustering is one of the typical features of OA cartilage (Clouet et al., 2009). Chondrocytes initially attempt to synthesize and replace degraded extracellular matrix (ECM) components such as collagen-2, -9, and -11, aggrecan, and pericellular collagen-4 (Buckwalter et al., 2007). This compensatory synthesis of ECM components is most evident among the deeper regions of articular cartilage (Fukui et al., 2008). Among the factors stimulating anabolism are insulin-like growth factor-1 (IGF-1), members of the transforming growth factor-β (TGF-β) superfamily, and fibroblast growth factors (FGFs) (Fukui et al., 2003; Hermansson et al., 2004). These attempt to offset the degradation caused by inflammatory mediators such as IL-1β, TNF-a, MMPs (e.g., MMP-1, MMP-3, MMP-8, MMP-13, and MMP-14), aggrecanases (e.g., ADAMTS-4 and ADAMTS-5), and other catabolic cytokines and chemokines.

As OA progresses, the synthetic balance shifts to favor catabolism, which leads to cartilage degradation. Significant heterogeneity in the synthetic capacity of articular chondrocytes occurs in OA cartilage. Overall gene activation is increased in the deep zone, but is decreased in the superficial zone and areas in the mid zone with degradation (Fukui et al., 2008). Evidence of phenotypic modulation of endochondral ossification, such as collagen-1, -3, -10, is found in osteoarthritic cartilage, which is not characteristic of normal adult articular cartilage (Sandell & Aigner, 2001). OA changes also occur in the subchondral bone that accompanies articular cartilage loss. Subchondral plate thickness increases, the tidemark advances, and angiogenesis invades an otherwise avascular structure (Lane et al., 1977). Apoptosis of the chondrocyte is seen in OA cartilage, which is mediated in part, by the caspases and inflammatory mediators such as IL-1 and Nitric Oxide (NO) (Kim & Blanco, 2007).

Another indication of aberrant behavior of osteoarthritic chondrocytes is the presence of collagen-10 (a marker of hypertrophic chondrocytes) and other differentiation markers, including annexin VI , alkaline phosphatase (Alp), osteopontin (Opn), and osteocalcin (Pfander et al., 2001; Pullig et al., 2000a; Pullig et al., 2000b; von der Mark et al., 1992), indicating that OA cartilage cannot maintain the characteristics of the permanent cartilage but adds those of the embryonic or growth plate cartilage. These observations suggest that chondrocyte maturation is likely to be deeply involved in the pathogenesis of OA. Recent findings on the regulatory effects of transcription/growth factors on the function of adult articular chondrocytes and their significance in the pathogenesis of OA are discussed below.

3. Regulation of articular chondrocyte function and its implication in pathogenesis of OA

Many governing factors that are critical for skeletal development have also been found to have a significant involvement in adult chondrocyte homeostasis and pathophysiology of OA. For instance, during skeletal development, chondrocytes in the growth plate undergo hypertrophic and apoptotic changes and cartilage is degraded and replaced by bone. One of the current hypotheses is that OA reflects the inappropriate recurrence of the hypertrophic pathway in articular chondrocytes. To better understand the regulatory mechanisms of various transcription and non-transcription factors in articular chondrocyte function, it is necessary to include their regulatory roles in chondrocyte differentiation, endochondral ossification, and joint formation during skeletal development here in this chapter.

3.1 Chondrocyte differentiation and joint formation during skeletal development
3.1.1 Chondrocyte differentiation and endochondral ossification
Both the chondrocyte (cartilage-forming cell) and osteoblast (bone-forming cell) are derived from a common mesenchymal stem cell referred to as the osteochondroprogenitor cell. Limb development first begins with the formation of mesenchymal condensations and the subsequent formation of a surrounding cartilaginous envelope called the perichondrium. The progenitor cells proceed to form the anlagen, or cartilaginous template of each bone. Cartilage cells undergo proliferation, differentiation to functional chondrocytes, hypertrophic differentiation, apoptosis, calcification of cartilage, invasion of cartilage tissue by capillaries and chondroclasts (osteoclasts), and eventual resorption and replacement by newly formed bone. This process of bone formation is called endochondral ossification. The

primary ossification center in the diaphysis of long bones is formed through endochondral ossification. A similar sequence of events occurs in the growth plate leading to rapid growth of the skeleton.

3.1.2 Joint formation

At the end of each long bone an interzone and secondary ossification center develop. The interzone is the first sign of joint development at each future joint location, which consists of closely associated mesenchymal cells. Articular chondrocytes may derive from a subset of interzone cells, especially from the intermediate layer. Physiological separation of the adjacent skeletal elements occurs with further development, which involves a process of cavitations within the interzone that leads to formation of a liquid-filled synovial space. Morphological and cytodifferentiation processes extending over developmental time eventually lead to maturation of the joint in which the proximal and distal ends acquire their reciprocal and interlocking shapes. The formation of hyaline articular cartilage and other joint-specific tissues makes the joint fully capable of providing its physiologic roles through life (Pacifici et al., 2005; Mitrovic, 1978).

3.1.3 Bone morphogenetic proteins (BMPs) and their antagonists in joint formation

BMPs are members of the TGF-β superfamily. BMP was originally identified as a secreted signaling molecule that could induce chondrocyte differentiation and endochondral bone formation. Subsequent molecular cloning studies have revealed that the BMP family consists of various molecules, including members of the growth and differentiation factor (GDF/Gdf) subfamily. BMP members have diverse biological activities during the development of various organs and tissues, as well as embryonic axis determination (Hogan, 1996; Sampath et al., 1990; Wozney et al., 1988). BMP2, BMP4, BMP7, and BMP14 (GDF5/Gdf5) are expressed in the perichondrium and are proposed to regulate cartilage formation and joint development (Francis-West et al., 1999; Macias et al., 1997; Zou et al., 1997; Tsumaki et al., 2002). Gdf5, also known as cartilage-derived morphogenetic protein 1 (CDMP-1), plays a role in chondrogenesis and chondrocyte metabolism, tendon and ligament tissue formation, and postnatal bone repair (Bos et al., 2008). Mutations of this gene are present in a number of developmental bone and cartilage diseases (Masuya et al., 2007; Bos et al., 2008). Gdf5 has at least two roles in skeletogenesis. At early stages, Gdf5 may stimulate recruitment and differentiation of chondrogenic cells when it is expressed throughout the condensations. At later stages, Gdf5 may promote interzone cell function and joint development when its expression becomes restricted to the interzone (Storm & Kingsley, 1999; Koyama et al., 2008).

Extracellular BMP antagonists such as Noggin and Chordin can block BMP signaling by binding to BMP and preventing BMP binding to specific cell surface receptors. *Noggin* is expressed in condensing limb mesenchyme in mouse embryos, and expression persists in differentiated chondrocytes. When the *Noggin* gene was ablated, the mesenchymal condensations became much larger and limb joints failed to form, indicating that *Noggin* is critical for normal development of both long bones and joints (Brunet et al., 1998). Subsequent work in chick embryos showed that expression of *Noggin, Chordin,* and BMP-2 characterizes the interzone once it is established, and that *Chordin* expression persists in older developing joints, while *Noggin* expression shifts to epiphyseal chondrocytes (Francis-West et al., 1999). These and other data are widely acknowledged to signify that the action of BMP antagonists is required to regulate the pace and extent of chondrogenesis in early developing long bones, and that sustained and more restricted expression and action of these factors in developing joints would maintain the mesenchymal character of interzone cells and permit normal progression of interzone function and joint formation (Hall & Miyake, 2000). Absence of joints in *Noggin*-null mice would thus be due to exuberant and nonphysiologic action by endogenous BMPs and, consequently, rapid and abnormal conversion of the entire mesenchymal condensations into chondrocytes. Though these conclusions are plausible and quite likely, what remains unclear is how the absence of *Noggin* leads to joint ablation; specifically, whether the interzone fails to form completely or whether it starts forming but cannot be sustained, whether other BMP inhibitors fail to be activated, or whether joint formation sites fail to respond to upstream patterning cues (Pacifici et al., 2005).

3.1.4 ERG regulates the differentiation of immature chondrocytes into permanent articular chondrocytes

The ERG (Ets-related gene) transcriptional activator belongs to the *Ets* gene family of transcription factors. ERG is not only expressed at the onset of joint formation, but persists once the articular layer has developed further. A variant of ERG named C-1-1 is expressed in most epiphyseal pre-articular/articular chondrocytes in developing long bones. When C-1-1 is mis-expressed in developing chick limbs, it is able to impose a stable and immature articular-like phenotype onto the entire limb chondrocyte population, effectively blocking maturation and endochondral ossification (Iwamoto et al., 2000). More recent studies found that limb long bone anlagen of transgenic mice expressing the ERG variant C-1-1 were entirely composed of chondrocytes actively expressing collagen-9 and aggrecan as well as articular markers such as Tenascin-C. Typical growth plates were absent and there was very low expression of maturation and hypertrophy markers, including Ihh, collagen-10, and Mmp13. There was a close spatio-temporal relationship in the expression of both ERG and GDF5 that is an effective inducer of ERG expression in developing mouse embryo joints. These results suggest that ERG is part of the molecular mechanisms driving the differentiation of immature chondrocytes into permanent articular chondrocytes, and may do so by acting downstream of GDF5 (Iwamoto et al., 2007).

These studies suggest that mesenchymal progenitor cells differentiate into two fundamentally distinct types of cartilage cells during skeletal development. The cartilage cells in the primary and secondary ossification centers and the growth plate undergo proliferation, differentiation to functional chondrocytes, hypertrophic differentiation, apoptosis, and eventual resorption and replacement by newly formed bone through the endochondral sequence of ossification. This type of cartilage is called temporal or replacement cartilage. In contrast, cartilage cells close to the surface of growing long bones divide and differentiate to form hyaline articular cartilage, which is termed permanent or persistent cartilage because articular chondrocytes normally do not undergo terminal differentiation or endochondral ossification and are not replaced by bone (Eames et al., 2004; Pacifici et al., 2005).

3.2 Transcriptional regulation of articular chondrocyte function

Factors that have been reported to regulate chondrocyte differentiation during development and articular chondrocyte function in the adult stage are discussed below.

3.2.1 Sox9

The transcription factor Sox9 is a member of the high mobility group (HMG) and appears to be an essential transcription factor driving chondrogenesis during development and growth (Bi et al., 1999). Sox9 is expressed predominantly by mesenchymal progenitor cells and proliferating chondrocytes, but is not found in hypertrophic chondrocytes or osteoblasts (Zou et al., 2006). Sox9 is critical for the differentiation of mesenchymal progenitor cells into chondrocytes during cartilage morphogenesis. Prechondrocytic mesenchymal cells lacking Sox9 are unable to differentiate into chondrocytes (Bi et al., 1999). Joint formation is defective in Sox9-deficient mouse embryos (Akiyama et al., 2002). Two other members of the Sox family, Sox5 and Sox6 may also be essential for cartilage formation (Smits et al., 2001). Sox9 up-regulates the expression of chondrocyte-specific marker genes encoding collagen-2, collagen-9, collagen-11, and aggrecan by binding to their enhancer sequences (Evangelou et al., 2009). Sox9 also acts cooperatively with Sox5 and Sox6, which are present after cell condensation during chondrocyte differentiation, to activate collagen-2 and aggrecan genes (Zou et al., 2006; Lefebvre et al., 1998; Leung et al., 1998). It has been reported that the Sox trio (Sox 5, Sox6, Sox9) inhibit terminal stages of chondrocyte differentiation (Ikeda et al., 2004; Saito et al., 2007); however, the precise underlying regulatory mechanism remains unclear. Recently, Amano *et al.* demonstrated that the Sox trio inhibited chondrocyte maturation and calcification by up-regulating parathyroid hormone related protein (PTHrP) (Amano et al., 2009). The anabolic effects of insulin-like growth factor-1 (IGF-1), bone morphogenetic protein-2 (BMP-2), and fibroblast growth factor-2 (FGF-2) on developing chondrocytes also appear to be mediated, in part, by Sox9 (Leung et al., 1998; Lefebvre et al., 1998; Goldring et al., 2008; Kolettas et al., 2001; Zehentner et al., 1999).

Despite the fact that Sox9 is critical for chondrocyte differentiation and cartilage morphogenesis during skeletal development (Bi et al., 1999), the expression and function of Sox9 in adult articular cartilage are controversial in literature. A gene expression study reported that Sox9 expression was lower in human OA cartilage (Brew et al., 2010). However, another study showed no significant difference in subcellular expression of Sox9 protein between osteoarthritic and normal control human cartilage. Sox9 overexpression did not correlate with collagen-2 expression in adult articular cartilage, suggesting that Sox9 is not a key regulator of collagen-2 expression in human adult articular chondrocytes (Aigner et al., 2003). Furthermore, *in vitro* studies showed that overexpression of Sox9 was unable to restore the chondrocyte phenotype of dedifferentiated osteoarthritic articular chondrocytes (Kypriotou et al., 2003). These studies suggest that although Sox9 plays a crucial role in chondrocyte differentiation during skeletal development, its regulatory effect on the function of adult articular chondrocytes and development of OA remains to be elucidated.

3.2.2 Runx2

The transcription factor Runx2 (also called Cbfa1, Osf2, or AML3) is a member of the Runt family of transcription factors. Runx2 has been identified as a master regulator of osteoblast differentiation. Runx2$^{-/-}$ mice died shortly after birth and exhibited a cartilaginous skeleton completely void of intramembranous and endochondral ossification due to the maturational arrest of osteoblasts. (Komori et al., 1999; Coffman, 2003; Takeda et al., 2001; Ducy et al., 1997; Komori et al., 1997; Otto et al., 1997). Histologic analyses of Runx2$^{-/-}$ mice have revealed delayed maturation of chondrocytes, indicating that Runx2 is involved in both osteogenesis and chondrogenesis (Inada et al., 1999). Eames et al. demonstrated the ability of Runx2 overexpression to change permanent cartilage (e.g., articular cartilage) to temporal cartilage (e.g., growth plate cartilage) (Eames et al., 2004). Among the chondrogenic phenotypes during endochondral ossification, Runx2 is expressed mainly in the prehypertrophic and, to a lesser extent, in the late hypertrophic chondrocytes (Takeda et al., 2001). Its expression coincides with Indian hedgehog (Ihh), collagen-10, and BMP-6. Matrix metalloproteinase-13 (MMP-13), which is expressed by terminal hypertrophic chondrocytes, is a downstream target of Runx2 (Hess et al., 2001). Growth arrest and DNA damage induceable-45β (GADD45β) has been described as a probable intermediate molecule in the interaction between Runx2 and MMP-13 (Goldring et al., 2006; Ijiri et al., 2008; Ijiri et al., 2005).

In adult mice, Runx2 is expressed in the articular cartilage of wild-type mice at the early stage of post-traumatic knee OA, induced by surgical transection of the medial collateral ligament and resection of the medial meniscus. In this mouse model of OA, Runx2 expression in osteoarthritic cartilage parallels collagen-10 expression but arises earlier than Mmp13. After induction of post-traumatic knee OA by the same surgical procedure, Runx2+/- mice displayed decreased cartilage destruction and osteophyte formation, along with reduced expression of collagen-10 and MMP13, as compared with wild-type mice (Kamekura et al., 2006). Human OA cartilage exhibits increased Runx2 expression when compared to control cartilage. Runx2 co-localizes with MMP13 in chondrocyte clusters of OA cartilage. Runx2 overexpression in cultured chondrocytes increases MMP 13 expression (Wang et al., 2004).

These findings suggest that Runx2 regulates chondrocyte differentiation both in the developmental and adult stages. Runx2 may stimulate the progression of OA by promoting articular chondrocyte hypertrophy (indicated by expression of Collagen-10) and expression of MMP13 in articular cartilage (**Figure 1**).

3.2.3 Nfat1

Nfat1 (NFAT1) is a member of the Nuclear Factor of Activated T-cells (NFAT) transcription factor family originally identified as a regulator of the expression of cytokine genes during the immune response (Hodge et al., 1996; Xanthoudakis et al., 1996). Recent studies have shown that Nfat1 plays an important role in maintaining the permanent cartilage phenotype in adult mice. Nfat1 knockout (*Nfat1-/-*) mice exhibited normal skeletal development, but displayed most of the features of human OA in load-bearing joints in adults (Wang et al., 2009; Rodova et al., 2011). *Nfat1-/-* articular cartilage shows overexpression of multiple specific proinflammatory cytokines (**Figure 2A-B**) and matrix-degrading proteinases (**Figure 3A**) at the initiation stage of OA (2-4 months of age). These initial changes are followed by articular chondrocyte clustering, formation of chondro-osteophytes, progressive articular surface destruction, formation of subchondral bone cysts, and exposure of thickened subchondral bone (Wang et al., 2009), all of which resemble human OA (Pritzker et al., 2006). The expression of mRNA for cartilage structural proteins (e.g., collagen-2, -9, and -11) was down-regulated but mRNA for collagen-10 was up-regulated at 2-4 months of age (**Figure 3B**). However, both collagen-2 and collagen-10 were up-regulated to varying degrees at 6 and 12 months, suggesting that early dysfunction of articular chondrocytes triggers repair activity within the degenerating cartilage (Rodova et al., 2011). These new findings revealed a previously unrecognized role of Nfat1 in maintaining the physiological function of differentiated adult articular chondrocytes by regulating the expression of specific matrix-degrading proteinases and proinflammatory cytokines.

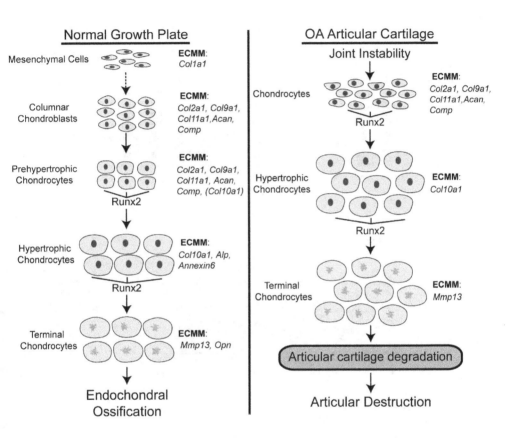

ECMM: Extracellular Matrix Markers, Acan: Aggrecan, Comp: Cartilage oligomeric matrix protein,
Alp: Alkaline phosphatase, Mmp13: Matrix metalloproteinase 13, Opn: Osteopontin

Fig. 1. A diagram shows Runx2 involvement in the chondrocyte differentiation pathways toward either physiological endochondral ossification in the growth plate or pathological chondrocyte hypertrophy in OA cartilage. Major morphological features and extracellular matrix markers for each step of chondrocyte differentiation are indicated.

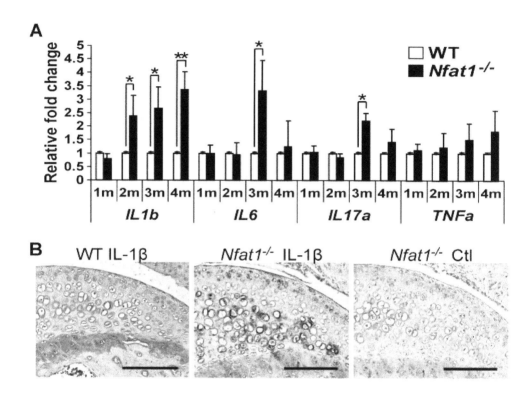

Fig. 2. Nfat1 deficiency causes dysfunction of adult articular chondrocytes with overexpression of specific proinflammatory cytokines. (**A**) Quantitative real-time PCR (qPCR) analyses indicate temporal changes in expression levels of various genes of proinflammatory cytokines in *Nfat1-/-* articular cartilage at 1-4 months (1-4m) of age. The expression level of each WT group has been normalized to "one". n = 3 pooled RNA samples, each prepared from the articular cartilage of 6-8 femoral heads. * $P < 0.05$; ** $P < 0.01$. (**B**) Immunohisto- chemical analyses using a polyclonal antibody against IL-1β (Santa Cruz) show substantially more intense expression of IL-1β (brown areas) in femoral head articular cartilage of 3-month-old *Nfat1-/-* mice compared to age-matched WT mice. *Nfat1-/-* Ctl represents a negative control using both IL-1β antibody and IL-1β blocking peptide (Santa Cruz) to validate the specificity of the immune reaction. Scale bar = 200 μm. Modified from the published figure (Wang, et al. J Pathol 2009; 219:163-72) with permission from the publisher.

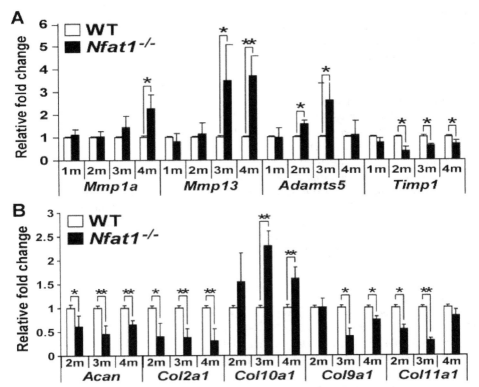

Fig. 3. Loss of Nfat1 leads to abnormal catabolic and anabolic activities of articular chondrocytes. (**A**) qPCR analyses demonstrate up-regulated expression of *Mmp1a,* *Mmp13, and Adamts5* and reduced expression of *Timp1* (tissue inhibitor of metalloproteinase-1) in femoral head articular cartilage of *Nfat1-/-* mice compared to age-matched WT mice at 1-4 months (1-4m) of age. (**B**) qPCR analyses indicate temporal changes in expression levels of various chondrocyte marker genes in *Nfat1-/-* articular cartilage at 2-4 months (2-4m) of age. The expression level of each WT group has been normalized to "one". n = 3 pooled RNA samples; * $P < 0.05$; ** $P < 0.01$. Modified from the published figure (Wang, et al. J Pathol 2009; 219:163-72) with permission from the publisher.

Thickening of subchondral bone is one of the characteristics of human OA. However, the precise biological mechanisms underlying the subchondral bone changes remain unclear. *Nfat1-/-* mouse joints display chondrocyte hypertrophy in the deep-calcified zones of articular cartilage, a feature of human OA cartilage. *Nfat1 -/-* mesenchymal cells derived from subchondral bone marrow cavities differentiate into chondrocytes which subsequently underwent hypertrophy and endochondral ossification, leading to thickening of both subchondral plate and subchondral trabecular bone (Wang et al., 2009). These findings suggest that Nfat1 may prevent chondrocyte hypertrophy in adult articular cartilage and endochondral ossification in subchondral bone, thereby maintaining the integrity of cartilage-bone structure of synovial joints.

3.2.4 c-Maf

Transcription factor c-Maf, a member of the basic leucine zipper (bZIP) superfamily, is required for normal chondrocyte differentiation during endochondral bone formation. C-Maf is expressed in hypertrophic chondrocytes during fetal development. There is an initial decrease in the number of mature hypertrophic chondrocytes in *c-Maf*-null mouse tibiae, with decreased expression domains of collagen-10 and osteopontin (Opn), markers of hypertrophic and terminal hypertrophic chondrocytes, respectively. However, terminal chondrocytes, which express Opn and MMP13, appear later and persist for a longer period of time in *c-Maf* -/- fetuses than in control littermates, resulting in expanded chondrocyte maturation zones and a delay in endochondral ossification. These results suggest that c-Maf may facilitate both the initiation of terminal differentiation and the completion of the chondrocyte differentiation program (MacLean et al., 2003).

A recent study demonstrated transcriptional activation of human MMP13 gene expression by c-Maf in osteoarthritic chondrocytes. C-Maf enhances MMP13 promoter activity and RNAi-mediated knockdown of c-Maf leads to a reduced expression of MMP13. Chromatin immunoprecipitation assays reveal that c-Maf binds to the MMP13 gene promoter, suggesting that MMP13 is a potential target of c-Maf in human articular chondrocytes (Li et al., 2010).

3.2.5 β-catenin

In the canonical Wnt signaling pathway, Wnts bind the transmembrane Frizzled receptor (FRZ) family and co-receptors LRP5/6. FRZ receptor activation recruits the cytoplasmic bridging molecule Dishevelled (Dsh) which inhibits glycogen synthase kinase-3β (GSK-3β). This interaction prevents GSK-3β from phosphorylating β-catenin to avoid degradation of β-catenin, thereby allowing β-catenin to accumulate in the cytoplasm and translocate to the nucleus as a co-transcriptional activator with lymphoid enhancing factor 1/T cell-specific transcription factor (LEF/TCF) at specific DNA binding sites to activate downstream genes (Zou et al., 2006; Deng et al., 2008). Thus, β-catenin is a key mediator of the canonical Wnt signaling. Non-canonical Wnt signaling pathway, which does not involve β-catenin (Logan & Nusse, 2004), is probably best studied in *Drosophila* and its function is not covered in this chapter.

The canonical Wnt signaling pathway is known to induce chondrocyte maturation and endochondral ossification during skeletal development. This signaling pathway stimulates the commitment of mesenchymal stem cells to the preosteoblast and mature osteoblast phenotype, and blocks chondrogenic differentiation (Zou et al., 2006). Activation of the canonical Wnt signaling cascade during development in the limb bud and growth plate chondrocytes stimulates chondrocyte hypertrophy, calcification, and expression of MMPs and vascular endothelial growth factor (VEGF) (Tamamura et al., 2005; Day et al., 2005; Kawaguchi, 2009). Wnt-14 overexpression in chick limb mesenchymal tissue cultures causes a severe inhibition of chondrogenesis. Wnt-14 is necessary for joint formation since it might maintain the mesenchymal nature of the interzone by preventing chondrogenesis. In addition to Wnt-14, the interzone expresses Wnt-4, Wnt-16, and β-catenin. Conditional ablation of β-catenin in chondrocytes leads to the absence of joints. Ectopic expression of activated β-catenin or Wnt-14 in chondrocytes leads to ectopic expression of joint markers (Tamamura et al., 2005; Hartmann & Tabin, 2001; Guo et al., 2004).

The canonical Wnt signaling is also important in susceptibility to OA. Recent studies revealed that Wnt/β-catenin is involved in chondrocyte maturation and endochondral ossification in adult chondrocytes. The inhibition of Dickkopf-1 (Dkk1), a negative regulator of the Wnt signal, has been reported to allow conversion of a mouse model of rheumatoid arthritis to OA, due to increased endochondral ossification (Diarra et al., 2007). The conditional activation of β-catenin in articular chondrocytes of adult mice caused OA-like cartilage degradation and osteophyte formation. These pathological changes were associated with accelerated chondrocyte maturation and Mmp expression (Zhu et al., 2009). Interestingly, the same group also reported that selective suppression of β-catenin signaling in articular chondrocytes also caused OA-like cartilage degradation in Col2a1-ICAT (inhibitor of β-catenin and T-cell factor) transgenic mice, and this was mediated by enhancement of apoptosis of the chondrocytes (Zhu et al., 2008). These results suggest that both excessive and insufficient β-catenin levels may impair the homeostasis of articular chondrocytes.

Transcription factors and transcriptional co-activators that may be responsible for the maintenance of the physiological function of adult articular chondrocytes and development of OA are presented in **Figure 4**.

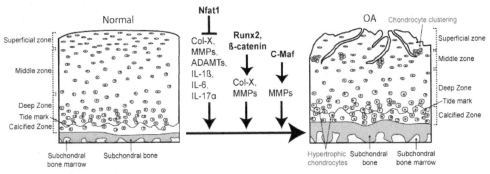

Fig. 4. A diagram demonstrates specific factors that may be responsible for the expression of catabolic molecules and collagen-X (Col-X, a marker of hypertrophic chondrocytes) during the development of OA.

3.3 Other factors that may regulate chondrocyte differentiation and function
3.3.1 BMPs

A variety of BMP members are present in articular cartilage. Among these BMPs, BMP-2 and BMP-7 (osteogenic protein-1, OP-1) are the two best studied BMPs with regard to cartilage homeostasis and OA. Both BMP-2 and BMP-7 have been shown to be capable of maintaining the chondrocyte phenotype. Inhibition of BMP-7 causes a reduction of aggrecan gene expression in chondrocytes. It has been reported that BMP-7 expression is decreased up to 9-fold in degenerated cartilage. In contrast to BMP-7, BMP-2 expression appears to increase with cartilage damage. In a study of BMPs in OA, BMP-2 is the only BMP member that demonstrates an increase in OA cartilage compared to cartilage from normal joints (Chubinskaya et al., 2007; Chubinskaya et al., 2000; Fukui et al., 2003; Sailor et al., 1996; Soder et al., 2005).

Multiple polymorphisms of the GDF-5 (BMP-14) gene have been found to produce an increased Odds Ratio of OA development, but the one that appears to have the most robust correlation is the rs143383 SNP in the 5'-UTR of GDF5. Miyamoto et al. reported a strong association between the rs143383 SNP of GDF5 and hip and knee OA in multiple Asian populations, with Odds Ratios ranging from 1.30-1.79 (Miyamoto et al., 2007). This association was confirmed in a large-scale meta-analysis; however, the magnitude of effect was less than previously reported (Evangelou et al., 2009). Interestingly, Egli *et al.* found that GDF5 expression imbalance was not limited to articular cartilage, but found in multiple joint tissues analyzed (synovium, fat pad, meniscus, ligaments) (Egli et al., 2009).

3.3.2 Insulin-like growth factor-1 (IGF-1)

IGF-1 is expressed in normal articular cartilage and is generally thought to be an important growth factor for maintenance of articular chondrocyte phenotype and articular cartilage repair (Fortier et al., 2002; Fortier et al., 2011). Chronic IGF-1 deficiency causes an increased severity of OA-like articular cartilage lesions in rat knee joints (Ekenstedt et al., 2006). Human OA cartilage responds to IGF-1 treatment by increasing proteoglycan synthesis; however, catabolism in OA cartilage is insensitive to IGF-1 treatment (Morales, 2008).

3.3.3 Indian hedgehog (Ihh)

Ihh is a member of the hedgehog proteins, and is essential for skeletal development. Ihh coordinates chondrocyte proliferation, chondrocyte differentiation, and osteoblast differentiation. Ihh is synthesized by prehypertrophic chondrocytes and by early hypertrophic chondrocytes during endochondral ossification. Ihh knockout (Ihh-/-) mice demonstrate abnormalities of chondrocyte differentiation and bone growth. Cartilage elements are small in Ihh-/- mice because of a marked decrease in chondrocyte proliferation. Ihh-/- chondrocytes leaving the pool of proliferating chondrocytes prematurely because Ihh-/- cartilage fails to synthesize parathyroid hormone-related protein (PTHrP) that acts primarily to keep proliferating chondrocytes in the proliferative pool. PTHrP, which is expressed by perichondral cells and early proliferative chondrocytes, down-regulates the expression of Ihh. This negative feedback loop mainly regulates the rate of chondrocyte differentiation and endochondral ossification. A third striking abnormality of Ihh-/- mice is the absence of osteoblasts in the primary spongiosa, suggesting that Ihh is required for osteoblast differentiation in endochondral bone formation (Kronenberg, 2003; Karp et al., 2000). Ihh is a critical and possibly direct regulator of joint development. In *Ihh-/-* mouse embryos, cartilaginous digit anlagen remained fused without interzones or mature joints (Koyama et al., 2007).

A recent study revealed that PTHrP may regulate articular chondrocyte maintenance in mice (Macica et al., 2011). In addition, parathyroid hormone (PTH) 1-34, a parathyroid hormone analog sharing the PTH receptor 1 with PTHrP, may inhibit the terminal differentiation of human articular chondrocytes *in vitro* and suppresses the progression of OA in rats (Chang et al., 2009).

3.3.4 Fibroblast growth factors (FGFs)

Recent evidence suggests that the FGF family plays an essential role in the proliferation and differentiation process of chondrocytes. The impact of many of these factors is not fully understood, but multiple FGF and FGFR (FGF receptor) genes are expressed at every stage of endochondral ossification. Within the chondrocyte pathway, FGFR3 is found in proliferating chondrocytes, FGFR1 in prehypertrophic and hypertrophic chondrocytes, and

FGFR2 is expressed among the earliest condensing mesenchyme (Ornitz & Marie, 2002). FGFs markedly enhance Sox9 expression in the early stages of development, likely through the mitogen-activated protein kinase (MAPK) pathway (Murakami et al., 2000).

The regulatory effects of FGF on adult articular chondrocytes are controversial in literature. A recent study showed that FGF-2 is an intrinsic chondroprotective agent that suppresses ADMTS5 and delays cartilage degradation in murine OA (Chia et al., 2009). However, other studies suggested that FGF-2 and FGF-23 may be involved in the progression of OA by stimulating MMP-13 expression through Runx2 (Orfanidou et al., 2009; Wang et al., 2004).

4. Future perspectives on pharmacological therapy

Over the past two decades, clinical trials applying a proinflammatory cytokine or proteinase inhibitor as a candidate disease-modifying OA drug (DMOAD) have been unsuccessful due to insufficient efficacy and/or severe side effects. A large number of candidate DMOADs have been tested but none have been approved (Hellio Le Graverand-Gastineau, 2009; Kawaguchi, 2009); suggesting that inhibition of a single catabolic molecule may not be sufficient for the treatment of OA because multiple catabolic factors are involved in its pathogenesis. Since specific transcriptional signaling molecules (e.g. Nfat1, Runx2, c-Maf, β-catenin) may regulate the expression of multiple catabolic and/or anabolic factors in articular chondrocytes, these regulatory factors may play more important roles in the development of OA than a single catabolic proteinase/cytokine. These findings have opened new avenues toward the development of DMOADs, using a more upstream factor as a molecular target than has been studied heretofore. In addition, OA not only affects articular cartilage but also involves other joint tissues such as the subchondral bone, synovium, capsule, menisci, and ligaments. Pathological changes in these joint tissues may affect the biological and mechanical properties of articular cartilage. Therefore, other joint tissues should not be ignored when designing pharmacological therapies. Furthermore, insufficient recognition of pathological changes in mechanical influence on the pathogenesis of OA may also negatively affect the efficacy of DMOAD candidates (Brandt et al., 2008). These recent research advances in the pathogenesis and treatment of OA may lead to the development of novel and effective therapeutic strategies using more up-stream pharmacological targets such as transcriptional signaling molecules, combined with biomechanical correction of abnormal joint loading if necessary, for the prevention and treatment of human OA.

5. Conclusion

OA is the most common form of joint disease and the major cause of chronic disability in middle-aged and older populations. All current pharmacological therapies are aimed at symptomatic control and have limited impacts on impeding or reversing the progression of OA, largely because the biological mechanisms of OA pathogenesis remain unclear. Previous studies have shown that overexpression of matrix-degrading proteinases and proinflammatory cytokines in articular cartilage is associated with osteoarthritic cartilage degradation. However, clinical trials applying an inhibitor of a proteinase or proinflammatory cytokine have been unsuccessful. Since multiple catabolic factors and pathological chondrocyte hypertrophy are involved in the development of OA, it is important to identify which upstream factors regulate the expression of catabolic molecules and/or chondrocyte hypertrophy in adult articular cartilage. This chapter summarizes the recent advances in the molecular regulation, with a main focus on transcriptional·regulation, of the function of adult articular chondrocytes and its implication in the pathogenesis and treatment of OA. Recent studies have revealed that biological and mechanical abnormalities may affect transcriptional activity of specific transcription factors in articular chondrocytes. Transcription factor Sox9 is critical for the formation of cartilage, including articular cartilage, but its role in maintenance of adult articular chondrocyte function remains to be elucidated. Transcription factor Nfat1 plays an important role in maintaining the physiological function of adult articular chondrocytes. Nfat1-deficient mice exhibit normal skeletal development but display most of the features of human OA in their adult stage, including chondrocyte hypertrophy with overexpression of specific matrix-degrading proteinases and proinflammatory cytokines in articular cartilage. Transcription factor Runx2 and β-catenin transcriptional signaling may also be involved in the pathogenesis of OA via regulating the expression of anabolic and catabolic molecules in articular chondrocytes. These novel findings may provide new insights into the pathogenesis and treatment of OA.

6. Acknowledgments

This work was supported in part by the United States National Institutes of Health (NIH) grants AR 052088 (to J. Wang) and AR 059088 (to J. Wang), the Mary Alice and Paul R. Harrington Distinguished Professorship Endowment (to J. Wang), and the University of Kansas Medical Center institutional funds. The authors would like to thank Jamie Crist, James Bernard, Brent Furomoto, and Clayton Theleman for their assistance in graphic design and editing.

7. References

Aigner, T., Gebhard, P. M., Schmid, E., Bau, B., Harley, V. & Poschl, E. (2003). SOX9 expression does not correlate with type II collagen expression in adult articular chondrocytes. *Matrix Biology*, 22, 363-72.

Akiyama, H., Chaboissier, M. C., Martin, J. F., Schedl, A. & de Crombrugghe, B. (2002). The transcription factor Sox9 has essential roles in successive steps of the chondrocyte differentiation pathway and is required for expression of Sox5 and Sox6. *Genes Dev.*, 16, 2813-28.

Amano, K., Hata, K., Sugita, A., Takigawa, Y., Ono, K., Wakabayashi, M., Kogo, M., Nishimura, R. & Yoneda, T. (2009). Sox9 family members negatively regulate maturation and calcification of chondrocytes through up-regulation of parathyroid hormone-related protein. *Mol Biol Cell*, 20, 4541-51.

Bi, W., Deng, J. M., Zhang, Z., Behringer, R. R. & de Crombrugghe, B. (1999). Sox9 is required for cartilage formation. *Nat. Genet.*, 22, 85-9.

Block, J. A. & Shakoor, N. (2009). The biomechanics of osteoarthritis: implications for therapy. *Curr. Rheumatol Rep*, 11, 15-22.

Borrelli, J., Jr., Silva, M. J., Zaegel, M. A., Franz, C. & Sandell, L. J. (2009). Single high-energy impact load causes posttraumatic OA in young rabbits via a decrease in cellular metabolism. *J. Orthop. Res.*, 27, 347-52.

Bos, S. D., Slagboom, P. E. & Meulenbelt, I. (2008). New insights into osteoarthritis: early developmental features of an ageing-related disease. *Curr Opin Rheumatol*, 20, 553-9.

Brandt, K. D., Dieppe, P. & Radin, E. L. (2008). Etiopathogenesis of osteoarthritis. *Rheum. Dis. Clin. North Am.*, 34, 531-59.

Brandt, K. D., Radin, E. L., Dieppe, P. A. & van de Putte, L. (2006). Yet more evidence that osteoarthritis is not a cartilage disease. *Ann Rheum Dis*, 65, 1261-4.

Brew, C. J., Clegg, P. D., Boot-Handford, R. P., Andrew, J. G. & Hardingham, T. (2010). Gene expression in human chondrocytes in late osteoarthritis is changed in both fibrillated and intact cartilage without evidence of generalised chondrocyte hypertrophy. *Ann. Rheum. Dis.*, 69, 234-40.

Brunet, L. J., McMahon, J. A., McMahon, A. P. & Harland, R. M. (1998). Noggin, cartilage morphogenesis, and joint formation in the mammalian skeleton. *Science*, 280, 1455-7.

Buckwalter, J. A., Einhorn, T. A., O'Keefe, R. J. & American Academy of Orthopaedic Surgeons. 2007. *Orthopaedic basic science : foundations of clinical practice*. Rosemont, IL: American Academy of Orthopaedic Surgeons.

Buckwalter, J. A., Saltzman, C. & Brown, T. (2004). The impact of osteoarthritis: implications for research. *Clinical Orthopaedics & Related Research*, S6-15.

Burrage, P., Mix, K. & Brinckerhoff, C. (2006). Matrix metalloproteinases: role in arthritis. *Front Biosci*, 11, 529-43.

Chang, J. K., Chang, L. H., Hung, S. H., Wu, S. C., Lee, H. Y., Lin, Y. S., Chen, C. H., Fu, Y. C., Wang, G. J. & Ho, M. L. (2009). Parathyroid hormone 1-34 inhibits terminal differentiation of human articular chondrocytes and osteoarthritis progression in rats. *Arthritis Rheum* 60, 3049-60.

Chia, S. L., Sawaji, Y., Burleigh, A., McLean, C., Inglis, J., Saklatvala, J. & Vincent, T. (2009). Fibroblast growth factor 2 is an intrinsic chondroprotective agent that suppresses ADAMTS-5 and delays cartilage degradation in murine osteoarthritis. *Arthritis Rheum*, 60, 2019-27.

Chubinskaya, S., Hurtig, M. & Rueger, D. C. (2007). OP-1/BMP-7 in cartilage repair. *Int Orthop*, 31, 773-81.

Chubinskaya, S., Merrihew, C., Cs-Szabo, G., Mollenhauer, J., McCartney, J., Rueger, D. C. & Kuettner, K. E. (2000). Human articular chondrocytes express osteogenic protein-1. *J Histochem Cytochem*, 48, 239-50.

Clouet, J., Vinatier, C., Merceron, C., Pot-vaucel, M., Maugars, Y., Weiss, P., Grimandi, G. & Guicheux, J. (2009). From osteoarthritis treatments to future regenerative therapies for cartilage. *Drug Discov Today*, 14, 913-25.

Coffman, J. A. (2003). Runx transcription factors and the developmental balance between cell proliferation and differentiation. *Cell Biol Int*, 27, 315-24.

Day, T. F., Guo, X., Garrett-Beal, L. & Yang, Y. (2005). Wnt/beta-catenin signaling in mesenchymal progenitors controls osteoblast and chondrocyte differentiation during vertebrate skeletogenesis. *Dev Cell*, 8, 739-50.

Deng, Z. L., Sharff, K. A., Tang, N., Song, W. X., Luo, J., Luo, X., Chen, J., Bennett, E., Reid, R., Manning, D., Xue, A., Montag, A. G., Luu, H. H., Haydon, R. C. & He, T. C. (2008). Regulation of osteogenic differentiation during skeletal development. *Front Biosci*, 13, 2001-21.

Diarra, D., Stolina, M., Polzer, K., Zwerina, J., Ominsky, M. S., Dwyer, D., Korb, A., Smolen, J., Hoffmann, M., Scheinecker, C., van der Heide, D., Landewe, R., Lacey, D.,

Richards, W. G. & Schett, G. (2007). Dickkopf-1 is a master regulator of joint remodeling. *Nat. Med.*, 13, 156-63.

Drewniak, E. I., Jay, G. D., Fleming, B. C. & Crisco, J. J. (2009). Comparison of two methods for calculating the frictional properties of articular cartilage using a simple pendulum and intact mouse knee joints. *J. Biomech.*, 42, 1996-9.

Ducy, P., Zhang, R., Geoffroy, V., Ridall, A. & Karsenty, G. (1997). Osf2/Cbfa1: a transcriptional activator of osteoblast differentiation. *Cell*, 89, 747-757.

Eames, B. F., Sharpe, P. T. & Helms, J. A. (2004). Hierarchy revealed in the specification of three skeletal fates by Sox9 and Runx2. *Dev. Biol.*, 274, 188-200.

Egli, R. J., Southam, L., Wilkins, J. M., Lorenzen, I., Pombo-Suarez, M., Gonzalez, A., Carr, A., Chapman, K. & Loughlin, J. (2009). Functional analysis of the osteoarthritis susceptibility-associated GDF5 regulatory polymorphism. *Arthritis Rheum*, 60, 2055-64.

Ekenstedt, K. J., Sonntag, W. E., Loeser, R. F., Lindgren, B. R. & Carlson, C. S. (2006). Effects of chronic growth hormone and insulin-like growth factor 1 deficiency on osteoarthritis severity in rat knee joints. *Arthritis Rheum*, 54, 3850-8.

Evangelou, E., Chapman, K., Meulenbelt, I., Karassa, F. B., Loughlin, J., Carr, A., Doherty, M., Doherty, S., Gomez-Reino, J. J., Gonzalez, A., Halldorsson, B. V., Hauksson, V. B., Hofman, A., Hart, D. J., Ikegawa, S., Ingvarsson, T., Jiang, Q., Jonsdottir, I., Jonsson, H., Kerkhof, H. J., Kloppenburg, M., Lane, N. E., Li, J., Lories, R. J., van Meurs, J. B., Nakki, A., Nevitt, M. C., Rodriguez-Lopez, J., Shi, D., Slagboom, P. E., Stefansson, K., Tsezou, A., Wallis, G. A., Watson, C. M., Spector, T. D., Uitterlinden, A. G., Valdes, A. M. & Ioannidis, J. P. (2009). Large-scale analysis of association between GDF5 and FRZB variants and osteoarthritis of the hip, knee, and hand. *Arthritis Rheum*, 60, 1710-21.

Fernandes, J. C., Martel-Pelletier, J. & Pelletier, J. P. (2002). The role of cytokines in osteoarthritis pathophysiology. *Biorheology*, 39, 237-46.

Fitzgerald, J. B., Jin, M., Dean, D., Wood, D. J., Zheng, M. H. & Grodzinsky, A. J. (2004). Mechanical compression of cartilage explants induces multiple time-dependent gene expression patterns and involves intracellular calcium and cyclic AMP. *J Biol Chem*, 279, 19502-11.

Fortier, L. A., Barker, J. U., Strauss, E. J., McCarrel, T. M. & Cole, B. J. (2011). The Role of Growth Factors in Cartilage Repair. *Clin Orthop Relat Res*, 2011/03/16 (Epub ahead of print].

Fortier, L. A., Mohammed, H. O., Lust, G. & Nixon, A. J. (2002). Insulin-like growth factor-I enhances cell-based repair of articular cartilage. *J. Bone Joint Surg. Br.*, 84 276-88.

Francis-West, P. H., Abdelfattah, A., Chen, P., Allen, C., Parish, J., Ladher, R., Allen, S., MacPherson, S., Luyten, F. P. & Archer, C. W. (1999). Mechanisms of GDF-5 action during skeletal development. *Development*, 126, 1305-15.

Fukui, N., Ikeda, Y., Ohnuki, T., Tanaka, N., Hikita, A., Mitomi, H., Mori, T., Juji, T., Katsuragawa, Y., Yamamoto, S., Sawabe, M., Yamane, S., Suzuki, R., Sandell, L. J. & Ochi, T. (2008). Regional differences in chondrocyte metabolism in osteoarthritis: a detailed analysis by laser capture microdissection. *Arthritis Rheum*, 58, 154-63.

Fukui, N., Zhu, Y., Maloney, W. J., Clohisy, J. & Sandell, L. J. (2003). Stimulation of BMP-2 expression by pro-inflammatory cytokines IL-1 and TNF-alpha in normal and osteoarthritic chondrocytes. *J Bone Joint Surg Am*, 85-A Suppl 3, 59-66.

Glasson, S. S., Askew, R., Sheppard, B., Carito, B., Blanchet, T., Ma, H. L., Flannery, C. R., Peluso, D., Kanki, K., Yang, Z., Majumdar, M. K. & Morris, E. A. (2005). Deletion of active ADAMTS5 prevents cartilage degradation in a murine model of osteoarthritis. *Nature,* 434, 644-8.

Goldring, M. B. (2001). Anticytokine therapy for osteoarthritis. *Expert Opinion on Biological Therapy,* 1, 817-29.

Goldring, M. B. & Goldring, S. R. (2007). Osteoarthritis. *J Cell Physiol,* 213, 626-34.

Goldring, M. B. & Marcu, K. B. (2009). Cartilage homeostasis in health and rheumatic diseases. *Arthritis Res Ther,* 11, 224.

Goldring, M. B., Otero, M., Tsuchimochi, K., Ijiri, K. & Li, Y. (2008). Defining the roles of inflammatory and anabolic cytokines in cartilage metabolism. *Ann Rheum Dis,* 67 Suppl 3, iii75-82.

Goldring, M. B., Tsuchimochi, K. & Ijiri, K. (2006). The control of chondrogenesis. *J Cell Biochem,* 97, 33-44.

Guo, X., Day, T. F., Jiang, X., Garrett-Beal, L., Topol, L. & Yang, Y. (2004). Wnt/beta-catenin signaling is sufficient and necessary for synovial joint formation. *Genes Dev,* 18, 2404-17.

Hall, B. K. & Miyake, T. (2000). All for one and one for all: condensations and the initiation of skeletal development. *Bioessays,* 22, 138-47.

Hartmann, C. & Tabin, C. J. (2001). Wnt-14 plays a pivotal role in inducing synovial joint formation in the developing appendicular skeleton. *Cell,* 104, 341-51.

Haudenschild, D. R., Nguyen, B., Chen, J., D'Lima, D. D. & Lotz, M. K. (2008). Rho kinase-dependent CCL20 induced by dynamic compression of human chondrocytes. *Arthritis Rheum.,* 58, 2735-42.

Hellio Le Graverand-Gastineau, M. P. (2009). OA clinical trials: current targets and trials for OA. Choosing molecular targets: what have we learned and where we are headed? *Osteoarthritis Cartilage,* 17, 1393-401.

Hermansson, M., Sawaji, Y., Bolton, M., Alexander, S., Wallace, A., Begum, S., Wait, R. & Saklatvala, J. (2004). Proteomic analysis of articular cartilage shows increased type II collagen synthesis in osteoarthritis and expression of inhibin betaA (activin A), a regulatory molecule for chondrocytes. *J Biol Chem,* 279, 43514-21.

Hess, J., Porte, D., Munz, C. & Angel, P. (2001). AP-1 and Cbfa/runt physically interact and regulate parathyroid hormone-dependent MMP13 expression in osteoblasts through a new osteoblast-specific element 2/AP-1 composite element. *J. Biol. Chem.,* 276, 20029-38.

Hodge, M., Ranger, A., Charles de la Brousse, F., Hoey, T., Grusby, M. & Glimcher, L. (1996). Hyperproliferation and dysregulation of IL-4 expression in NF-ATp-deficient mice. *Immunity,* 4, 397-405.

Hogan, B. L. (1996). Bone morphogenetic proteins: multifunctional regulators of vertebrate development. *Genes Dev.,* 10, 1580-94.

Ijiri, K., Zerbini, L. F., Peng, H., Correa, R. G., Lu, B., Walsh, N., Zhao, Y., Taniguchi, N., Huang, X. L., Otu, H., Wang, H., Wang, J. F., Komiya, S., Ducy, P., Rahman, M. U., Flavell, R. A., Gravallese, E. M., Oettgen, P., Libermann, T. A. & Goldring, M. B. (2005). A novel role for GADD45beta as a mediator of MMP-13 gene expression during chondrocyte terminal differentiation. *J Biol Chem,* 280, 38544-55.

Ijiri, K., Zerbini, L. F., Peng, H., Otu, H. H., Tsuchimochi, K., Otero, M., Dragomir, C., Walsh, N., Bierbaum, B. E., Mattingly, D., van Flandern, G., Komiya, S., Aigner, T., Libermann, T. A. & Goldring, M. B. (2008). Differential expression of GADD45beta in normal and osteoarthritic cartilage: potential role in homeostasis of articular chondrocytes. *Arthritis Rheum,* 58, 2075-87.

Ikeda, T., Kamekura, S., Mabuchi, A., Kou, I., Seki, S., Takato, T., Nakamura, K., Kawaguchi, H., Ikegawa, S. & Chung, U. I. (2004). The combination of SOX5, SOX6, and SOX9 (the SOX trio) provides signals sufficient for induction of permanent cartilage. *Arthritis Rheum*, 50, 3561-73.

Inada, M., Yasui, T., Nomura, S., Miyake, S., Deguchi, K., Himeno, M., Sato, M., Yamagiwa, H., Kimura, T., Yasui, N., Ochi, T., Endo, N., Kitamura, Y., Kishimoto, T. & Komori, T. (1999). Maturational disturbance of chondrocytes in Cbfa1-deficient mice. *Dev Dyn*, 214, 279-90.

Iwamoto, M., Higuchi, Y., Koyama, E., Enomoto-Iwamoto, M., Kurisu, K., Yeh, H., Abrams, W. R., Rosenbloom, J. & Pacifici, M. (2000). Transcription factor ERG variants and functional diversification of chondrocytes during limb long bone development. *J. Cell Biol.*, 150, 27-40.

Iwamoto, M., Tamamura, Y., Koyama, E., Komori, T., Takeshita, N., Williams, J. A., Nakamura, T., Enomoto-Iwamoto, M. & Pacifici, M. (2007). Transcription factor ERG and joint and articular cartilage formation during mouse limb and spine skeletogenesis. *Dev. Biol.*, 305, 40-51.

June, R. K. & Fyhrie, D. P. (2008). Molecular NMR T2 values can predict cartilage stress-relaxation parameters. *Biochem. Biophys. Res. Commun.*, 377, 57-61.

Kamekura, S., Kawasaki, Y., Hoshi, K., Shimoaka, T., Chikuda, H., Maruyama, Z., Komori, T., Sato, S., Takeda, S., Karsenty, G., Nakamura, K., Chung, U. I. & Kawaguchi, H. (2006). Contribution of runt-related transcription factor 2 to the pathogenesis of osteoarthritis in mice after induction of knee joint instability. *Arthritis Rheum.*, 54, 2462-70.

Karp, S. J., Schipani, E., St-Jacques, B., Hunzelman, J., Kronenberg, H. & McMahon, A. P. (2000). Indian hedgehog coordinates endochondral bone growth and morphogenesis via parathyroid hormone related-protein-dependent and - independent pathways. *Development,* 127, 543-8.

Karsenty, G. (2005). An aggrecanase and osteoarthritis. *New England Journal of Medicine,* 353, 522-3.

Kawaguchi, H. (2009). Regulation of osteoarthritis development by Wnt-beta-catenin signaling through the endochondral ossification process. *J. Bone Miner. Res.*, 24, 8-11.

Kim, H. A. & Blanco, F. J. (2007). Cell death and apoptosis in osteoarthritic cartilage. *Curr Drug Targets*, 8, 333-45.

Kolettas, E., Muir, H. I., Barrett, J. C. & Hardingham, T. E. (2001). Chondrocyte phenotype and cell survival are regulated by culture conditions and by specific cytokines through the expression of Sox-9 transcription factor. *Rheumatology (Oxford)*, 40, 1146-56.

Komori, H., Ichikawa, S., Hirabayashi, Y. & Ito, M. (1999). Regulation of intracellular ceramide content in B16 melanoma cells. Biological implications of ceramide glycosylation. *J Biol Chem*, 274, 8981-7.

Komori, T., Yagi, H., Nomura, S., Yamaguchi, A., Sasaki, K., Deguchi, K., Shimizu, Y., Bronson, R., Gao, Y., Inada, M., Sato, M., Okamoto, R., Kitamura, Y., Yoshiki, S. & Kishimoto, T. (1997). Targeted disruption of Cbfa1 results in a complete lack of bone formation owing to maturational arrest of osteoblasts. *Cell*, 89, 755-64.

Koyama, E., Ochiai, T., Rountree, R. B., Kingsley, D. M., Enomoto-Iwamoto, M., Iwamoto, M. & Pacifici, M. (2007). Synovial joint formation during mouse limb skeletogenesis: roles of Indian hedgehog signaling. *Ann. N Y Acad. Sci.*, 1116, 100-12.

Koyama, E., Shibukawa, Y., Nagayama, M., Sugito, H., Young, B., Yuasa, T., Okabe, T., Ochiai, T., Kamiya, N., Rountree, R. B., Kingsley, D. M., Iwamoto, M., Enomoto-Iwamoto, M. & Pacifici, M. (2008). A distinct cohort of progenitor cells participates in synovial joint and articular cartilage formation during mouse limb skeletogenesis. *Dev. Biol.*, 316, 62-73.

Kronenberg, H. M. (2003). Developmental regulation of the growth plate. *Nature*, 423, 332-6.

Kurz, B., Lemke, A. K., Fay, J., Pufe, T., Grodzinsky, A. J. & Schunke, M. (2005). Pathomechanisms of cartilage destruction by mechanical injury. *Ann Anat*, 187, 473-85.

Kypriotou, M., Fossard-Demoor, M., Chadjichristos, C., Ghayor, C., de Crombrugghe, B., Pujol, J. P. & Galera, P. (2003). SOX9 exerts a bifunctional effect on type II collagen gene (COL2A1) expression in chondrocytes depending on the differentiation state. *DNA Cell. Biol.*, 22, 119-29.

Lane, L. B., Villacin, A. & Bullough, P. G. (1977). The vascularity and remodelling of subchondrial bone and calcified cartilage in adult human femoral and humeral heads. An age- and stress-related phenomenon. *J Bone Joint Surg Br*, 59, 272-8.

Lefebvre, V., Li, P. & de Crombrugghe, B. (1998). A new long form of Sox5 (L-Sox5), Sox6 and Sox9 are coexpressed in chondrogenesis and cooperatively activate the type II collagen gene. *EMBO J*, 17, 5718-33.

Leung, K. K., Ng, L. J., Ho, K. K., Tam, P. P. & Cheah, K. S. (1998). Different cis-regulatory DNA elements mediate developmental stage- and tissue-specific expression of the human COL2A1 gene in transgenic mice. *J Cell Biol*, 141, 1291-300.

Li, T., Xiao, J., Wu, Z., Qiu, G. & Ding, Y. (2010). Transcriptional activation of human MMP-13 gene expression by c-Maf in osteoarthritic chondrocyte. *Connect Tissue Res*, 51, 48-54.

Loeser, R. F. & Shakoor, N. (2003). Aging or osteoarthritis: which is the problem? *Rheum Dis Clin North Am*, 29, 653-73.

Logan, C. Y. & Nusse, R. (2004). The Wnt signaling pathway in development and disease. *Annu. Rev. Cell Dev. Biol.*, 20, 781-810.

Lotz, M. (1999). The role of nitric oxide in articular cartilage damage. *Rheum. Dis. Clin. North Am.*, 25, 269-82.

Lotz, M. K. & Kraus, V. B. (2010). New developments in osteoarthritis. Posttraumatic osteoarthritis: pathogenesis and pharmacological treatment options. *Arthritis Res Ther*, 12, 211.

Macias, D., Ganan, Y., Sampath, T. K., Piedra, M. E., Ros, M. A. & Hurle, J. M. (1997). Role of BMP-2 and OP-1 (BMP-7) in programmed cell death and skeletogenesis during chick limb development. *Development*, 124, 1109-17.

Macica, C., Liang, G., Nasiri, A. & Broadus, A. E. (2011). Genetic evidence that parathyroid hormone-related protein regulates articular chondrocyte maintenance. *Arthritis Rheum*, 2011 Jun 23. doi: 10.1002/art.30515. [Epub ahead of print].

MacLean, H. E., Kim, J. I., Glimcher, M. J., Wang, J., Kronenberg, H. M. & Glimcher, L. H. (2003). Absence of transcription factor c-maf causes abnormal terminal differentiation of hypertrophic chondrocytes during endochondral bone development. *Dev. Biol.*, 262, 51-63.

Masuya, H., Nishida, K., Furuichi, T., Toki, H., Nishimura, G., Kawabata, H., Yokoyama, H., Yoshida, A., Tominaga, S., Nagano, J., Shimizu, A., Wakana, S., Gondo, Y., Noda,

T., Shiroishi, T. & Ikegawa, S. (2007). A novel dominant-negative mutation in Gdf5 generated by ENU mutagenesis impairs joint formation and causes osteoarthritis in mice. *Hum Mol Genet*, 16, 2366-75.

Mitrovic, D. (1978). Development of the diarthrodial joints in the rat embryo. *Am. J. Anat.*, 151, 475-85.

Miyamoto, Y., Mabuchi, A., Shi, D., Kubo, T., Takatori, Y., Saito, S., Fujioka, M., Sudo, A., Uchida, A., Yamamoto, S., Ozaki, K., Takigawa, M., Tanaka, T., Nakamura, Y., Jiang, Q. & Ikegawa, S. (2007). A functional polymorphism in the 5' UTR of GDF5 is associated with susceptibility to osteoarthritis. *Nat Genet*, 39, 529-33.

Mobasheri, A., Richardson, S., Mobasheri, R., Shakibaei, M. & Hoyland, J. A. (2005). Hypoxia inducible factor-1 and facilitative glucose transporters GLUT1 and GLUT3: putative molecular components of the oxygen and glucose sensing apparatus in articular chondrocytes. *Histol Histopathol*, 20, 1327-38.

Morales, T. I. (2008). The quantitative and functional relation between insulin-like growth factor-I (IGF) and IGF-binding proteins during human osteoarthritis. *J Orthop Res*, 26, 465-74.

Murakami, S., Kan, M., McKeehan, W. L. & de Crombrugghe, B. (2000). Up-regulation of the chondrogenic Sox9 gene by fibroblast growth factors is mediated by the mitogen-activated protein kinase pathway. *Proc Natl Acad Sci U S A*, 97, 1113-8.

Orfanidou, T., Iliopoulos, D., Malizos, K. N. & Tsezou, A. (2009). Involvement of SOX-9 and FGF-23 in RUNX-2 regulation in osteoarthritic chondrocytes. *J Cell Mol Med*, 13, 3186-94.

Ornitz, D. M. & Marie, P. J. (2002). FGF signaling pathways in endochondral and intramembranous bone development and human genetic disease. *Genes Dev*, 16, 1446-65.

Otto, F., Thornell, A. P., Crompton, T., Denzel, A., Gilmour, K. C., Rosewell, I. R., Stamp, G. W., Beddington, R. S., Mundlos, S., Olsen, B. R., Selby, P. B. & Owen, M. J. (1997). Cbfa1, a candidate gene for cleidocranial dysplasia syndrome, is essential for osteoblast differentiation and bone development. *Cell* 89, 765-71.

Pacifici, M., Koyama, E. & Iwamoto, M. (2005). Mechanisms of synovial joint and articular cartilage formation: recent advances, but many lingering mysteries. *Birth Defects Research Part C, Embryo Today: Reviews*, 75, 237-48.

Pelletier, J. P., Jovanovic, D. V., Lascau-Coman, V., Fernandes, J. C., Manning, P. T., Connor, J. R., Currie, M. G. & Martel-Pelletier, J. (2000). Selective inhibition of inducible nitric oxide synthase reduces progression of experimental osteoarthritis in vivo: possible link with the reduction in chondrocyte apoptosis and caspase 3 level. *Arthritis & Rheumatism*, 43, 1290-9.

Pfander, D., Swoboda, B. & Kirsch, T. (2001). Expression of early and late differentiation markers (proliferating cell nuclear antigen, syndecan-3, annexin VI, and alkaline phosphatase) by human osteoarthritic chondrocytes. *Am. J. Pathol.*, 159, 1777-83.

Piscoya, J., Fermor, B., Kraus, V., Stabler, T. & Guilak, F. (2005). The influence of mechanical compression on the induction of osteoarthritis-related biomarkers in articular cartilage explants. *Osteoarthritis Cartilage*, 13, 1092-1099.

Pritzker, K. P., Gay, S., Jimenez, S. A., Ostergaard, K., Pelletier, J. P., Revell, P. A., Salter, D. & van den Berg, W. B. (2006). Osteoarthritis cartilage histopathology: grading and staging. *Osteoarthritis Cartilage*, 14, 13-29.

Pullig, O., Weseloh, G., Gauer, S. & Swoboda, B. (2000a). Osteopontin is expressed by adult human osteoarthritic chondrocytes: protein and mRNA analysis of normal and osteoarthritic cartilage. *Matrix Biol.,* 19, 245-55.

Pullig, O., Weseloh, G., Ronneberger, D., Kakonen, S. & Swoboda, B. (2000b). Chondrocyte differentiation in human osteoarthritis: expression of osteocalcin in normal and osteoarthritic cartilage and bone. *Calcif. Tissue Int.,* 67, 230-40.

Rodova, M., Lu, Q., Li, Y., Woodbury, B. G., Crist, J. D., Gardner, B. M., Yost, J. G., Zhong, X. B., Anderson, H. C. & Wang, J. (2011). Nfat1 regulates adult articular chondrocyte function through its age-dependent expression mediated by epigenetic histone methylation. *J Bone Miner Res,* 26, 1974-1986.

Ross, M. H. & Pawlina, W. 2006. Cartilage. In *Histology, 5th Edition,* eds. M. H. Ross & W. Pawlina, pp 182-201. Philadelphia: Lippincott Williams & Wilkins.

Rothschild, B. M. & Panza, R. K. (2007). Lack of bone stiffness/strength contribution to osteoarthritis--evidence for primary role of cartilage damage. *Rheumatology (Oxford),* 46, 246-9.

Sailor, L. Z., Hewick, R. M. & Morris, E. A. (1996). Recombinant human bone morphogenetic protein-2 maintains the articular chondrocyte phenotype in long-term culture. *J Orthop Res,* 14, 937-45.

Saito, T., Ikeda, T., Nakamura, K., Chung, U. I. & Kawaguchi, H. (2007). S100A1 and S100B, transcriptional targets of SOX trio, inhibit terminal differentiation of chondrocytes. *EMBO Rep,* 8, 504-9.

Sampath, T. K., Coughlin, J. E., Wheststone, R. M., Banach, D., Corbett, C., Ridge, R. J., Ozkaynak, E., Oppermann, H. & Rueger, D. C. (1990). Bovine osteogenic protein is composed of dimers of OP-1 and BMP-2A, two members of the transforming growth factor b superfamily. *J. Biol. Chem.,* 265, 13198-13205.

Sandell, L. J. & Aigner, T. (2001). Articular cartilage and changes in arthritis. An introduction: cell biology of osteoarthritis. *Arthritis Res,* 3, 107-13.

Segal, N. A., Anderson, D. D., Iyer, K. S., Baker, J., Torner, J. C., Lynch, J. A., Felson, D. T., Lewis, C. E. & Brown, T. D. (2009). Baseline articular contact stress levels predict incident symptomatic knee osteoarthritis development in the MOST cohort. *J. Orthop. Res.,* 27, 1562-8.

Smits, P., Li, P., Mandel, J., Zhang, Z., Deng, J. M., Behringer, R. R., de Crombrugghe, B. & Lefebvre, V. (2001). The transcription factors L-Sox5 and Sox6 are essential for cartilage formation. *Dev. Cell* 1, 277-90.

Soder, S., Hakimiyan, A., Rueger, D. C., Kuettner, K. E., Aigner, T. & Chubinskaya, S. (2005). Antisense inhibition of osteogenic protein 1 disturbs human articular cartilage integrity. *Arthritis Rheum,* 52, 468-78.

Stanton, H., Rogerson, F. M., East, C. J., Golub, S. B., Lawlor, K. E., Meeker, C. T., Little, C. B., Last, K., Farmer, P. J., Campbell, I. K., Fourie, A. M. & Fosang, A. J. (2005). ADAMTS5 is the major aggrecanase in mouse cartilage in vivo and in vitro. *Nature,* 434, 648-52.

Storm, E. E. & Kingsley, D. M. (1999). GDF5 coordinates bone and joint formation during digit development. *Dev Biol,* 209, 11-27.

Takeda, S., Bonnamy, J., Owen, M. J., Ducy, M. & Karsenty, G. (2001). Continuous expression of Cbfa1 in nonhypertrophic chondrocytes uncovers its ability to induce hypertrophic chondrocyte differentiation and partially rescues Cbfa1-deficient mice. *Genes Dev.,* 15, 467-81.

Tamamura, Y., Otani, T., Kanatani, N., Koyama, E., Kitagaki, J., Komori, T., Yamada, Y., Costantini, F., Wakisaka, S., Pacifici, M., Iwamoto, M. & Enomoto-Iwamoto, M. (2005). Developmental regulation of Wnt/beta-catenin signals is required for growth plate assembly, cartilage integrity, and endochondral ossification. *J Biol Chem*, 280, 19185-95.

Tsumaki, N., Nakase, T., Miyaji, T., Kakiuchi, M., Kimura, T., Ochi, T. & Yoshikawa, H. (2002). Bone morphogenetic protein signals are required for cartilage formation and differently regulate joint development during skeletogenesis. *J. Bone Miner. Res.*, 17, 898-906.

van der Meulen, M. C. & Huiskes, R. (2002). Why mechanobiology? A survey article. *J. Biomech.*, 35, 401-14.

Verzijl, N., DeGroot, J., Ben, Z. C., Brau-Benjamin, O., Maroudas, A., Bank, R. A., Mizrahi, J., Schalkwijk, C. G., Thorpe, S. R., Baynes, J. W., Bijlsma, J. W., Lafeber, F. P. & TeKoppele, J. M. (2002). Crosslinking by advanced glycation end products increases the stiffness of the collagen network in human articular cartilage: a possible mechanism through which age is a risk factor for osteoarthritis. *Arthritis Rheum*, 46, 114-23.

von der Mark, K., Kirsch, T., Nerlich, A., Kuss, A., Weseloh, G., Gluckert, K. & Stoss, H. (1992). Type X collagen synthesis in human osteoarthritic cartilage. Indication of chondrocyte hypertrophy. *Arthritis Rheum.*, 35, 806-11.

Wang, J., Gardner, B. M., Lu, Q., Rodova, M., Woodbury, B. G., Yost, J. G., Roby, K. F., Pinson, D. M., Tawfik, O. & Anderson, H. C. (2009). Transcription factor NFAT1 deficiency causes osteoarthritis through dysfunction of adult articular chondrocytes. *J. Pathol.*, 219, 163-72.

Wang, X., Manner, P. A., Horner, A., Shum, L., Tuan, R. S. & Nuckolls, G. H. (2004). Regulation of MMP-13 expression by RUNX2 and FGF2 in osteoarthritic cartilage. *Osteoarthritis Cartilage*, 12, 963-73.

Wilkins, R. J., Browning, J. A. & Ellory, J. C. (2000). Surviving in a matrix: membrane transport in articular chondrocytes. *J Membr Biol*, 177, 95-108.

Wozney, J. M., Rosen, V., Celeste, A. J., Mitsock, L. M., Whitters, M. J., Kritz, R. W., Hewick, R. M. & Wang, E. A. (1988). Novel regulators of bone formation: molecular clones and activities. *Science*, 242, 528-1534.

Xanthoudakis, S., Viola, J., Shaw, K., Luo, C., Wallace, J., Bozza, P., Luk, D., Curran, T. & Rao, A. (1996). An enhanced immune response in mice lacking the transcription factor NFAT1. *Science*, 272, 892-895.

Zehentner, B. K., Dony, C. & Burtscher, H. (1999). The transcription factor Sox9 is involved in BMP-2 signaling. *J Bone Miner Res*, 14, 1734-41.

Zhu, M., Chen, M., Zuscik, M., Wu, Q., Wang, Y. J., Rosier, R. N., O'Keefe, R. J. & Chen, D. (2008). Inhibition of beta-catenin signaling in articular chondrocytes results in articular cartilage destruction *Arthritis Rheum.*, 58, 2053-64.

Zhu, M., Tang, D., Wu, Q., Hao, S., Chen, M., Xie, C., Rosier, R. N., O'Keefe, R. J., Zuscik, M. & Chen, D. (2009). Activation of beta-catenin signaling in articular chondrocytes leads to osteoarthritis-like phenotype in adult beta-catenin conditional activation mice. *J. Bone Miner. Res.*, 24, 12-21.

Zou, H., Wieser, R., Massague, J. & Niswander, L. (1997). Distinct roles of type I bone morphogenetic protein receptors in the formation and differentiation of cartilage. *Genes Dev.*, 11, 2191-203.

Zou, L., Zou, X., Li, H., Mygind, T., Zeng, Y., Lu, N. & Bunger, C. (2006). Molecular mechanism of osteochondroprogenitor fate determination during bone formation. *Adv Exp Med Biol*, 585, 431-41.

8

The Cholinergic System Can Be of Unexpected Importance in Osteoarthritis

Sture Forsgren

Department of Integrative Medical Biology, Anatomy Section, Umeå University, Umeå, Sweden

1. Introduction

The main belief is that joints such as the knee and ankle joints are not innervated by nerves with a cholinergic function. That includes the assumption that these joints are not innervated by the vagus nerve (van Maanen et al., 2009a, see also Grimsholm et al., 2008). Accordingly, there is actually no morphologic proof of a cholinergic innervation of the knee joint, nor of the ankle joint. Despite this fact, it is shown that electrical and pharmacological stimulation of the vagus nerve has a diminishing effect on carragenan-induced paw inflammation in rats (Borovikova et al., 2000a) and that interference with the effects of the vagus nerve leads to effects on the knee joint arthritis as seen experimentally (van Maanen et al., 2009b). There are also other findings which show the potential effects that interference with vagal effects has on joint inflammation. These will be discussed below.

It is actually strange that interference with cholinergic effects, as via manipulations of the vagus nerve, has effects in knee joint inflamed synovium without presence of a vagal nerve innervation. One possibility is that the effects are indirect, via an occurrence of vagal effects on other sites such as the spleen (Huston et al., 2006, see also van Maanen et al., 2009a). However, another possibility is that there is a non-neuronal production of acetylcholine (ACh) within the synovial tissue itself. This has actually been shown to be the case (Grimsholm et al., 2008) (see further in paragraph 3).

2. Non-neuronal ACh production – General aspects

It is nowadays known that there is a production of ACh in non-neuronal cells. The information has especially emerged via studies on expressions of the ACh-producing enzyme choline acetyltransferase (ChAT), but new knowledge on this topic has also become evident via studies of expressions of vesicular acetylcholine transporter (VAChT), carnitine acetyltransferase (CarAT), and the high-affinity choline transporter (CHT1). It is likely that the ACh produced in non-neuronal cells is released directly after synthesis, in contrast to the nerve-related ACh which is released via exocytosis.

Cell types for which ACh production has been shown are cells in the airways (Wessler et al., 2003, 2007), the keratinocytes of the skin (Grando et al., 1993, 2006), cells of the intestinal epithelium (Klapproth et al., 1997; Ratcliffe et al., 1998; Jönsson et al., 2007), cells of the urinary bladder wall (Lips et al., 2007; Yoshida et al., 2008), cells in blood vessel walls (Kirkpatrick et al., 2003; Lips et al., 2003) and certain cancer cells (Song et al., 2003, 2008;

Paleari et al., 2008). A further celltype for which there is evidence of ACh production is the tenocyte of human patellar (Danielson et al., 2006, 2007) and Achilles (Bjur et al., 2008) tenocytes. It was hereby found that the evidence was much stronger for chronic painful (tendinosis) tendons than normal pain-free tendons (Danielson et al., 2006, 2007; Bjur et al., 2008). Existence of a non-neuronal cholinergic system has also recently been shown for osteoblast-like cells (En-Nosse et al., 2009) and hepatocytes (Delbro et al., 2011).

Of special interest with respect to what will be discussed below, is the fact that inflammatory cells (Kawashima & Fuji, 2004) and fibroblasts (Fisher et al., 1993; Lips et al., 2003) show production of ACh. It should here be remembered that the tenocytes of human tendons in principle have fibroblast-like appearances.

3. Non-neuronal ACh production in synovium

It has previously been unclear as to whether there is a non-neuronal cholinergic system in synovial tissues. However, studies performed during recent years have provided evidence of ACh production in the synovial tissue of the human knee joint (Grimsholm et al., 2008). That was shown both via immunohistochemistry and in situ hybridization and was related to findings of ChAT expression in mononuclear-like as well as fibroblast-like cells (Grimsholm et al., 2008). The findings were shown both for synovial tissue of patients with rheumatoid arthritis (RA) as well as patients with osteoarthritis (OA). The occurrence of ChAT expression in mononuclear-like cells in OA synovium is shown below (Fig 1).

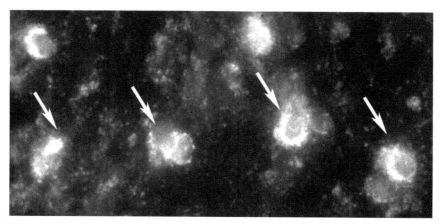

Fig. 1. Figure showing the expression of ChAT in mononuclear-like cells in the OA synovial tissue. Some of the immunoreactive cells are indicated with arrows.

4. Functions of non-neuronally produced ACh

The effects of the non-neuronal cholinergic system include functions on growth/differentiation and secretion and barrier functions (c.f. Wessler & Kirkpatrick, 2001, 2008). ACh has e.g. well-known effects on angiogenesis (Jacobi et al., 2002; Cooke et al., 2007). It is also known that an increased cell proliferation occurs in response to cholinergic stimulation (Mayerhofer & Fritz, 2002; Metzen et al., 2003; Oben et al., 2003). That includes proliferative effects on human fibroblasts (Matthiesen et al., 2006). Interestingly, it is also frequently emphasized that ACh not only is produced in immune cells but that it also has effects on these cells, ACh hereby modulating the activity of the immune cells via auto- and paracrine loops (Kawashima & Fuji, 2003, 2008). The findings that ACh hereby has anti-inflammatory effects, findings wich will be considered below, are especially interesting, but it is also possible that acute ACh stimulation can lead to proinflammatory effects (cf. Kawashima & Fuji, 2003).

5. Cholinergic anti-inflammatory pathway

A newly recognized concept is the "cholinergic anti-inflammatory pathway" (Borovikova et al., 2000b; Pavlov & Tracey, 2005; Tracey 2007). It is related to the occurrence of immunomodulatory effects of ACh released from cholinergic nerves. For example, as is commented on above, there occurs a suppression of the inflammation in the carrageenan paw edema in the rat in response to activation of this anti-inflammatory pathway via pharmalogic or electrical stimulation of the vagus nerve (Borovikova et al., 2000a). There is furthermore an attenuation in macrophage activation in response to electrical stimulation of the vagus nerve (de Jonge et al., 2005) and stimulation of the vagus nerve does on the whole improve survival in animal models of inflammation (e.g. Bernik et al., 2002). Neural inputs to immune cells can control cytokine production (Tracey, 2007). Concerning joints, there is evidence of a role of the cholinergic anti-inflammatory pathway in the murine CIA model of RA (van Maanen et al., 2010). Studies on the synovium in RA do nevertheless suggest that the cholinergic anti-inflammatory pathway might be suppressed in this condition (Goldstein et al., 2007).

It can be asked as to whether ACh originating from non-neuronal cells can be involved in the anti-inflammatory pathway. This can actually be the case. It is thus possible that neuronally released ACh triggers the release of ACh from these non-neuronal cells (Wessler & Kirkpatrick., 2008) and that effects via the non-neuronal cholinergic system even can occur independently of actions via cholinergic nerves (Kawashima & Fuji, 2003). Further evidence is the finding that ACh-induced modulation of immune functions in peripheral leukocytes occurs independently of neuronal innervation (Neumann et al., 2007). The non-neuronal ACh production in synovial tissue might therefore be of importance in the regulation of the processe that occur in this tissue in various forms of arthritis, including OA.

6. Involvement of the α7nAChR in anti-inflammatory effects

The nicotinic acetylcholine receptor AChRα7 (α7nAChR) is considered to be important in the cholinergic anti-inflammatory pathway (Wang et al., 2003; Kawashima & Fuji, 2008). The α7nAChR is thus shown to contribute to anti-inflammatory effects of ACh in several models (Tracey, 2002; Ulloa, 2005; de Jonge & Ulloa, 2007). α7nAChR agonists are furthermore shown to suppress the production of TNF alpha, IL-1, IL-6 and IL-8 and various other cytokines in macrophages after challenge with lipopolysaccharide (Borovikova et al., 2000a; Wang et al., 2003). An α7nAChR agonist is also shown to decrease the production of IL-6 by IL-1 stimulated fibroblast-like synoviocytes (Waldburger et al., 2008). The results of still other studies show that specific α7nAChR agonists can reduce TNFalpha-induced IL-6 as well as IL-8 production by fibroblast-like synoviocytes (van Maanen et al., 2009c).

7. Current study: Expression of α7nAChR in osteoarthritis

7.1 Introduction

Except for effects in the autonomic nervous system, ACh is reported to have proliferative and growth-promoting effects, effects in cancer progression and anti-inflammatory effects. As ACh has anti-inflammatory effects and effects in relation to growth/proliferation, it is of interest to consider its importance in arthritic processes. The findings that mononuclear- as well as fibroblast-like cells in the synovium of the knee joints of patients with RA as well as OA show ChAT, favouring ACh production, is therefore of interest (Grimsholm et al., 2008). The receptor through which the inflammatory-mediating effects of ACh is reported to be mainly mediated is the α7nAChR (Kawashima & Fuji., 2008). It is therefore of interest to note that expression of α7nAChR has been shown for the synovial tissue of patients with RA and psoriatic arthritis (van Maanen et al., 2009a; Westman et al., 2009) . The receptor was also to some extent noted for the synovium of healthy individuals (Westman et al., 2009). In studies on synovial tissue from 3 patients with OA, as well 3 patients with RA, it was shown that the α7nAChR was expressed in the synovial intimal lining (Waldburger et al., 2008). The details of receptor expression at the tissue level concerning OA has not been further studied. More information is therefore welcome concerning the situation in OA.

Therefore, the expression pattern of the α7nAChR in the knee synovial joint of patients with OA was examined in the present study.

7.2 Materials & methods

7.2.1 Patient material

Synovial biopsies were collected from the knee joint of six patients with OA. Four of these were females (range 58-81 years; mean age 68 years) and two were males (50 and 62 years of age). The biopsies were obtained during prosthesis operations. They thus corresponded to samples of cases with advanced and long-lasting OA. The OA patients fullfilled the criteria of Altman and co-writers (Altman et al., 1986). All study protocols were approved by the Regional Ethical Review Board in Umeå (EPN) (project nr. 05-016M). The experiments were conducted according to the principles expressed in the Declaration of Helsinki. Informed consent was obtained from all individuals.

7.2.2 Fixation and sectioning

Directly after the surgical procedures, the tissue samples were transported to the laboratory. They were fixed in 4% formaldehyde in 0.1 M phosphate buffer (pH 7.0) at 4°C for 24 h and were then washed in Tyrode's solution (pH 7.2) containing 10% (w/v) sucrose for 24 h, mounted on thin cardboard with OCT embedding medium (Miles Laboratories, Naperville, IL, USA) and frozen in propane chilled by liquid N_2. A series of 7 μm thick sections were cut on a cryostat and mounted on slides coated with chrome-alum gelatine for immunohistochemistry. Some of the sections were stained with haematoxylin-eosin (htx-eosin) for delineating tissue morphology.

7.2.3 Immunofluorescence staining

The sections were mounted in Vectashield hard set microscopy mounting medium (Dakopatts, Denmark). The immunohistochemical procedures were in principle as previously described (Bjur et al., 2008). In order to enhance specific immunoreactions, treatment with KMnO$_4$ was applied in accordance with developed procedures in the laboratory (Hansson & Forsgren., 1995).

The sections were incubated for 20 min in a 1% solution of Triton X-100 (Kebo lab, Stockholm) in 0.01 M phosphate buffer saline (PBS), pH 7.2, containing 0,1% sodium azide as preservative, and thereafter rinsed in PBS three times, 5 min each time. The sections were then incubated with 5% normal donkey serum in PBS. The sections were thereafter incubated with the primary antibody, diluted in PBS, in a humid environment. Incubation was performed for 60 min at 37°C. After incubation with specific antiserum, and three 5 min washes in PBS, another incubation in normal donkey serum followed, after which the sections were incubated with secondary antibody. As secondary antibody, a FITC-conjugated donkey anti-goat IgG (Jackson Immunoresearch, West Grove, PA), diluted 1:100, was used. Incubation with secondary antibody was performed for 30 min at 37°C. The sections were thereafter washed in PBS and then mounted in Vectashield Mounting Medium (H-1000) (Vector Laboratories, Burlingame, CA, USA). Examination was carried out in a Zeiss Axioscope 2 plus microscope equipped with an Olympus DP70 digital camera. The primary antibody was an antibody against the nicotinic acetylcholine receptor AChRα7 (α7nAChR). This antibody is an affinity purified goat polyclonal antibody raised against a peptide mapping at the C-terminus of α7nAChR of human origin (Santa Cruz Biotechnology; sc-1447, dilution used 1:100). The outcome of immunostaining using the used protocol, including the currently used secondary antiserum, with primary antibody being substituted by PBS or normal serum, has been previously evaluated for human tissue (Danielson et al 2006a; Bjur et al., 2008) (control stainings). Sections of fixed rabbit muscle/inflammatory tissue were furthermore processed in parallel for control purposes, the same procedures as used here for demonstration of α7nAChR immunoreactions in the synovial tissue being used. It was hereby found that the inflammatory cells in the muscle inflammation (myositis) showed distinct α7nAChR immunoreactions, whilst the muscle tissue did not (not shown). Occurrence of α7nAChR immunoreactions for inflammatory cells in muscle inflammation (myositis) is a well-known fact (Leite et al., 2010).

7.3 Results

Mononuclear-like and fibroblast-like cells occurred to varying extents in the synovial samples. They mainly lay scattered in the tissue. The degree of the inflammatory response varied greatly.

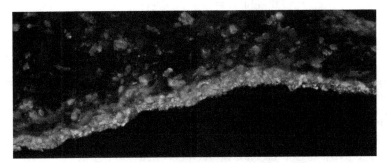

Fig. 2. Figure showing existence of marked α7nAChR immunoreactions in the synovial lining layer.

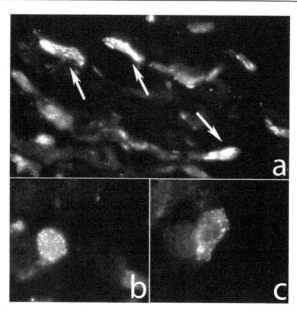

Fig. 3. Figure showing presence of α7nAChR immunoreactions in fibroblast-like (a) and mononuclear-like (b,c) cells in the synovial tissue. Arrows at fibroblast-like cells in (a).

Marked α7nAChR immunoreactions (IR) were seen in the synovial lining layer (Fig 2). α7nAChR IR were also seen for mononuclear-like and fibroblast-like cells (Fig 3).

7.4 Discussion

The observations show that there indeed is immunolabelling for the α7nAChR in the synovial tissue of patients with advanced OA. The findings are in line with recent findings of α7nAChR immunoreactions in the synovial lining layer for RA patients (van Maanen et al., 2009a) and similar findings made in another recent study on patients with RA and psoriatic arthritis (Westman et al., 2009). The observations are also in line with the findings of scattered cells showing fibroblast-like and mononuclear-like appearances exhibiting α7nAChR immunoreactions in RA and psoriatric arthritis (Westman et al., 2009). Furthermore, cultured RA fibroblast-like synoviocytes have been found to express α7nAChR (van Maanen et al., 2009a).

OA synovial intimal lining as well as cultured fibroblast-like synoviocytes obtained from synovial tissue from 3 OA patients express the α7nAChR (Waldburger et al., 2008). The present study thus extends the current knowledge in showing the expression patterns for mononuclear-like and fibroblast-like cells within the OA synovial tissue and is complementary concerning the delineation of the expression pattern for the synovial lining layer.

The existence of not only ACh production (Grimsholm et al., 2008) but also α7nAChR in fibroblast-like cells in the OA synovial tissue can be of functional importance. Stimulation of ACh receptors on pulmonary fibroblasts leads to an increase in collagen accumulation (Sekhon et al., 2002). It can also not be excluded that the α7nAChR may be related to attempts for repair. In studies on skin wound healing, it was thus shown that the α7nAChR is time-dependently expressed in distinct skin cell types, which may be closely involved in the repair processes of the skin wound (Fan et al., 2011). The α7nAChR is also described to contribute to the wound repair of respiratory epithelium (Tournier et al., 2006). Furthermore, an up-regulation of the cholinergic system is reported to be involved in the stimulation of collagen deposition during wound healing (Jacobi et al., 2002). The occurrence of anti-inflammatory effects via cholinergic effects on inflammatory cells is frequently doumented (e.g. Kawashima and Fuji., 2008). The in vitro studies performed by Waldburger and collaborators showed that both synovial fibroblast-like cells and peripheral macrophages respond to cholinergic stimulation leading to inhibition of pro-inflammatory cytokines (Waldburger et al., 2008).

8. Conclusion

The present study adds new information on the expression patterns of the α7nAChR for synovial tissue, namely for this tissue in OA. The results presented here, coupled to the finding that there is evidence favouring the occurrence of synthesis of ACh in OA synovial tissue (Grimsholm et al., 2008), imply that the non-neuronal cholinergic system should be further considered for the OA affected joint. It is likely that non-neuronal ACh can have its effects on the α7nAChR in the OA synovial tissue. Similarly, it is considered that the locally produced ACh in the airways targets ACh receptors located in the airway region where the ACh is produced (Racké et al., 2006).

One possibility is that the production of ACh in non-neuronal cells is related to the occurrence of a great demand on the tissue. That is discussed as one possibility to explain the much more marked ChAT expression in tenocytes of patients with chronic painful tendons than in tendons of normal subjects (Forsgren et al., 2009). Tissue organization and function is hereby influenced. Concerning OA, it would therefore be of interest to know if there is a cholinergic component concerning the cartilage destruction that occurs. It can hereby be noted that less cartilage destruction, as well as on the whole a milder arthritis, was observed for mice lacking the α7nAChR in studies on collagen-induced arthritis (Westman et al., 2010). It might be that the increased production of ACh in the tissue initially is an attempt to "rescue" the tissue, but that long-standing cholinergic upregulation can contribute to deterioration of the tissue. That was suggested to be the case for the chronic painful tendons (Forsgren et al., 2009). Effects of ACh on fibroblasts and myofibroblasts in chronic obstructive pulmonary disease are considered to be involved in remodelling of the tissue (Haag et al., 2008; Racké et al., 2008).

Interference with the effects of ACh, mainly via influences on the α7nAChR, may be a new strategy of value in the treatment of arthritis (van Maanen et al 2009b,c; Westman et al., 2009; Bruchfeld et al., 2010; Pan et al., 2010; Zhang et al., 2010). There are several lines of evidence which suggest that α7nAChR agonists can inhibit the proinflammatory cascade that occurs in arthritis. Selective α7nAChR agonist decreases the production of IL-6 by IL-6 stimulated fibroblast-like synoviocytes and the reduction of production from these cells of several cytokines/chemokines via ACh was blocked by a α7nAChR antagonist (Waldburger et al., 2008). It, however, remains to be clarified as to wheter α7nAChR agonist treatment is valuable in the chronic long-lasting stages of arthritis.

The overwhelming part of the studies favouring a functional importance of the cholinergic system and the possible usefulness of interfering with the α7nAChR are performed on RA. It should here be recalled that some RA specimens from chronic stages of severe RA contained an abundance of ChAT immunoreactive cells (fibroblast-like and monuclear-like cells) in our previous study (Grimsholm et al., 2008). The present study reinforces that a non-neuronal cholinergic system, including presence of the α7nAChR in the synovium, should be further considered also for OA.

9. Acknowledgements

The technical support of Ms. Ulla Hedlund is greatly acknowledged. Dr. Tore Dalén is gratefully acknowledged for supply of the samples. Professor Solbritt Rantapää-Dahlqvist and PhD Ola Grimsholm are acknowledged for the colloborative research in the initial studies on the non-neuronal cholinergic system of human synovium. Financial support has been given by the Faculty of Medicine, Umeå University.

10. References

Altman, R.; Asch, E.; Bloch, D.; Bole, G.; Borenstein, D.; Brandt, K.; Christy, W.; Cooke, TD.; Greenwald, R.; Hochberg, M.; et al. (1986). Development of criteria for the classification and reporting of osteoarthritis. Classification of osteoarthritis of the knee. Diagnostic and Therapeutic Criteria Committee of the American Rheumatism Association. *Arthritis and Rheumatism*, Vol.29, pp.1039-1049.

Bernik, TR.; Friedman, SG.; Ochani, M.; DiRaimo, R.; Ulloa, L.; Yang, H.; Sudan, S.; Czura, CJ.; Ivanova, SM. & Tracey KJ. (2002). Pharmalogical stimulation of the cholinergic anti-inflammatory patyhway. *Journal of Experimental Medicine*, Vol.195, pp. 781-788

Bjur, D.; Danielson, P.; Alfredson, H. & Forsgren, S. (2008). Presence of a non-neuronal cholinergic system and occurrence of up- and down-regulation of M2 muscarinic acetylcholine receptors: new aspects of importance regarding Achilles tendon tendinosis (tendinopathy). *Cell and Tissue Research*, Vol.331, pp. 385-400

Borovikova, LV.; Ivanova, S.; Zhang, M.; Yang, H.; Botchina, GI.; Watkins, LR.;Wang, H.; Abumrad, N.; Eaton, JW. & Tracey, KJ. (2000a). Vagus nerve stimulation attenuates the systemic inflammatory response to endotoxin. *Nature*, Vol.405, pp. 458-462

Borovikova, LV.; Ivanova, S.; Nardi, D.; Zhang, M.; Yang, H.; Ombrellino, M. & Tracey KJ. (2000b). Role of vagus nerve signaling in CNI-1493-mediated suppression of acute inflammation. *Autonomic Neuroscience* 2000, 85, 141-147

Bruchfeld, A.; Goldstein, RS.; Chavan, S.; Patel NB.;Rosas-Ballina, M.; Kohn, N.; Qureshi AR. & Tracey, KJ. (2010). Whole blood cytokine attenuation by cholinergic agionists ex vivo and relationship to vaghus nerve activity in rheumatoid arthritis. *Journal of Internal Medicine*, Vol.268, pp. 94-101

Cooke, JP. (2007). Angiogenesis and the role of the endothelial acetylcholine receptor. *Life Sciences*, Vol.80, pp. 2347-2351

Danielson, P.; Alfredson, H. & Forsgren, S. (2006). Immunohistochemical and histochemical findings favoring the occurrence of autocrine/paracrine as well as nerve-related cholinergic effects in chronic patellar tendon tendinosis. *Microscoscopy Research and Technique*, Vol.69, pp. 808-819

Danielson, P.; Alfredson, H. & Forsgren, S. (2007). In situ hybridization studies confirming recent findings of the existence of a local non-neuronal catecholamine production in human patellar tendinosis. *Microscopy Research and Technique*, Vol.70, pp. 908-911.

de Jonge, W.; van der Zanden, E.; The, FO.; Bijlsma, MF.; van Westerloo, DJ.; Bennink, RJ.; Barthoud, HR.; Uematsau, S.; Akira, S.; van den Wijngaard, RM. & Boeckxstaens, GE. (2005). Stimulation of the vagus nerve attenuates macrophage activation by activating the Jak2-STAT3 signaling pathway. *Nature Immunology*, Vol.6, pp. 844-851

de Jonge, WJ. & Ulloa, L. (2007). The α7 nicotinic acetylcholine receptor as a pharmalogical target for inflammation. *British Journal of Pharmacology*, Vol.151, pp. 915-929

Delbro, DS.; Hallsberg, L.; Wallin, M.; Gustafsson, BI. & Friman, S. (2011). Expression of the non-neuronal cholinergic system in rat liver. *APMIS*, Vol.119, pp. 227-228

En-Nosse, M.; Hartmann, S.; Trinkaus, K.; Alt, V.; Stigler, B.; Heiss, C.; Kilian, O.; Schnettler, R. & Lips, KS. (2009). Expression of non-neuronal cholinergic system in osteoblast-like cells and its involvement in osteogenesis. *Cell and Tissue Research*, Vol.338, pp. 203-215

Fan, YY.; Yu, TS.; Wang, T.; Liu, WW.; Zhao, R.; Zhang, ST.; Ma, WX.; Zheng, JL. & Guan, DW. (2011). Nicotinic acetylcholine receptor alpha7 subunit is time-dependently expressed in distinct cell types during skin wound healing in mice. *Histochemistry and Cell Biology*, publ online

Fisher, LJ.; Schinstine, M.; Salvaterra, P.; Dekker, AJ.; Thal, L. & Gage, FH. (1993). In vivo production and release of acetylcholine from primary fibroblasts genetically modified to express choline acetyltransferase. *Journal of Neurochemistry*, Vol.61, pp. 1323-1332.

Forsgren, S.; Grimsholm, O.; Jönsson, M.; Alfredson, H. & Danielson, P. (2009) New insight into the non-neuronal cholinergic system via studies on chronically painful tendons and inflammatory situations. Life Sciences, Vol.84, pp. 865-870

Grando, SA.; Kist, DA.; Qi, M. & Dahl, MV. (1993). Human keratinocytes synthesize, secrete, and degrade acetylcholine. *Journal of Investigative Dermatology*, Vol.101, pp. 32-36.

Grando, SA.; Pittelko, MR. & Schallreuter, KU. (2006). Adrenergic and cholinergic control in the biology of epidermis: physiological and clinical significance. *Journal of Investigative Dermatology*, Vol.126, pp. 1948-1965.

Goldstein, RS.; Bruchfeld, A.; Yang, L.; Qureshi, AR.; Gallowitsch-Puerta, M.; Patel NB.; Huston, BJ.; Chavan, S.; Rosas-Ballina, M.; Gregersen, PK.; Czura, CJ.; Sloan, RP.; Sama, AE. & Tracey, KJ. (2007) Cholinergic anti-inflammatory pathway activity and High Mobility Group Box-1 (HMGB1) serum levels in patients with rheumatoid arthritis. *Molecular Medicine*, Vol.13, pp. 210-215

Grimsholm, O.; Rantapää-Dahlqvist, S.; Dalén, T. & Forsgren, S. (2008). Unexpected findings of a marked non-neuronal cholinergic system in human knee joint synovial tissue. *Neuroscience Letters*, Vol.442, pp. 128-133

Haag, S.; Matthiesen, S.; Juergens, UR. & Racké, K. (2008). Muscarinic receptors mediate stimulation of collagen synthesis in human lung fibroblasts. *European Respiration Journal*, publ. online, 10.1183/09031936.00129307

Hansson, M. & Forsgren, S. (1995). Immunoreactive atrial and brain natriuretic peptides are co-localized in Purkinje fibres but not in the innervation of the bovine heart conduction system,. *Histochemical Journal*, Vol.27, pp. 222-230

Huston, JM.; Ochani, M.; Rosas-Ballina, M.; Liao, H.; Ochani, K.; Pavlov, VA.; Gallawitsch-Puerta, M.; Ashok, M.; Czura, CJ.; Foxwell, B.; Tracey. & Ulloa, L. (2006).

Splenectomy inactivates the cholinergic antiinflammatory pathway during lethal endotoxemia and polymicrobial sepsis. *Journal of Experimental Medicine*, vol.203, pp. 1623-1628

Jacobi, J.; Jang, JJ.; Sundram, U.; Dayoub, H.; Fajardo, LF. & Cooke, JP. (2002). Nicotine accelerates angiogenesis and wound healing in genetically diabetic mice. *American Journal of Pathology*, Vol.161, pp. 97-104

Jönsson, M.; Norrgård, Ö. & Forsgren, S. (2007). Presence of a marked non-neuronal cholinergic system in the human colon - Studies on the normal colon and the colon in ulcerative colitis. *Inflammatory Bowel Diseases*, Vol.13, pp. 1347-1356

Kawashima, K. & Fuji, T. (2003). The lymphocytic cholinergic system and its contribution to the regulation of immune activity. *Life Sciences*, Vol.74, pp. 675-696

Kawashima, K. & Fuji, T. (2004). Expression of non-neuronal acetylcholine in lymphocytes and its contribution to the regulation of immune function. *Frontieres in Biosciences*, Vol.9, pp. 2063-2085.

Kawashima, K. & Fuji, T. (2008). Basic and clinical aspects of non-neuronal acetylcholine: Overview of non-neuronal cholinergic systems and their biological significance. Forum Minireview. *Journal of Pharmacological Sciences*, Vol.106, pp. 167-173

Kirkpatrick, CJ.; Bittinger, F.; Nozadze, K. & Wessler, I. (2003). Expression and function of the non-neuronal cholinergic ystem in endothelial cells. *Life Sciences*, Vol.72, pp. 2111-2116

Klapproth, H.; Reinheimer, T.; Metzen, J.; Münch, M.; Bittinger, F.; Kirkpatrick, CJ.; Höhle, KD.; Schermann, M.; Racke, K. & Wessler, I. (1997). Non-neuronal acetylcholine, a signaling molecule synthezised by surface cells of rat and man. *Naunyn-Schmiedeberg´s Archieves in Pharmacology*, Vol.355, pp. 515-523

Leite, PE.; Lagrota-Candido, J.; Moraes, L.; D´Elia, L.; Pinheiro, DF.; da Silva, RF.; Yamasaki, EN & Quirico-Santos, T. (2010). Nicotinic acetylcholine receptor activation reduces skeletal muscle inflammation of mdx mice. *Journal of Neuroimmunology*, Vol. 227, pp. 44-51

Lips, KS.; Pfeil, U.; Reiners, K.; Rimasch, C.; Kuchelmeister, K.; Braun-Dullaeus, RC.; Haberberger, RV.; Schmidt, R. & Kummer, W. (2003). Expression of the high-affinity choline transporter CHT1 in rat and human arteries. *Journal of Histochemistry and Cytochemistry*, Vol. 51, pp. 1645-1654

Lips, KS.; Wunsch, J.; Zargooni, S.; Bschleipfer, T.; Schukowski, K.; Weidner, M.; Wessler, I.; Schwantes, U.; Koepsell, H. & Kummer, W. (2007). Acetylcholine and Molecular Components of its Synthesis and Release Machinery in the Urothelium. *European Journal of Urology*, Vol.51, pp. 1042-1053

Matthiesen, S.; Bahulayan, A.; Kempkens, S.; Haag, S.; Fuhrmann, M.; Stichnote, C.; Juergens, UR. & Racke, K. (2006). Muscarinic receptors mediate stimulation of human lung fibroblast proliferation. *American Journal of Respiration and Cell Molecular Biology*, Vol. 35, pp. 621-627

Mayerhofer, A. & Fritz, S. (2002). Ovarian acetylcholine and muscarinic receptors: hints of a novel intrinsic ovarian regulatory system. *Microscoscopy Research and Technique*, Vol.59, pp. 503-508

Metzen, J.; Bittinger, F.; Kirkpatrick, J.; Kilbinger, H. & Wessler, I. (2003). Proliferative effect of acetylcholine on rat trachea epithelial cells is mediated by nicotinic receptors and muscarinic receptors of the M1-subtype. *Life Sciences*, Vol.72, pp. 2075-2080

Neumann, S.; Razen, M.; Habermehl, P.; Meyer, CU.; Zepp, F.; Kirkpatrick, CJ. & Wessler, I. (2007). The non-neuronal cholinergic system in peripheral blood cells: effects of nicotinic and muscarinic antagonists on phagocytosis, respiratory burst and migration. *Life Sciences,* Vol.80, pp. 2361-2364

Oben, JA.; Yang, S.; Lin, H.; Ono, M. & Diehl, AM. (2003). Acetylcholine promotes the proliferation and collagen gene expression of hepatic myofibroblastic stellate cells. *Biochemical and Biophysical Research Communications,* Vol.300, pp. 172-177

Pan, XH.; Zhang, J.; Yu, X.; Qin, L.; Kang, L. & Zhang, P. (2010). New therapeutic approaches for the treatment of rheumatoid arthritis may rise from the cholinergic anti-inflammatory pathway and antinociceptive pathway. *ScientificWorldJournal,* Vol.10, pp. 2248-2253

Paleari, L.; Grozio, A.; Cesario, A. & Russo, P. (2008). The cholinergic system and cancer. *Semininars in Cancer Biology,* Vol.18, pp. 211-217

Pavlov, VA. & Tracey, KJ. (2005). The cholinergic anti-inflammatory pathway. *Brain Behaviour Immunology,* Vol.19, pp. 493-499

Racké, K.; Juergens, UR. & Matthiesen, S. (2006). Control by cholinergic mechanisms. *European Journal of Pharmacology,* Vol.533, pp. 57-68

Racké, K.; Haag, S.; Bahulayan, A. & Warnken, M. (2008). Pulmonary fibroblasts, an emerging target for anti-obstructive drugs. *Naunyn Schmiedebergs Archives in Pharmacology,* Vol.378, pp. 193-201.

Ratcliffe, EM.; de Sa, DJ.; Dixon, MF. & Stead, RH. (1998). Choline acetyltransferase (ChAT) immunoreactivity in paraffin sections of normal and diseased intestines. *Journal of Histochemistry and Cytochemistry,* Vol.46, pp. 1223-1231

Sekhon, HS.; Keller, JA.; Proskocil, BJ.; Martin, EL. & Spindel, ER. (2002). Maternal nicotine exposure upregulates collagen gene expression in fetal monkey lung. Association with alpha7 nicotinic acetylcholine receptors. *American Journal of Respiration and Cell Molecular Biology,* Vol.26, pp. 31-41.

Song, P.; Sekhon, HS.; Keller, JA.; Blusztajn, JK.; Mark, GP. & Spindel, ER. (2003). Acetylcholine is synthesized by and acts as an autocrine growth factor for small cell lung carcinoma. *Cancer Research,* Vol. 63, 214-221.

Song, P. & Spindel, ER. (2008). Basic and clinical aspects of non-neuronal acetylcholine: expression of non-neuronal acetylcholine in lung cancer provides a new target for cancer therapy. *Journal of Pharmacological Sciences,* Vol.106, pp. 180-185.

Tournier, JM.; Maoche, K.; Coraux, C.; Zahm, JM.; Cloez-Tayarani, I.; Nawrocki-Raby, B.; Bonnomet, A.; Burlet, H.; Lebargy, F.; Polette, M. & Birembaut, P. (2006). Alpha3alpha5beta2-nicotinic acetylcholine receptor contributes to the wound repair of the respiratory epithelium by modulating intracellular calcium in migrating cells. *American Journal of Pathology,* Vol.168, pp. 55-68.

Tracey, KJ. (2002). The inflammatory reflex. *Nature,* Vol.420, pp. 853-859

Tracey, KJ. (2007). Physiology and immunology of the cholinergic antiinflammatory pathway. *Journal of Clinical Investigation,* Vol.117, pp. 289-296.

Ulloa, L. (2005). The vagus nerve and the nicotinic anti-inflammatory pathway. *Nature Review of Drug Discovery,* Vol.4, pp. 673-784

Van Maanen, MA.; Stoof, S.; Esmerij, P.; van der Zanden EP.; de Jonge, WJ.; Janssen, RA.; Fischer, DF.; Vandeghinste, N.; Brys, R.; Vervoordeldonk, MJ. & Tak, PP. (2009a). The alpha7 nicotinic acetylcholine receptor on fibroblast-like synoviocytes and in synovial tissue from rheumatoid arthritis patients: a possible role for a key neurotransmitter in synovial inflammation. *Arthritis and Rheumatism*, Vol.60, pp. 1272-1281

Van Maanen, MA.; Lebre, MC.; van der Poll, T.; LaRosa, GJ.; Elbaum, D.; Vervoordeldonk, MJ. & Tak, PP. (2009b). Stimulation of nicotinic acetylcholine receptors attenuates collagen-induced arthritis in mice. *Arthritis and Rheumatism*, Vol.60, pp. 114-122

Van Maanen, MA.; Vervoordeldonk, MJ. & Tak, PP. (2009c) The cholinergic anti-inflammatory pathway: towards innovative treatment of rheumatoid arthrits. *Nature Review in Rheumatology*, Vol.5, pp. 229-232

Van Maanen, MA.; Stoof, S.; LaRosa, G.; Vervoordeldonk, M. & Tak, PP. (2010). Role of the cholinergic system in rheumatoid arthritis: aggravation of arthritis in nicotinic acetylcholine receptor α7 subunit gene knockout mice. *Annals of Rheumatic Diseases*, Vol.69, pp. 1717-1723

Waldburger, JM.; Boyle, DL.; Pavlov, VA.; Tracey, KJ. & Firestein, GS. (2008). Acetylcholine regulation of synoviocyte expression by the alpha7 nicotinic receptor. *Arthritis and Rheumatism*, Vol.58, pp. 3439-3449

Wang, H.; Yu, M.; Ochani, M.; Amella, CA.; Tanovic, M.; Susarla, S.; Li, JH.; Wang, H.; Yang H.; Ulloa, L.; Al-Abed, Y.; Czura, CJ. & Tracey, KJ. (2003). Nicotinic acetylcholine receptor alpha7 subunit is an essential regulator of inflammation. *Nature*, vol.421, pp. 384-388

Westman, M.; Engström, M.; Catrina, AI. & Lampa, J. (2009). Cell specific synovial expression of nicotinic alpha 7 acetylcholine receptor in rheumatoid arthritis and psoriatic arthritis. *Scandinavian Journal of Immunology*, Vol.70, pp. 136-140

Westman, M.; Saha, S.; Morshed, M. & Lampa, J. (2010). Lack of acetylcholine nicotine alpha 7 receptor suppresses development of collagen-induced arthritis and adaptive immunity. *Clinical and Experimental Immunology*, Vol. 162, pp. 62-67

Wessler, I. & Kirkpatrick, CJ. (2001). The Non-neuronal cholinergic system: an emerging drug target in the airways. *Pulmonary Pharmacology and Therapy*, Vol.14, pp. 423-434

Wessler, I.; Kilbinger, H.; Bittinger, F.; Unger, R. & Kirkpatrick, J. (2003). The non-neuronal cholinergic system in humans: Expression, function and pathophysiology. *Life Sciences*, Vol.72, pp. 2055-2061

Wessler, I.; Bittinger, F.; Kamin, W.; Zepp, F.; Meyer, E.; Schad, A. & Kirkpatrick, CJ. (2007). Dysfunction of the non-neuronal cholinergic system in the airways and blood cells of patients with cystic fibrosis. *Life Sciences*, Vol.80, pp. 2253-2258

Wessler, I. & Kirkpatrick, CJ. (2008). Acetylcholine beyond neurons: the non-neuronal cholinergic system in humans. Review. *British Journal of Pharmacology*, Vol.154, pp. 1558-1571

Yoshida, M.; Masunaga, K.; Satoji, Y.; Maeda, Y.; Nagata, T. & Inadome, A. (2008). Basic and clinical aspects of non-neuronal acetylcholine: expression of non-neuronal acetylcholine in urothelium and its clinical significance. *Journal of Pharmacological Sciences*, Vol.106, pp. 193-198.

Zhang, P.; Qin, L. & Zhang, G. (2010). The potential application of nicotinic acetylcholine receptor agonists for the treatment of rheumatoid arthritis. *Inflammation Research*, publ online 2010

9

TGF-β Action in the Cartilage in Health and Disease

Kenneth W. Finnson, Yoon Chi and Anie Philip

Division of Plastic Surgery, Department of Surgery, Montreal General Hospital,
McGill University, Montreal, QC,
Canada

1. Introduction

Transforming growth factor-β (TGF-β) is a pleiotropic cytokine that plays a critical role in the maintenance of healthy cartilage [1-4]. Aberrant TGF-β signaling has been implicated in a number of cartilage-related disorders including gout [5-6], lupus [7-8], rheumatoid arthritis [9] and osteoarthritis (OA) [1-3]. Although much progress has been made in understanding the molecular mechanism of TGF-β action in normal and OA cartilage, this knowledge has not translated into the development of a therapeutic strategy to slow or reverse the progression of the disease. In this chapter, we will highlight recent advances in understanding the role of TGF-β signaling in normal cartilage, the changes that occur in the TGF-β signaling pathway components in OA and the potential of targeting the TGF-β signaling pathway as a therapeutic strategy for the treatment of this disease.

2. TGF-β signaling

Members of the TGF-β superfamily, including TGF-βs, activins and bone morphogenetic proteins (BMPs), are critical for development and homeostasis [10-12]. They regulate diverse cellular processes including proliferation, differentiation and migration as well as extracellular matrix (ECM) production [11-14]. The three mammalian TGF-β isoforms (TGF-β1, -β2, -β3) share significant sequence (approximately 75% identity) and structural similarity [15-19]. However, the phenotypes of TGF-β isoform knockout mice do not overlap [20] and the isoforms exhibit distinct spatial and temporal expression in developing/regenerating tissues and in pathologic responses [21], suggesting distinct functions *in vivo*.

TGF-β is synthesized as a homo-dimeric pro-protein (pro-TGF-β) and is processed in the trans-Golgi network by furin-like enzymes. Cleavage by furin results in the formation of a mature TGF-β dimer along with its pro-peptide, known as latency associated peptide (LAP). TGF-β remains non-covalently associated with LAP and is in an inactive state. In most cases, this small latent complex associates with the latent TGF-β binding protein (LTBP) which forms a disulphide bond with LAP, giving rise to a large latent complex. Once secreted, the large latent complex becomes attached to the ECM by covalent cross-linking of LTBP with ECM proteins which is catalyzed by a transglutaminase [22-25].

TGF-β activation involves its dissociation from the latent complex which is necessary for TGF-β binding to its receptors and for mediating its biological effects [25]. Latent TGF-β can be activated by physical processes including acidification, alkalization and heat denaturation, and biological processes involving proteolysis or protein-protein interactions [22, 24-26]. Many serine proteases such as plasmin and thrombin, and several matrix metalloproteinases (MMPs) such as MMP-2, -9, -13 and -14 have been implicated in TGF-β activation [24]. In addition, thrombospondin-1 (TSP-1) has been shown to bind LAP directly and is thought to cause a conformational change in LAP that leads to activation of latent TGF-β [27]. Although the precise mechanisms of TGF-β activation *in vivo* in different tissues remain to be determined, it is likely to be a critical step for regulating TGF-β bioavailability [22, 24-26].

TGF-β signals through a pair of transmembrane serine/threonine kinases known as the type I (TβRI, also known as activin receptor-like kinase-5 or ALK5) and type II (TβRII) TGF-β receptors [10-12]. TGF-β binds TβRII, a constitutively active kinase, which then phosphorylates and activates TβRI/ALK5 [28-29]. Activated ALK5 phosphorylates intracellular Smad2 and Smad3 proteins, which then bind to Smad4 and accumulate in the nucleus where they interact with various co-activators, co-repressors and transcription factors to regulate gene expression [30-31]. TGF-β has also been shown to activate another TGF-β type I receptor known as ALK1 which phosphorylates Smad-1, -5 and -8 [32-34]. In addition, TGF-β activates several non-Smad pathways including mitogen-activated protein (MAP) kinase pathways (ERK, JNK and p38), Rho-like GTPase pathways and phosphatidylinositol-3-kinase (PI3K)/Akt pathways [35-36].

3. Regulation of TGF-β signaling

Intracellular regulation of TGF-β signaling involves the interplay of many cytoplasmic proteins including FKBP12, TRIP-1, STRAP, TRAP-1, SARA, HSP90 [37] and nuclear proteins such as TGIF, c-Ski, SnoN and Evi-1 [31]. The inhibitory Smads or I-Smads, which include Smad6 and Smad7, play critical roles in negative feedback regulation of TGF-β/BMP signaling by forming stable complexes with the activated type I receptors thereby blocking Smad phosphorylation [38-39]. Smad6 and Smad7 also act as adaptor proteins that recruit E3 ubiquitin ligases such as Smurf1 and Smurf2 to the TGF-β type I receptors and induce their ubiquitination and proteosomal degradation [40].

Extracellular control of TGF-β signaling is orchestrated by many factors including those that regulate activation of latent TGF-β as described in Section 2. In addition, several ECM components such as decorin and biglycan bind TGF-β and regulate its bioavailability [41]. Other extracellular molecules such as lipoproteins have been shown to sequester TGF-β ligand into an inactive pool [42]. TGF-β co-receptors such as endoglin, betaglycan and CD109 are emerging as important factors that regulate many aspects of TGF-β signaling in health and disease.

Endoglin (CD105) is a single-pass transmembrane homo-dimeric glycoprotein that is expressed mainly in endothelial cells. It binds TGF-β1 and TGF-β3 with high affinity in the presence of TβRII but does not bind the TGF-β2 isoform [43]. Endoglin has been shown to (i) alter TβRII and TβRI (ALK1 and ALK5) phosphorylation status, (ii) promote TGF-β/ALK1 signaling, (iii) suppress TGF-β/ALK5/Smad2/3 signaling and (iv) antagonize TGF-β-induced MAP kinase signaling through a β-arrestin-2-dependent mechanism [44-45].

Betaglycan, also known as TGF-β type III receptor, is a homologue of endoglin and is a more ubiquitously expressed transmembrane glycoprotein. It binds all three TGF-β isoforms (TGF-β1, -β2, -β3) with high affinity and enhances their binding to the signaling receptors, especially that of the TGF-β2 isoform [43, 46-47]. Betaglycan has been shown to direct clathrin-mediated endocytosis of TβRII and ALK5 [48], and enhance TGF-β signaling via Smad and MAP kinase pathways [49-51]. Conversely, betaglycan has also been reported to promote β-arrestin2-dependent TGF-β receptor internalization and down-regulation of TGF-β signaling [52].

CD109 is a glycosyl phosphatidylinostol (GPI)-anchored protein and a member of the α2-macroglobulin/complement family. It is found on activated T-cells and platelets, endothelial cells and many human cancer cell lines [53-56]. We have recently identified CD109 as a TGF-β co-receptor which binds TGF-β1 with high affinity, forms a heteromeric complex with the TGF-β signaling receptors and inhibits Smad2/3 signaling in different cell types [57-58]. Recent results indicate that CD109 inhibits TGF-β signaling by promoting TGF-β receptor internalization and degradation in a Smad7/Smurf2-dependent manner [57, 59]. Taken together, these studies demonstrate that the TGF-β co-receptors endoglin, betaglycan and CD109 play critical roles in regulating TGF-β signaling.

4. TGF-β and cartilage

Articular cartilage is an avascular tissue that receives its nutrients from synovial fluid, a thin layer of fluid surrounding the cartilage. The only cell type found in cartilage is the chondrocyte which are embedded in an extensive ECM made of mainly collagens and proteoglycans [60]. Type II collagen is the main collagen found in articular cartilage and is important for providing tensile strength [61-62]. Aggrecan is the main proteoglycan of articular cartilage and provides structural support by retaining water in the matrix [63]. Articular cartilage is commonly divided into four distinct zones, namely the superficial zone, middle zone, deep zone and calcified cartilage [60]. The zones differ in collagen organization, proteoglycan content and chondrocyte morphologies [60].

TGF-β plays a number of roles in the development, growth and maintenance of articular cartilage. During cartilage development, TGF-β stimulates chondrogenic condensation [64-65], chondroprogenitor cell proliferation and chondrocyte differentiation [66-67]. TGF-β also inhibits terminal differentiation or "hypertrophy" of chondrocytes thereby blocking endochondral bone formation [68-69] and allowing formation of articular cartilage at the end of the long bones [70]. The maintenance of mature articular cartilage is dependent on the action of TGF-β which not only stimulates production of ECM proteins such as type II collagen and aggrecan, but also blocks degradation of ECM proteins by increasing production of protease inhibitors such as tissue inhibitor of metalloproteases (TIMPs) [69, 71]. TGF-β also counteracts the catabolic effects of interleukin (IL)-1 and tumor necrosis factor (TNF)-α on cartilage[69, 71].

The potent anabolic effects of TGF-β on articular cartilage *in vivo* in animal models are well known. TGF-β injected into the periosteum of rat or mouse femur induces chondrocyte differentiation and cartilage formation [72-73]. Local administration of TGF-β into murine knee joints stimulated articular cartilage repair [74] and healing of full-thickness cartilage defects [75-76]. Conversely, blocking endogenous TGF-β using a soluble form of TβRII impaired articular cartilage repair in a murine model of experimental OA [77]. In addition, expression of a dominant negative TβRII in cartilage resulted in an OA-like phenotype in the mouse [78]. Furthermore, Smad3 knockout mice develop degenerative joint disease resembling human OA [70]. In addition, decreased TGF-β expression and Smad2 phosphorylation are associated with a reduced protective effect during OA progression [79]. Evidence for a causal relationship between TGF-β and OA in the human is further supported by the identification of asporin (a proteoglycan that sequesters TGF-β in the ECM and inhibits TGF-β function) as an OA susceptibility gene [80-83]. However, TGF-β also has been shown to have undesirable effects on cartilage. A number of studies have reported that TGF-β treatment of normal murine joints is associated with osteophyte outgrowth, inflammation and synovial fibroplasia [84-86]. Thus, normal cartilage function may dependent on a narrow range of bioactive TGF-β levels, and concentrations above or below this level may lead to alterations in TGF-β signaling, resulting in abnormal cartilage function.

5. Altered expression and function of TGF-β pathway components in osteoarthritis

OA is a chronic degenerative joint disease characterized by articular cartilage degradation, subchondral bone alterations and synovial inflammation [87-88]. The cause of OA is unknown but risk factors include aging, obesity, abnormal mechanical loading and anatomical abnormalities [89]. Subchondral bone alterations contribute to the initiation and/or progression of OA by producing catabolic factors that degrade the overlying cartilage [90]. Synovial inflammation is thought to be induced by cartilage matrix degradation products that are phagocytosed by macrophages of the synovial lining. The macrophages, in turn, secrete pro-inflammatory mediators into the synovial fluid that diffuse into the cartilage, thereby creating a vicious circle of synovial inflammation and cartilage degradation [90]. The current chapter focuses on the role of TGF-β signaling in articular cartilage homeostasis and its deregulation in OA.

5.1 TGF-β ligands and their activation

Several studies suggest that TGF-β isoform (TGF-β1, -β2, -β3) levels are down-regulated in OA cartilage. For example, TGF-β1 protein levels were shown to be decreased in human OA cartilage [91-92] and TGF-β3 levels were shown to be reduced in both spontaneous (STR/Ort) and collagenase-induced mouse models of OA [79]. In addition, TGF-β1 and TGF-β2 levels were moderately decreased in rabbit OA cartilage [93]. In constrast, a number of studies have demonstrated that TGF-β isoform expression is up-regulated in OA cartilage. TGF-β1, -β2 and -β3 levels were found to be increased in human OA [94-96] and TGF-β1 and -β3 levels were elevated in a papain-induced mouse model of OA [77]. Furthermore, TGF-β2 was increased in a surgically-induced model of early OA in rats [97]. One possible explanation for these discrepancies is that TGF-β isoform expression may vary during the course of OA. For instance, TGF-β levels might increase in the early stages of OA to counteract the catabolic effects of inflammatory cytokines such as IL-1β or TNF-α [98-99]. However, with the progressive loss of TGF-β receptor expression (see Section 5.2), chondrocytes may eventually lose their responsiveness to TGF-β, leading to a decrease in TGF-β levels due to the loss of TGF-β auto-induction [100]. Future studies using age-, race- and gender- matched normal and OA human articular cartilage and a better characterization of TGF-β isoform expression in the different animal models during OA progression will be needed to resolve this issue.

Although TGF-β isoform levels are altered in OA, it is not known whether these changes represent active TGF-β levels. Moreover, accumulating evidence suggests that components of the large latent complex may be disrupted in OA. For example, both LTBP-1 and LTBP-2 were shown to be increased in human OA cartilage [97, 101-102] and in experimental models of OA [97, 101]. Although LTBP-1 [103-104] and LTBP-2 [105] knockout mice do not display an OA phenotype suggesting that these proteins may not contribute to the OA process, LTBP-3 knockout mice develop an OA phenotype and display features resembling those of mice with impaired TGF-β signaling [106-107]. These results suggest that LTBP-3 might have a protective effect against OA progression. It is also possible that studies using LTBP-1 and LTBP-2 knockout mice in an experimental OA setting may reveal a role for these proteins in OA progression. Interestingly, the levels of TGF-β activators are also upregulated in human OA and in a variety of animal models of OA. Transglutaminase-2 (TG-2), the predominant transglutaminase subtype in hypertrophic chondrocytes, are higher in knee [108-109] and femoral [110] cartilage in human OA and in experimental OA models [97, 101, 111]. Whether the enhanced TG-2 expression in OA correlates with increased TGF-β activation or LTBP cross-linking to ECM remains to be determined. In addition, TSP-1 levels are increased in the cartilage in mild and moderate OA, but decreased in severe OA [112]. Intra-articular gene transfer of TSP-1 was shown to reduce disease progression in a collagen- or anterior cruciate ligament transection-induced OA in rats [113-114]. This is consistent with the notion that TSP-1 mediates latent TGF-β activation in OA cartilage and that the up-regulation of TSP-1 is an adaptive response in an attempt to increase cartilage repair.

5.2 TGF-β receptors

Increasing evidence indicates that TGF-β receptor expression levels are altered in OA. TβRII levels were shown to be decreased in human OA cartilage [92] and in a rabbit OA model [93]. In addition, TβRII mRNA expression was decreased in cultured human OA chondrocytes as compared to normal chondrocytes in vitro [115]. These results suggest that loss of TβRII during OA might represent an intrinsic defect of human OA chondrocytes. The notion that loss of TβRII might contribute to the initiation and/or progression of OA is supported by a study showing that a truncated, kinase-defective TβRII expressed in mouse skeletal tissue was associated terminal chondrocyte differentiation and the development of OA-like features [78]. A more recent study has shown that conditional expression of dominant negative TβRII inhibits cartilage formation in mice [116]. Thus, loss of TβRII expression and/or activity may not only promote an OA-like phenotype but may also contribute to OA progression by limiting the ability of cartilage to repair itself. Future studies using cartilage-specific knockout of TβRII may provide further insight into the role of this TGF-β receptor in OA pathogenesis.

Emerging evidence indicates that the expression of TGF-β type I receptors is also altered in OA. Our group has shown that in addition to the canonical TGF-β type I receptor ALK5, human chondrocytes also express ALK1 [34]. Both ALK5 and ALK1 are required for TGF-β-induced Smad1/5 phosphorylation whereas only ALK5 is essential for TGF-β-induced Smad3 phosphorylation in these cells [34]. We also demonstrated that ALK1 inhibits whereas ALK5 potentiates the expression of type II collagen and PAI-1 in chondrocytes, indicating that ALK1 and ALK5 elicit opposite efffects in chondrocytes [34]. More recent data suggest that both ALK5 and ALK1 levels are decreased in mouse models of OA, but that ALK1 expression decreases to a lesser extent than that of ALK5, suggesting that the ratio of ALK1/ALK5 increases during OA [117]. Interestingly, ALK1 has been identified as one of the genes upregulated in a mensical tear rat model of OA [101] whereas ALK5 levels were dramatically reduced in partial meniscectomy and post-surgery training rat model of OA [118]. These two latter studies are consistent with the notion that the ALK1/ALK5 ratio increases during OA. In human OA cartilage, ALK1 mRNA expression highly correlates with MMP-13 levels whereas ALK5 mRNA levels correlate with aggrecan and collagen type II levels [117]. Collectively, these data suggest that alterations in the expression of TGF-β signaling receptors (TβRII and ALK5/ALK1) play an important role in OA pathogenesis and that an increase in the TGF-β/ALK1 pathway activation relative to that of the TGF-β/ALK5 pathway activation is likely to be a critical event in the OA disease progression.

5.3 Smads

Since TGF-β receptor levels are altered in OA, it can be anticipated that activities of downstream signaling mediators such as Smad2 and Smad3 are also altered. Indeed, Smad2 phosphorylation levels are reduced in cartilage during OA progression in both spontaneous- (STR/Ort) and collagenase-induced mouse models of OA [79] and in cartilage of old mice as compared to young mice [119]. Although Smad3 phosphorylation was not examined in these models, a recent study has reported decreased Smad3 phosphorylation levels in the Smurf-2 transgenic mice which spontaneously develop an OA-like phenotype [120]. Together, these studies suggest that OA is associated with reduced TGF-β/ALK5/Smad2/3 signaling.

The potential importance of Smad3 in OA is further underscored by the finding that Smad3 knockout mice develop a degenerative joint disease resembling human OA [70] and intervertebral disc degeneration [121]. Moreover, several genetic studies in humans suggest that mutations in the Smad3 gene may be an important factor in OA. A missense mutation in the Smad3 gene was found in a patient with knee OA and was associated with elevated serum MMP-2 and MMP-9 levels [122]. A single nucleotide polymorphism (SNP) mapping to the Smad3 intron 1 was shown to be involved in risk of both hip and knee OA in European populations [123]. Furthermore, several mutations in the Smad3 gene were found in individuals that presented early-onset OA [124]. Although the functional significance of these mutations in Smad3 remains to be determined, these studies suggest that alteration in Smad3 function may play a role in the pathogenesis of OA.

A shift in the balance of signaling from Smad2/3 towards Smad1/5 is thought to play an important role in OA pathogenesis. TGF-β signals through both of these pathways in human chondrocytes with the Smad1/5 pathway opposing the Smad2/3 pathway [34]. This is consistent with the findings in endothelial cells [32-33], skin fibroblasts [125] and in chondrocyte terminal differentiation [126]. Although Smad-1, -5 and -8 expression levels and subcellular localization in human OA cartilage did not differ significantly from that of normal cartilage, two Smad1 gene splice variants of unknown significance were reduced in OA cartilage [127]. When the reported decrease in ALK5 expression and Smad2/3 signaling (see above) in OA cartilage is taken into account, it is possible to envision that a shift in TGF-β signaling away from the ALK5/Smad2/3 pathway and towards the ALK1/Smad1/5/8 pathway may occur, contributing to OA progression. However, whether such a shift is an adaptive response without a causal relationship to OA progression cannot be ruled out at this time.

As mentioned above, Smad7/Smurf2-mediated TGF-β receptor degradation is an important mechanism for the termination of TGF-β signaling [38-39]. Although Smad7 expression levels in human OA cartilage did not significantly differ from that of normal cartilage [128] it did show an age-related increased expression in murine cartilage [119] suggesting that age might be an important factor to consider when comparing Smad7 expression levels in OA versus normal cartilage. In addition, Smurf2 is increased in human OA cartilage as compared to normal cartilage [129] and Smurf2-transgenic mice spontaneously develop an OA-like phenotype [129]. Because Smad7 and Smurf-2 work in concert to promote TGF-β receptor degradation, these data suggest that increased Smad7/Smurf2 action resulting in decreased TGF-β receptor levels might be involved in OA pathogenesis.

5.4 MAP kinases

In addition to the Smad pathway, TGF-β also activates several non-Smad pathways including MAPK kinase (ERK, p38, JNK) pathways, Rho-like GTPase signaling pathways and PI3K/Akt pathways [35-36]. TGF-β-activated kinase-1 (TAK1), a MAP3 kinase activated by TGF-β and other pathways, plays a critical role in cartilage development and function [130]. TGF-β signaling via TAK-1 stimulates type II collagen synthesis in chondrocytes in a Smad3-independent manner [131]. On the other hand, activation of MAPK kinase activity by cytokines such as IL-1β or TNF-α decreases Smad3/4 DNA binding and ECM production in chondrocytes [132]. In addition, activating transcription factor (ATF)-2 works synergistically with Smad3 to mediate TGF-βs inhibition of chondrocyte maturation [133]. These studies suggest extensive cross-talk between Smad and non-Smad pathways in chondrocytes which should be taken into account when considering the role of aberrant TGF-β signaling in OA.

5.5 TGF-β co-receptors

TGF-β co-receptors such as endoglin, betaglycan and CD109 have emerged as important regulators of TGF-β signaling and responses with critical roles in diseases such as cancer and organ fibrosis [43, 47, 54, 58, 134-136]. This section focuses on the available information on these TGF-β co-receptors in cartilage health and disease.

Endoglin (CD105): We have previously shown that endoglin is detected in human articular cartilage *in vivo* and in primary human articular chondrocytes *in vitro* [137]. We have also demonstrated that endoglin enhances TGF-β-induced Smad1/5 signaling and suppresses Smad2/3 signaling and ECM production in human chondrocytes [138]. Importantly, we found that endoglin protein levels are increased in human OA cartilage as compared to normal cartilage [138]. These results are in agreement with the microarray data showing that endoglin mRNA levels are increased in human OA cartilage [102] and in a rat model of OA [97]. Interestingly, elevated circulating and synovial fluid endoglin are associated with primary knee OA severity, suggesting that endoglin may be a useful biomarker for determining disease severity and/or play a causative role in OA pathogenesis [139].

Betaglycan: Our group has shown that betaglycan is expressed in human chondrocytes and that it forms a complex with the signaling receptors and endoglin in a ligand- and TβRII-independent manner [137]. Betaglycan levels in damaged versus intact human OA cartilage were similar [140] although normal cartilage was not analyzed in this study. Furthermore, betaglycan levels did not change in a rat model of OA [97]. However, betaglycan expression was shown to be increased in adult human articular cartilage in response to mechanical injury [141]. These results suggest that elevated betaglycan expression might be important in secondary OA when joint trauma is involved. Interestingly, betaglycan expression was shown to be increased in mesenchymal stem cells from the femur channel [142] and in trabecular bone from the iliac crest [143] of OA patients. These studies suggest that altered betaglycan expression or function in bone might play a role in OA pathogenesis.

CD109: Information available on CD109 expression or function in cartilage is limited. CD109 was detected in conditioned media of human articular chondrocytes in monolayer culture [144-145] and in that of bovine cartilage explants treated with IL-1β or TNF-α [146]. These studies suggest that CD109 is released from the chondrocyte cell surface which is in agreement with our previous studies on skin cells [58, 147]. We have detected CD109 protein in conditioned media and cell lysates of human OA and normal human articular chondrocytes cultured in monolayer (Finnson and Philip, unpublished data). Recently, CD109 was detected in peripheral circulation and synovial fluid as a component of CD146-positive lymphocytes in patients with various musculoskeletal diseases [148]. The precise mechanisms by which TGF-β co-receptors may contribute to deregulation of TGF-β action in OA remain to be determined.

6. Targeting the TGF-β pathway for osteoarthritis therapy

Several components of the TGF-β signaling pathway display altered expression in human OA cartilage and in experimental models of OA. Genetic manipulation of some of the TGF-β pathway components in mice leads to OA-like phenotypes or to delayed OA progression in experimental OA models. These findings suggest that targeting specific components of the TGF-β pathway may represent a suitable therapeutic strategy for the treatment of OA. Many groups have studied the effect of exogenous TGF-β to promote cartilage repair and/or prevent cartilage degradation. Early studies showed that intra-articular injection of recombinant TGF-β1 into murine joints conferred protection against IL-induced articular cartilage destruction [149-150] although this effect was not observed in older mice [150-151]. Subsequently, exogenous delivery of TGF-β1 was shown to restore depleted proteoglycans in arthritic murine joints [74] and to stimulate proteoglycan synthesis and content in normal murine joints [152]. In addition, TGF-β injected into the osteoarthritic temporomandibular joint of rabbits was shown to have a protective effect on articular cartilage degradation [153]. Although these studies support the notion that TGF-β promotes cartilage repair, its use has been hampered by undesirable side effects including inflammation, synovial hyperplasia and osteophyte formation [84-86, 152, 154]. In this regard, several studies suggest that adjuvant therapies might be used to circumvent the undesirable effects TGF-βs on the osteoarthritic joint. For example, TGF-β was shown to stimulate cartilage repair and the resulting synovial fibrosis could be blocked by Smad7 overexpression in the synovial lining [155]. Such findings suggest that strategies designed to take advantage of the beneficial effects of TGF-β on cartilage repair and simultaneously block its unwanted side effects will be a fruitful avenue for the development of this molecule for OA therapy.

Another important factor to consider when developing a TGF-β-based strategy for OA therapy is that TGF-β may have differential effects on the chondrocyte itself, depending on the cellular context. We have shown that TGF-β signaling in chondrocytes occurs through two different TGF-β type I receptors, ALK5 and ALK1, with ALK1/Smad1/5 pathway opposing ALK5/Smad2/3 signaling and ECM production in human chondrocytes [34]. These data suggest that ALK1 signaling might interfere with the chondroprotective effects of TGF-β. Furthermore, others have shown that ALK1 expression is highly correlated with MMP-13 expression in human OA cartilage and that ALK1 stimulates MMP13 expression in chondrocytes [117]. Thus, a better approach for OA therapy might involve treatment with TGF-β while simultaneously blocking ALK1 activity in chondrocytes. Alternatively, targeting molecules that tip the balance of signaling away from ALK1 and towards ALK5 in OA chondrocytes might also prove to be beneficial. However, there are others who argue that the critical transition from a non-reparative to a reparative cell phenotype involves switching from ALK5-mediated fibrogenic signaling to ALK1-mediated chondrogenic signaling [156]. Therefore, further research on understanding the role of ALK5 and ALK1 signaling pathways in regulating chondrocyte phenotype is needed.

Targeting TGF-β co-receptors for the treatment of human diseases is an attractive concept. Endoglin, betaglycan and CD109 exist both as membrane-anchored and soluble forms due to enzymatic shedding of their ectodomains [134-135, 157-158] and soluble forms of these proteins have been shown to bind and neutralize TGF-β [58, 159, 160, 2001 #587]. One way that these soluble proteins might be used in combination with TGF-β for OA therapy would be to restrict TGF-β expression to the OA chondrocytes. For example, one can use an adenoviral vector containing a type II collagen-specific promoter to drive TGF-β expression in the cartilage while blocking the adverse side effects (synovial fibrosis) of exogenous TGF-β in the joint by co-administration of a soluble co-receptor protein into the synovial fluid. The soluble co-receptor because of its higher molecular weight would not readily diffuse into the cartilage from the synovial fluid [161-162] to block TGF-β action in chondrocytes but would sequester any TGF-β that diffuses from the cartilage into the synovial fluid. Alternatively, TGF-β co-receptor expression in chondrocytes might be targeted directly to promote cartilage repair. Our results indicate that endoglin inhibits TGF-β-induced ALK5-Smad2/3 signaling and ECM production and enhances TGF-β-induced ALK1-Smad1/5 signaling in human chondrocytes [138]. These findings suggest that reducing endoglin expression in OA chondrocytes might promote cartilage repair.

7. Concluding remarks

TGF-β is a critical regulator of articular cartilage development, maintenance and repair. Studies to date indicate that several extracellular, cell surface and intracellular components of the TGF-β pathway display altered expression or activity in OA suggesting that they might represent potential targets for therapeutic treatment of this disease. TGF-β has been shown to promote cartilage repair and its therapeutic use might be improved by "compartmentalized" inhibition of TGF-β activity in synovial tissues to halt or reverse synovial fibrosis and osteophyte formation. Targeting TGF-β co-receptors such as endoglin, betaglycan and CD109 represent new opportunities to explore aberrant TGF-β signaling in OA and to discover new strategies for manipulating the TGF-β pathway for OA therapy.

8. List of abbreviations

ALK, activin receptor-like kinase; ATF, activating transcription factor; ECM, extracellular matrix; ERK, extracellular signal-regulated kinase; Evi-1, ecotropic virus integration site 1 protein homologue; FKBP, FK506 binding protein; GPI, glycosyl phosphatidylinositol; HSP, heat shock protein; IL, interleukin; JNK, c-jun N-terminal kinase/stress-activated protein kinase; kDa, kilodalton; LAP, latency associated peptide; LTBP, latent TGF-β binding protein; MMP, matrix metalloproteinase; OA, osteoarthritis; PI3K, phosphatidylinositol 3-kinase; SARA, Smad anchor for receptor activation; Ski, Sloan Kettering Institute proto-oncogene; Sno, ski-related novel protein; SNP, single nucleotide polymorphism; Smurf, Smad ubiquitin regulatory factor; STRAP, serine-threonine kinase receptor-associated protein; TAK, TGF-β activated kinase; TG, transglutaminase; TGF-β, transforming growth factor-beta; TGIF, TGF-β-induced factor; TIMP, tissue inhibitor of metalloproteinase; TSP, thrombospondin; TNF, tumor necrosis factor; TRAP, TGF-β receptor-associated protein; TRIP, TGF-β receptor-interacting protein.

9. References

[1] van der Kraan PM, Goumans MJ, Blaney Davidson E, Ten Dijke P. Age-dependent alteration of TGF-β signalling in osteoarthritis. Cell Tissue Res 2011.

[2] van den Berg WB. Pathomechanisms of OA: 2010 in review. Osteoarthritis Cartilage 2011; 19: 338-341.

[3] Finnson K, Chi Y, Bou-Gharios G, Leask A, Philip A. TGF-β signaling in cartilage homeostasis and osteoarthritis. Front Biosci 2011; S4: 261-268.

[4] Song B, Estrada KD, Lyons KM. Smad signaling in skeletal development and regeneration. Cytokine Growth Factor Rev 2009; 20: 379-388.

[5] Chang SJ, Chen CJ, Tsai FC, Lai HM, Tsai PC, Tsai MH, et al. Associations between gout tophus and polymorphisms 869T/C and -509C/T in transforming growth factor β1 gene. Rheumatology (Oxford) 2008; 47: 617-621.

[6] Dalbeth N, Pool B, Gamble GD, Smith T, Callon KE, McQueen FM, et al. Cellular characterization of the gouty tophus: a quantitative analysis. Arthritis Rheum 2010; 62: 1549-1556.

[7] Kriegel MA, Li MO, Sanjabi S, Wan YY, Flavell RA. Transforming growth factor-β: recent advances on its role in immune tolerance. Curr Rheumatol Rep 2006; 8: 138-144.

[8] Kim EY, Moudgil KD. Regulation of autoimmune inflammation by pro-inflammatory cytokines. Immunol Lett 2008; 120: 1-5.

[9] Pohlers D, Brenmoehl J, Loffler I, Muller CK, Leipner C, Schultze-Mosgau S, et al. TGF-β and fibrosis in different organs - molecular pathway imprints. Biochim Biophys Acta 2009; 1792: 746-756.

[10] Heldin CH, Moustakas A. Role of Smads in TGFβ signaling. Cell Tissue Res 2011; DOI: 10.1007/s00441-011-1190-x.

[11] Wu MY, Hill CS. TGF-β superfamily signaling in embryonic development and homeostasis. Dev Cell 2009; 16: 329-343.

[12] Wharton K, Derynck R. TGF-β family signaling: novel insights in development and disease. Development 2009; 136: 3691-3697.

[13] Moustakas A, Heldin CH. The regulation of TGFβ signal transduction. Development 2009; 136: 3699-3714.

[14] Heldin C, Landstrom M, Moustakas A. Mechanism of TGF-β signaling to growth arrest, apoptosis, and epithelial-mesenchymal transition. Current Opinion in Cell Biology 2009; 21: 166-176.

[15] Schlunegger MP, Grutter MG. An unusual feature revealed by the crystal structure at 2.2 A resolution of human transforming growth factor-β2. Nature 1992; 358: 430-434.

[16] Mittl PR, Priestle JP, Cox DA, McMaster G, Cerletti N, Grutter MG. The crystal structure of TGF-β3 and comparison to TGF-β2: implications for receptor binding. Protein Sci 1996; 5: 1261-1271.

[17] Hinck AP, Archer SJ, Qian SW, Roberts AB, Sporn MB, Weatherbee JA, et al. Transforming growth factor β1: three-dimensional structure in solution and comparison with the X-ray structure of transforming growth factor β2. Biochemistry 1996; 35: 8517-8534.

[18] Daopin S, Piez KA, Ogawa Y, Davies DR. Crystal structure of transforming growth factor-β2: an unusual fold for the superfamily. Science 1992; 257: 369-373.

[19] Radaev S, Zou Z, Huang T, Lafer EM, Hinck AP, Sun PD. Ternary complex of TGF-β1 reveals isoform-specific ligand recognition and receptor recruitment in the superfamily. J Biol Chem 2010; 285: 14806-14814.

[20] Bottinger EP, Letterio JJ, Roberts AB. Biology of TGF-β in knockout and transgenic mouse models. Kidney Int 1997; 51: 1355-1360.

[21] Roberts AB, Sporn MB. Differential expression of the TGF-β isoforms in embryogenesis suggests specific roles in developing and adult tissues. Mol Reprod Dev 1992; 32: 91-98.

[22] Ramirez F, Rifkin DB. Extracellular microfibrils: contextual platforms for TGFβ and BMP signaling. Curr Opin Cell Biol 2009; 21: 612-622.

[23] Hynes RO. The extracellular matrix: not just pretty fibrils. Science 2009; 326: 1216-1219.

[24] Jenkins G. The role of proteases in transforming growth factor-β activation. Int J Biochem Cell Biol 2008; 40: 1068-1078.

[25] Annes JP, Munger JS, Rifkin DB. Making sense of latent TGF-β activation. Journal of Cell Science 2003; 116: 217-224.

[26] Wipff PJ, Hinz B. Integrins and the activation of latent transforming growth factor β1 - An intimate relationship. Eur J Cell Biol 2008; 87: 601-615.

[27] Murphy-Ullrich JE, Poczatek M. Activation of latent TGF-β by thrombospondin-1: mechanisms and physiology. Cytokine Growth Factor Rev 2000; 11: 59-69.

[28] Massague J, Gomis RR. The logic of TGF-β signaling. FEBS Lett 2006; 580: 2811-2820.

[29] Shi Y, Massague J. Mechanisms of TGF-β signaling from cell membrane to the nucleus. Cell 2003; 113: 685-700.

[30] Schmierer B, Hill CS. TGFβ-Smad signal transduction: molecular specificity and functional flexibility. Nat Rev Mol Cell Biol 2007; 8: 970-982.

[31] Ross S, Hill CS. How the Smads regulate transcription. Int J Biochem Cell Biol 2008; 40: 383-408.

[32] Goumans M, Valdimarsdottir G, Itoh S, Rosendahl A, Sideras P, ten Dijke P. Balancing the activation state of the endothelium via two distinct TGF-β type I receptors. Embo J 2002; 21: 1743-1753.

[33] Goumans MJ, Valdimarsdottir G, Itoh S, Lebrin F, Larsson J, Mummery C, et al. Activin receptor-like kinase (ALK)1 is an antagonistic mediator of lateral TGF-β/ALK5 signaling. Mol Cell 2003; 12: 817-828.

[34] Finnson KW, Parker WL, ten Dijke P, Thorikay M, Philip A. ALK1 opposes ALK5/Smad3 signaling and expression of extracellular matrix components in human chondrocytes. J Bone Miner Res 2008; 23: 896-906.

[35] Mu Y, Gudey SK, Landstrom M. Non-Smad signaling pathways. Cell Tissue Res 2011; DOI: 10.1007/s00441-011-1201-y.

[36] Zhang YE. Non-Smad pathways in TGF-β signaling. Cell Res 2008; 19: 128-139.

[37] Wrighton KH, Lin X, Feng XH. Phospho-control of TGF-β superfamily signaling. Cell Res 2009; 19: 8-20.

[38] Yan X, Chen YG. Smad7: not only a regulator, but also a cross-talk mediator of TGF-β signalling. Biochem J 2011; 434: 1-10.

[39] Briones-Orta MA, Tecalco-Cruz AC, Sosa-Garrocho M, Caligaris C, Macias-Silva M. Inhibitory Smad7: Emerging Roles in Health and Disease. Curr Mol Pharmacol 2011; 4: 141-153.

[40] Inoue Y, Imamura T. Regulation of TGF-β family signaling by E3 ubiquitin ligases. Cancer Sci 2008.

[41] Macri L, Silverstein D, Clark RA. Growth factor binding to the pericellular matrix and its importance in tissue engineering. Adv Drug Deliv Rev 2007; 59: 1366-1381.

[42] Grainger DJ, Byrne CD, Witchell CM, Metcalfe JC. Transforming growth factor β is sequestered into an inactive pool by lipoproteins. J Lipid Res 1997; 38: 2344-2352.

[43] Bernabeu C, Lopez-Novoa JM, Quintanilla M. The emerging role of TGF-β superfamily co-receptors in cancer. Biochim Biophys Acta 2009; 1792: 954-973.

[44] Pardali E, ten Dijke P. Transforming growth factor-β signaling and tumor angiogenesis. Front Biosci 2009; 14: 4848-4861.

[45] ten Dijke P, Goumans MJ, Pardali E. Endoglin in angiogenesis and vascular diseases. Angiogenesis 2008; 11: 79-89.

[46] Bilandzic M, Stenvers KL. Betaglycan: A multifunctional accessory. Mol Cell Endocrinol 2011; 339: 180-189.

[47] Gatza CE, Oh SY, Blobe GC. Roles for the type III TGF-β receptor in human cancer. Cell Signal 2010; 22: 1163-1174.

[48] McLean S, Di Guglielmo GM. TβRIII directs clathrin-mediated endocytosis of TGFβ type I and II receptors. Biochem J 2010; 429: 137-145

[49] Finger EC, Lee NY, You HJ, Blobe GC. Endocytosis of the type III TGF-β receptor through the clathrin-independent/lipid raft pathway regulates TGF-β signaling and receptor downregulation. J Biol Chem 2008; 283: 34808-34818.

[50] Santander C, Brandan E. Betaglycan induces TGF-β signaling in a ligand-independent manner, through activation of the p38 pathway. Cell Signal 2006; 18: 1482-1491.

[51] You HJ, Bruinsma MW, How T, Ostrander JH, Blobe GC. The type III TGF-β receptor signals through both Smad3 and the p38 MAP kinase pathways to contribute to inhibition of cell proliferation. Carcinogenesis 2007; 28: 2491-2500.

[52] Chen W, Kirkbride KC, How T, Nelson CD, Mo J, Frederick JP, et al. β-arrestin 2 mediates endocytosis of type III TGF-β receptor and down-regulation of its signaling. Science 2003; 301: 1394-1397.

[53] Solomon KR, Sharma P, Chan M, Morrison PT, Finberg RW. CD109 represents a novel branch of the α2-macroglobulin/complement gene family. Gene 2004; 327: 171-183.

[54] Hashimoto M, Ichihara M, Watanabe T, Kawai K, Koshikawa K, Yuasa N, et al. Expression of CD109 in human cancer. Oncogene 2004; 23: 3716-3720.

[55] Schuh AC, Watkins NA, Nguyen Q, Harmer NJ, Lin M, Prosper JYA, et al. A tyrosine703serine polymorphism of CD109 defines the Gov platelet alloantigens. Blood 2002; 99: 1692-1698.

[56] Lin M, Sutherland DR, Horsfall W, Totty N, Yeo E, Nayar R, et al. Cell surface antigen CD109 is a novel member of the alpha 2 macroglobulin/C3, C4, C5 family of thioester-containing proteins. Blood 2002; 99: 1683-1691.

[57] Bizet AA, Liu K, Tran-Khanh N, Saksena A, Vorstenbosch J, Finnson KW, Buschmann MD, Philip A. The TGF-β co-receptor, CD109, promotes internalization and degradation of TGF-β receptors. Biochim Biophys Acta 2011; 1813: 742-753.

[58] Finnson KW, Tam BY, Liu K, Marcoux A, Lepage P, Roy S, et al. Identification of CD109 as part of the TGF-β receptor system in human keratinocytes. FASEB J 2006; 20: 1525-1527.

[59] Bizet AA, Tran-Khanh N, Saksena A, Liu K, Buschmann MD, Philip A. CD109-mediated degradation of the TGF-β receptors and inhibition of TGF-β responses involve regulation of Smad7 and Smurf2 localization and function. Journal of Cellular Biochemistry 2011; doi: 10.1002/jcb.23349

[60] Bhosale AM, Richardson JB. Articular cartilage: structure, injuries and review of management. Br Med Bull 2008; 87: 77-95.

[61] Eyre DR. Collagens and cartilage matrix homeostasis. Clin Orthop Relat Res 2004: S118-122.

[62] Eyre DR, Weis MA, Wu JJ. Articular cartilage collagen: an irreplaceable framework? Eur Cell Mater 2006; 12: 57-63.

[63] Heinegard D. Proteoglycans and more--from molecules to biology. Int J Exp Pathol 2009; 90: 575-586.

[64] Goldring MB, Tsuchimochi K, Ijiri K. The control of chondrogenesis. J Cell Biochem 2006; 97: 33-44.

[65] Onyekwelu I, Goldring MB, Hidaka C. Chondrogenesis, joint formation, and articular cartilage regeneration. J Cell Biochem 2009; 107: 383-392.

[66] Kawakami Y, Rodriguez-Leon J, Izpisua Belmonte JC. The role of TGF-βs and Sox9 during limb chondrogenesis. Curr Opin Cell Biol 2006; 18: 723-729.

[67] Quintana L, zur Nieden NI, Semino CE. Morphogenetic and regulatory mechanisms during developmental chondrogenesis: new paradigms for cartilage tissue engineering. Tissue Eng Part B Rev 2009; 15: 29-41.

[68] van der Kraan PM, Blaney Davidson EN, van den Berg WB. A role for age-related changes in TGF-β signaling in aberrant chondrocyte differentiation and osteoarthritis. Arthritis Res Ther 2010; 12: 201.

[69] van der Kraan PM, Blaney Davidson EN, Blom A, van den Berg WB. TGF-β signaling in chondrocyte terminal differentiation and osteoarthritis: modulation and integration of signaling pathways through receptor-Smads. Osteoarthritis Cartilage 2009; 17: 1539-1545.

[70] Yang X, Chen L, Xu X, Li C, Huang C, Deng C-X. TGF-β/Smad3 signals repress chondrocyte hypertrophic differentiation and are required for maintaining articular cartilage. J. Cell Biol. 2001; 153: 35-46.

[71] Blaney Davidson E, van der Kraan P, van den Berg W. TGF-β and osteoarthritis. Osteoarthritis Cartilage 2007; 15: 597-604.

[72] Chimal-Monroy J, Diaz de Leon L. Differential effects of transforming growth factors β1, β2, β3 and β5 on chondrogenesis in mouse limb bud mesenchymal cells. Int J Dev Biol 1997; 41: 91-102.

[73] Joyce ME, Roberts AB, Sporn MB, Bolander ME. Transforming growth factor-β and the initiation of chondrogenesis and osteogenesis in the rat femur. J Cell Biol 1990; 110: 2195-2207.

[74] Glansbeek HL, van Beuningen HM, Vitters EL, van der Kraan PM, van den Berg WB. Stimulation of articular cartilage repair in established arthritis by local administration of transforming growth factor-β into murine knee joints. Lab Invest 1998; 78: 133-142.

[75] Hunziker EB. Growth-factor-induced healing of partial-thickness defects in adult articular cartilage. Osteoarthritis Cartilage 2001; 9: 22-32.

[76] Hunziker EB, Rosenberg LC. Repair of partial-thickness defects in articular cartilage: cell recruitment from the synovial membrane. J Bone Joint Surg Am 1996; 78: 721-733.

[77] Scharstuhl A, Glansbeek HL, van Beuningen HM, Vitters EL, van der Kraan PM, van den Berg WB. Inhibition of endogenous TGF-β during experimental osteoarthritis prevents osteophyte formation and impairs cartilage repair. J Immunol 2002; 169: 507-514.

[78] Serra R, Johnson M, Filvaroff EH, LaBorde J, Sheehan DM, Derynck R, et al. Expression of a truncated, kinase-defective TGF-β type II receptor in mouse skeletal tissue promotes terminal chondrocyte differentiation and osteoarthritis. J. Cell Biol. 1997; 139: 541-552.

[79] Blaney Davidson EN, Vitters EL, van der Kraan PM, van den Berg WB. Expression of transforming growth factor-β (TGFβ) and the TGFβ signalling molecule Smad-2P in spontaneous and instability-induced osteoarthritis: role in cartilage degradation, chondrogenesis and osteophyte formation. Ann Rheum Dis 2006; 65: 1414-1421.

[80] Loughlin J. The genetic epidemiology of human primary osteoarthritis: current status. Expert Rev Mol Med 2005; 7: 1-12.

[81] Ikegawa S. New gene associations in osteoarthritis: what do they provide, and where are we going? Curr Opin Rheumatol 2007; 19: 429-434.

[82] Ikegawa S. Expression, regulation and function of asporin, a susceptibility gene in common bone and joint diseases. Curr Med Chem 2008; 15: 724-728.

[83] Dai J, Ikegawa S. Recent advances in association studies of osteoarthritis susceptibility genes. J Hum Genet 2010; 55: 77-80.

[84] van Beuningen HM, van der Kraan PM, Arntz OJ, van den Berg WB. Transforming growth factor-β1 stimulates articular chondrocyte proteoglycan synthesis and induces osteophyte formation in the murine knee joint. Lab Invest 1994; 71: 279-290.

[85] van Beuningen HM, Glansbeek HL, van der Kraan PM, van den Berg WB. Osteoarthritis-like changes in the murine knee joint resulting from intra-articular transforming growth factor-β injections. Osteoarthritis Cartilage 2000; 8: 25-33.

[86] Bakker AC, van de Loo FA, van Beuningen HM, Sime P, van Lent PL, van der Kraan PM, et al. Overexpression of active TGF-β1 in the murine knee joint: evidence for synovial-layer-dependent chondro-osteophyte formation. Osteoarthritis Cartilage 2001; 9: 128-136.

[87] Alcaraz MJ, Megias J, Garcia-Arnandis I, Clerigues V, Guillen MI. New molecular targets for the treatment of osteoarthritis. Biochem Pharmacol 2010; 80: 13-21.

[88] Goldring MB, Goldring SR. Articular cartilage and subchondral bone in the pathogenesis of osteoarthritis. Ann N Y Acad Sci 2010; 1192: 230-237.

[89] Zhang Y, Jordan JM. Epidemiology of Osteoarthritis. Clin Geriatr Med 2010; 26: 355-369.

[90] Martel-Pelletier J, Pelletier JP. Is osteoarthritis a disease involving only cartilage or other articular tissues? Eklem Hastalik Cerrahisi 2010; 21: 2-14.

[91] Wu J, Liu W, Bemis A, Wang E, Qiu Y, Morris EA, et al. Comparative proteomic characterization of articular cartilage tissue from normal donors and patients with osteoarthritis. Arthritis Rheum 2007; 56: 3675-3684.

[92] Verdier MP, Seite S, Guntzer K, Pujol JP, Boumediene K. Immunohistochemical analysis of transforming growth factor β isoforms and their receptors in human cartilage from normal and osteoarthritic femoral heads. Rheumatol Int 2005; 25: 118-124.

[93] Boumediene K, Conrozier T, Mathieu P, Richard M, Marcelli C, Vignon E, et al. Decrease of cartilage transforming growth factor-β receptor II expression in the rabbit experimental osteoarthritis-potential role in cartilage breakdown. Osteoarthritis Cartilage 1998; 6: 146-149.

[94] Xiao J, Li T, Wu Z, Shi Z, Chen J, Lam SK, et al. REST corepressor (CoREST) repression induces phenotypic gene regulation in advanced osteoarthritic chondrocytes. J Orthop Res 2010; 28: 1569-1575.

[95] Pombo-Suarez M, Castano-Oreja MT, Calaza M, Gomez-Reino JJ, Gonzalez A. Differential up-regulation of the three TGF-β isoforms in human osteoarthritic cartilage. Ann Rheum Dis 2009; 68: 568-571.

[96] Nakajima M, Kizawa H, Saitoh M, Kou I, Miyazono K, Ikegawa S. Mechanisms for asporin function and regulation in articular cartilage. J. Biol. Chem. 2007; 282: 32185-32192.

[97] Appleton CT, Pitelka V, Henry J, Beier F. Global analyses of gene expression in early experimental osteoarthritis. Arthritis Rheum 2007; 56: 1854-1868.

[98] Malemud CJ. Anticytokine therapy for osteoarthritis: evidence to date. Drugs Aging 2010; 27: 95-115.

[99] Pujol JP, Chadjichristos C, Legendre F, Bauge C, Beauchef G, Andriamanalijaona R, et al. Interleukin-1 and transforming growth factor-β1 as crucial factors in osteoarthritic cartilage metabolism. Connect Tissue Res 2008; 49: 293-297.

[100] Kim SJ, Angel P, Lafyatis R, Hattori K, Kim KY, Sporn MB, et al. Autoinduction of transforming growth factor β1 is mediated by the AP-1 complex. Mol Cell Biol 1990; 10: 1492-1497.

[101] Wei T, Kulkarni NH, Zeng QQ, Helvering LM, Lin X, Lawrence F, et al. Analysis of early changes in the articular cartilage transcriptisome in the rat meniscal tear model of osteoarthritis: pathway comparisons with the rat anterior cruciate transection model and with human osteoarthritic cartilage. Osteoarthritis Cartilage 2010; 18: 992-1000.

[102] Aigner T, Fundel K, Saas J, Gebhard PM, Haag J, Weiss T, et al. Large-scale gene expression profiling reveals major pathogenetic pathways of cartilage degeneration in osteoarthritis. Arthritis Rheum 2006; 54: 3533-3544.

[103] Todorovic V, Frendewey D, Gutstein DE, Chen Y, Freyer L, Finnegan E, et al. Long form of latent TGF-beta binding protein 1 (Ltbp1L) is essential for cardiac outflow tract septation and remodeling. Development 2007; 134: 3723-3732.

[104] Drews F, Knobel S, Moser M, Muhlack KG, Mohren S, Stoll C, et al. Disruption of the latent transforming growth factor-β binding protein-1 gene causes alteration in facial structure and influences TGF-β bioavailability. Biochim Biophys Acta 2008; 1783: 34-48.

[105] Shipley JM, Mecham RP, Maus E, Bonadio J, Rosenbloom J, McCarthy RT, et al. Developmental expression of latent transforming growth factor beta binding protein 2 and its requirement early in mouse development. Mol Cell Biol 2000; 20: 4879-4887.

[106] Dabovic B, Chen Y, Colarossi C, Obata H, Zambuto L, Perle MA, et al. Bone abnormalities in latent TGF-β binding protein (LTBP)-3-null mice indicate a role for LTBP-3 in modulating TGF-β bioavailability. J Cell Biol 2002; 156: 227-232.

[107] Dabovic B, Chen Y, Colarossi C, Zambuto L, Obata H, Rifkin DB. Bone defects in latent TGF-β binding protein (LTBP)-3 null mice; a role for LTBP in TGF-β presentation. J Endocrinol 2002; 175: 129-141.

[108] Johnson K, Hashimoto S, Lotz M, Pritzker K, Terkeltaub R. Interleukin-1 induces pro-mineralizing activity of cartilage tissue transglutaminase and factor XIIIa. Am J Pathol 2001; 159: 149-163.

[109] Heinkel D, Gohr CM, Uzuki M, Rosenthal AK. Transglutaminase contributes to CPPD crystal formation in osteoarthritis. Front Biosci 2004; 9: 3257-3261.

[110] Orlandi A, Oliva F, Taurisano G, Candi E, Di Lascio A, Melino G, et al. Transglutaminase-2 differently regulates cartilage destruction and osteophyte formation in a surgical model of osteoarthritis. Amino Acids 2009; 36: 755-763.

[111] Huebner JL, Johnson KA, Kraus VB, Terkeltaub RA. Transglutaminase 2 is a marker of chondrocyte hypertrophy and osteoarthritis severity in the Hartley guinea pig model of knee OA. Osteoarthritis Cartilage 2009; 17: 1056-1064.

[112] Pfander D, Cramer T, Deuerling D, Weseloh G, Swoboda B. Expression of thrombospondin-1 and its receptor CD36 in human osteoarthritic cartilage. Ann Rheum Dis 2000; 59: 448-454.

[113] Jou IM, Shiau AL, Chen SY, Wang CR, Shieh DB, Tsai CS, et al. Thrombospondin 1 as an effective gene therapeutic strategy in collagen-induced arthritis. Arthritis Rheum 2005; 52: 339-344.

[114] Hsieh JL, Shen PC, Shiau AL, Jou IM, Lee CH, Wang CR, et al. Intra-articular gene transfer of thrombospondin-1 suppresses the disease progression of experimental osteoarthritis. J Orthop Res 2010; 28: 1300-1306.

[115] Dehne T, Karlsson C, Ringe J, Sittinger M, Lindahl A. Chondrogenic differentiation potential of osteoarthritic chondrocytes and their possible use in matrix-associated autologous chondrocyte transplantation. Arthritis Res Ther 2009; 11: R133.

[116] Hiramatsu K, Iwai T, Yoshikawa H, Tsumaki N. Expression of dominant negative TGF-β receptors inhibits cartilage formation in conditional transgenic mice. J Bone Miner Metab 2011.

[117] Blaney Davidson EN, Remst DF, Vitters EL, van Beuningen HM, Blom AB, Goumans MJ, et al. Increase in ALK1/ALK5 ratio as a cause for elevated MMP-13 expression in osteoarthritis in humans and mice. J Immunol 2009; 182: 7937-7945.

[118] Gomez-Camarillo MA, Kouri JB. Ontogeny of rat chondrocyte proliferation: studies in embryo, adult and osteoarthritic (OA) cartilage. Cell Res 2005; 15: 99-104.

[119] Blaney Davidson EN, Scharstuhl A, Vitters EL, van der Kraan PM, van den Berg WB. Reduced transforming growth factor-β signaling in cartilage of old mice: role in impaired repair capacity. Arthritis Res Ther 2005; 7: R1338-1347.

[120] Wu Q, Huang JH, Sampson ER, Kim KO, Zuscik MJ, O'Keefe RJ, et al. Smurf2 induces degradation of GSK-3β and upregulates β-catenin in chondrocytes: a potential mechanism for Smurf2-induced degeneration of articular cartilage. Exp Cell Res 2009; 315: 2386-2398.

[121] Li CG, Liang QQ, Zhou Q, Menga E, Cui XJ, Shu B, et al. A continuous observation of the degenerative process in the intervertebral disc of Smad3 gene knock-out mice. Spine (Phila Pa 1976) 2009; 34: 1363-1369.

[122] Yao JY, Wang Y, An J, Mao CM, Hou N, Lv YX, et al. Mutation analysis of the Smad3 gene in human osteoarthritis. Eur J Hum Genet 2003; 11: 714-717.

[123] Valdes AM, Spector TD, Tamm A, Kisand K, Doherty SA, Dennison EM, et al. Genetic variation in the Smad3 gene is associated with hip and knee osteoarthritis. Arthritis Rheum 2010; 62: 2347-2352.

[124] van de Laar IM, Oldenburg RA, Pals G, Roos-Hesselink JW, de Graaf BM, Verhagen JM, et al. Mutations in SMAD3 cause a syndromic form of aortic aneurysms and dissections with early-onset osteoarthritis. Nat Genet 2011; 43: 121-126.

[125] Pannu J, Nakerakanti S, Smith E, Dijke Pt, Trojanowska M. Transforming growth factor-β receptor type I dependent fibrogenic gene program is mediated via activation of Smad1 and ERK1/2 pathways. J. Biol. Chem. 2007; 282: 10405–10413.

[126] Valcourt U, Gouttenoire J, Moustakas A, Herbage D, Mallein-Gerin F. Functions of transforming growth factor-β family type I receptors and Smad proteins in the hypertrophic maturation and osteoblastic differentiation of chondrocytes. J Biol Chem 2002; 277: 33545-33558.

[127] Bau B, Haag J, Schmid E, Kaiser M, Gebhard PM, Aigner T. Bone morphogenetic protein-mediating receptor-associated Smads as well as common Smad are expressed in human articular chondrocytes but not up-regulated or down-regulated in osteoarthritic cartilage. J Bone Miner Res 2002; 17: 2141-2150.

[128] Kaiser M, Haag J, Soder S, Bau B, Aigner T. Bone morphogenetic protein and transforming growth factor beta inhibitory Smads 6 and 7 are expressed in human adult normal and osteoarthritic cartilage in vivo and are differentially regulated in vitro by interleukin-1β. Arthritis Rheum 2004; 50: 3535-3540.

[129] Wu Q, Kim KO, Sampson ER, Chen D, Awad H, O'Brien T, et al. Induction of an osteoarthritis-like phenotype and degradation of phosphorylated Smad3 by Smurf2 in transgenic mice. Arthritis Rheum 2008; 58: 3132-3144.

[130] Gunnell LM, Jonason JH, Loiselle AE, Kohn A, Schwarz EM, Hilton MJ, et al. TAK1 regulates cartilage and joint development via the MAPK and BMP signaling pathways. J Bone Miner Res 2010; 25: 1784-1797.

[131] Qiao B, Padilla SR, Benya PD. TGF-β activated kinase 1 (TAK1) mimics and mediates TGF-β-induced stimulation of type II collagen synthesis in chondrocytes

independent of Col2a1 transcription and Smad3 signaling. J. Biol. Chem. 2005; 280: 17562-17571.

[132] Roman-Blas JA, Stokes DG, Jimenez SA. Modulation of TGF-β signaling by proinflammatory cytokines in articular chondrocytes. Osteoarthritis Cartilage 2007; 15: 1367-1377.

[133] Ionescu AM, Schwarz EM, Zuscik MJ, Drissi H, Puzas JE, Rosier RN, et al. ATF-2 cooperates with Smad3 to mediate TGF-β effects on chondrocyte maturation. Exp Cell Res 2003; 288: 198-207.

[134] Hagiwara S, Murakumo Y, Mii S, Shigetomi T, Yamamoto N, Furue H, et al. Processing of CD109 by furin and its role in the regulation of TGF-β signaling. Oncogene 2010; 29: 2181-2191.

[135] Hockla A, Radisky DC, Radisky ES. Mesotrypsin promotes malignant growth of breast cancer cells through shedding of CD109. Breast Cancer Res Treat 2009; 124: 27-38.

[136] Leask A. Targeting the TGFβ, endothelin-1 and CCN2 axis to combat fibrosis in scleroderma. Cell Signal 2008; 20: 1409-1414.

[137] Parker WL, Goldring MB, Philip A. Endoglin is expressed on human chondrocytes and forms a heteromeric complex with betaglycan in a ligand and type II TGFβ receptor independent manner. J Bone Miner Res 2003; 18: 289-302.

[138] Finnson KW, Parker WL, Chi Y, Hoemann C, Goldring MB, Antoniou J, et al. Endoglin differentially regulates TGF-β-induced Smad2/3 and Smad1/5 signalling and its expression correlates with extracellular matrix production and cellular differentiation state in human chondrocytes. Osteoarthritis Cartilage 2010; 18: 1518-1527.

[139] Honsawek S, Tanavalee A, Yuktanandana P. Elevated circulating and synovial fluid endoglin are associated with primary knee osteoarthritis severity. Arch Med Res 2009; 40: 590-594.

[140] Tsuritani K, Takeda J, Sakagami J, Ishii A, Eriksson T, Hara T, et al. Cytokine receptor-like factor 1 is highly expressed in damaged human knee osteoarthritic cartilage and involved in osteoarthritis downstream of TGF-β. Calcif Tissue Int 2010; 86: 47-57.

[141] Dell'accio F, De Bari C, Eltawil NM, Vanhummelen P, Pitzalis C. Identification of the molecular response of articular cartilage to injury, by microarray screening: Wnt-16 expression and signaling after injury and in osteoarthritis. Arthritis Rheum 2008; 58: 1410-1421.

[142] Rollin R, Alvarez-Lafuente R, Marco F, Garcia-Asenjo JA, Jover JA, Rodriguez L, et al. Abnormal transforming growth factor-β expression in mesenchymal stem cells from patients with osteoarthritis. J Rheumatol 2008; 35: 904-906.

[143] Sanchez-Sabate E, Alvarez L, Gil-Garay E, Munuera L, Vilaboa N. Identification of differentially expressed genes in trabecular bone from the iliac crest of osteoarthritic patients. Osteoarthritis Cartilage 2009; 17: 1106-1114.

[144] Polacek M, Bruun JA, Elvenes J, Figenschau Y, Martinez I. The secretory profiles of cultured human articular chondrocytes and mesenchymal stem cells: implications for autologous cell transplantation strategies. Cell Transplant 2011; 20:1381-93.

[145] Polacek M, Bruun JA, Johansen O, Martinez I. Differences in the secretome of cartilage explants and cultured chondrocytes unveiled by SILAC technology. J Orthop Res 2010; 28: 1040-1049.

[146] Stevens AL, Wishnok JS, Chai DH, Grodzinsky AJ, Tannenbaum SR. A sodium dodecyl sulfate-polyacrylamide gel electrophoresis-liquid chromatography tandem mass spectrometry analysis of bovine cartilage tissue response to mechanical compression injury and the inflammatory cytokines tumor necrosis factor-α and interleukin-1β. Arthritis Rheum 2008; 58: 489-500.

[147] Tam B, Larouche D, Germain L, Hooper N, Philip A. Characterization of a 150 kDa accessory receptor for TGF-β1 on keratinocytes: direct evidence for a GPI anchor and ligand binding of the released form. Journal of Cellular Biochemistry 2001; 83: 494-507.

[148] Dagur PK, Tatlici G, Gourley M, Samsel L, Raghavachari N, Liu P, et al. CD146+ T lymphocytes are increased in both the peripheral circulation and in the synovial effusions of patients with various musculoskeletal diseases and display pro-inflammatory gene profiles. Cytometry B Clin Cytom 2010; 78B: 88-95.

[149] van Beuningen HM, van der Kraan PM, Arntz OJ, van den Berg WB. Protection from interleukin 1 induced destruction of articular cartilage by transforming growth factor β: studies in anatomically intact cartilage in vitro and in vivo. Ann Rheum Dis 1993; 52: 185-191.

[150] van Beuningen HM, van der Kraan PM, Arntz OJ, van den Berg WB. In vivo protection against interleukin-1-induced articular cartilage damage by transforming growth factor-β1: age-related differences. Ann Rheum Dis 1994; 53: 593-600.

[151] Scharstuhl A, van Beuningen HM, Vitters EL, van der Kraan PM, van den Berg WB. Loss of transforming growth factor counteraction on interleukin 1 mediated effects in cartilage of old mice. Ann Rheum Dis 2002; 61: 1095-1098.

[152] van Beuningen HM, Glansbeek HL, van der Kraan PM, van den Berg WB. Differential effects of local application of BMP-2 or TGF-β1 on both articular cartilage composition and osteophyte formation. Osteoarthritis Cartilage 1998; 6: 306-317.

[153] Man C, Zhu S, Zhang B, Hu J. Protection of articular cartilage from degeneration by injection of transforming growth factor-β in temporomandibular joint osteoarthritis. Oral Surg Oral Med Oral Pathol Oral Radiol Endod 2009; 108: 335-340.

[154] Blaney Davidson E, Vitters E, van Beuningen HM, van de Loo F, van den Berg W, van der Kraan P. Resemblance of osteophytes in experimental osteoarthritis to transforming growth factorβ-induced osteophytes: limited role of bone morphogenetic protein in early osteoarthritic osteophyte formation. Arthritis Rheum 2007; 56: 4065-4073.

[155] Blaney Davidson EN, Vitters EL, van den Berg WB, van der Kraan PM. TGFβ-induced cartilage repair is maintained but fibrosis is blocked in the presence of Smad7. Arthritis Res Ther 2006; 8: R65.

[156] Plaas A, Velasco J, Gorski DJ, Li J, Cole A, Christopherson K, et al. The relationship between fibrogenic TGFβ1 signaling in the joint and cartilage degradation in post-injury osteoarthritis. Osteoarthritis Cartilage 2011.

[157] Velasco-Loyden G, Arribas J, Lopez-Casillas F. The shedding of betaglycan is regulated by pervanadate and mediated by membrane type matrix metalloprotease-1. J Biol Chem 2004; 279: 7721-7733.

[158] Hawinkels LJ, Kuiper P, Wiercinska E, Verspaget HW, Liu Z, Pardali E, et al. Matrix metalloproteinase-14 (MT1-MMP)-mediated endoglin shedding inhibits tumor angiogenesis. Cancer Res 2010; 70: 4141-4150.

[159] Vilchis-Landeros MM, Montiel JL, Mendoza V, Mendoza-Hernandez G, Lopez-Casillas F. Recombinant soluble betaglycan is a potent and isoform-selective transforming growth factor-β neutralizing agent. Biochem J 2001; 355: 215-222.

[160] Venkatesha S, Toporsian M, Lam C, Hanai J, Mammoto T, Kim YM, et al. Soluble endoglin contributes to the pathogenesis of preeclampsia. Nat Med 2006; 12: 642-649.

[161] Urech DM, Feige U, Ewert S, Schlosser V, Ottiger M, Polzer K, et al. Anti-inflammatory and cartilage-protecting effects of an intra-articularly injected anti-TNF{alpha} single-chain Fv antibody (ESBA105) designed for local therapeutic use. Ann Rheum Dis 2010; 69: 443-449.

[162] van Lent PL, van den Berg WB, Schalkwijk J, van de Putte LB, van den Bersselaar L. The impact of protein size and charge on its retention in articular cartilage. J Rheumatol 1987; 14: 798-805.

Part 2

Cellular Aspects of Osteoarthritis

10

How Important are Innate Immunity Cells in Osteoarthritis Pathology

Petya Dimitrova and Nina Ivanovska
Department of Immunology, Institute of Microbiology
Bulgaria

1. Introduction

Osteoarthritis (OA) is a chronic degenerative bone disorder leading to cartilage loss, frequently associated with the aging process. It is widely spread in society and often causes disability. Joint swelling which attends OA is due to osteophyte formation or to synovial fluid accumulation. Pathologically, focal damage of cartilage in load-bearing areas are observed together with the formation of new bone at the joint margins, as well as with changes in subchondral bone, and synovitis. Current diagnosis of OA is based on the clinical history and on the radiographical data which occur late at the disease and are very irreversible. Ideally, we wish to detect osteoarthritis at an early stage by following the changes in expression of particular molecular markers, assuming that these markers are sufficiently sensitive, specific, and quantitative for the disease. OA is no longer considered an exclusively degenerative joint disorder because it is related to changes in the synovial membrane as a result of more or less exerted inflammation (Hedbom & Hauselmann, 2002). Trauma or some mechanical problem might be the primary reason for OA initiation. The initiation and progression of OA is sometimes associated with synovial inflammation and the production of proinflammatory and destructive mediators from the synovium causing the invasion of chondrocytes into the cartilage. In early OA the influx of mononuclear cells is enhanced simultaneously with overexpression of inflammatory molecules compared with late OA (Benito et al., 2005). A fundamental question is which cell populations in OA contribute to and maintain synovial inflammation and cartilage destruction.

2. Neutrophils as the main participants in the development of OA

2.1 Phenotype of OA neutrophils

Neutrophils are an essential part of the innate immune system, triggering the initial inflammatory response and the development of host defense mechanisms. During inflammation they leave the circulation and enter the tissues in which they are under the influence of various local factors such as cytokines, endogenous growth factors, microbial products etc. In a result, neutrophils adopt effector functions of great importance for initiation and maintaining of many chronic inflammatory diseases (Duan et al., 2001; Edwards & Hallett, 1997; Mitsuyama et al., 1994).

Neutrophils develop from progenitor cells in bone marrow. They have short lifespans of several hours and then die via apoptosis. Constitutive apoptosis of neutrophils is regulated by two transcription factors: hypoxia-inducible factor 1 (HIF1) and forkhead box O3A. When certain stimuli such as granulocyte-macrophage colony-stimulating factor (GM-CSF), TNF-α, IL-8 and IFN-γ are provided, the lifespan of blood neutrophils is significantly prolonged (Brach et al., 1992; Kilpatrick et al., 2006). Increased neutrophil survival is related with an enhanced expression of anti-apoptotic genes (Marshall et al., 2007) and by death-inducing receptors belonging to the tumor necrosis factor (TNF)/nerve growth factor (NGF) receptor super-family, such as Fas, TNF-related apoptosis-inducing ligand (TNFSF10) receptors, TNFRSF9 (CD137), and the type I TNF receptor (Simon et al., 2003).

It has been shown that RA synovial fluid counteracts neutrophil apoptosis and leads to prolonged survival (Ottonello et al., 2002). Such inhibited apoptosis is characteristic for the earliest phase of RA in contrast to other early arthritides (Raza et al., 2006), suggesting that the suppression of apoptosis in RA patients at high risk is a possible therapeutic approach. RA neutrophils are also functionally different from healthy neutrophils as it has been demonstrated by up-regulated expression of complement receptors CR1, CR3 and CR4 (Felzmann et al., 1991). They show an increased chemotaxis to synovium (Pronai et al., 1991) promoted by TNF-α, IL-17, IL-20 and IL-24 (Kragstrup et al., 2008; Shen et al., 2005). Reports about apoptosis of neutrophils in OA are few and controversial. Bell et al. showed that synovial fluid from OA patients contains factors inhibiting neutrophil survival (Bell et al., 1995). There is also a hypothesis that pyrophosphate dihydrate (CPPD) and basic calcium phosphate (BCP) crystals present in the OA joint fluid and tissue can activate Ca2+ signal in neutrophils thereby prolonging their survival and reducing their apoptosis (Rosenthal, 2011). Chakravarti et al. isolated a subset of blood neutrophils which represents 8–17% of the total neutrophil population and persists beyond 72 h after an exposure to GM-CSF, TNF-α and IL-4. These neutrophils secrete IL-1, IL-1Ra and IL-8, and interact strongly with resident stromal cells (Chakravarti et al., 2009). The phenotype of "long-lived" neutrophils also differs from that of the circulating neutrophils. Although they express the common neutrophil cell surface markers CD32, CD18 and CD11b, they acquire new surface markers, such as HLA-DR and the co-stimulation molecule CD80 (Cross et al., 2003).

Neutrophils participate actively in joint inflammation as proven by their depletion in an experimental model of arthritis (Santos et al., 1997). They affect chemotaxis of macrophages and dendritic cells by cleaving prochemerin to chemerin. Neutrophils produce TNF-α and other cytokines like IL-1, IL-6 that drive the differentiation and activation of dendritic cells and macrophages. The destructive potential of neutrophils is related with their ability to release reactive oxygen species and granules with myeloperoxidase, defensins and MMP-8, MMP-9, MMP-25. MMPs are secreted in response to IL-8 and through ERK1/2 and Src-family kinase pathways (Chakrabarti & Patel, 2005).

2.2 RANKL expression on OA neutrophils

The uncoordinated bone remodeling events in OA results from the impaired balance between bone resorption mediated by mature osteoclasts and bone formation mediated by osteoblasts. The receptor activator of nuclear factor-κB ligand (RANKL) and its receptor RANK are actively involved in osteoclast formation (Yasuda et al., 1998). Immature osteoblasts express RANKL which binds to RANK on osteoclasts, initiating the recruitment of osteoclast precursors in bone marrow and promoting their differentiation.

Intracellularly, RANK interacts with TNF receptor-associated factor 6 (TRAF6), which unlocks signaling through NF-κB, p38 kinase, and c-Jun N-terminal kinase (Teitelbaum, 2000). OPG is released by osteoblasts and stromal cells and is expressed by macrophages in synovial lining layer. Bone resorption is controlled by the balance between RANKL, RANK and osteoprotegerin (Crotti et al., 2002). The inhibition of RANKL in serum transfer model (Ji et al., 2002), in TNF-α-induced model (Keffer et al., 1991) and in autoimmune type II collagen-induced arthritis (Kamijo et al., 2006) resulted in amelioration of bone destruction.

Recently, Poubelle and co-workers reported that RA neutrophils express RANKL and are activated through RANK/RANKL interaction (Poubelle et al., 2007). Despite the studies in RA, there are no investigations showing the involvement of RANKL positive neutrophils in the pathogenesis of OA. A little is known about the expression of RANKL in active or inactive stages of OA. We have conducted a study on RANKL expression by neutrophils in OA patients and in mouse models. OA patients have been divided into two groups depending on the presence of active inflammatory process. The first group, with active OA had swelling, local hyperthermia of one or more joints and high erythrocyte sedimentation rate (ESR). The second group with inactive OA lacked above mentioned painful swelling and local hyperthermia. A number of healthy controls have also been included (Table 1).

	healthy controls	active OA	inactive OA
No. of subjects (women/men)	10 (4/6)	12 (5/7)	14 (6/8)
Duration (years)	not assessed	4.5 ± 1.2	2.5 ± 1.2
ESR (mm/h)	<20	24.8 ± 6.2	14.0 ± 3.6
RF	not assessed	<20	<20
CRP	<0.01	58.9 ± 30.4	<0.01

CRP – C reactive protein; ESR-erythrocyte sedimentation rate; OA-osteoarthritis; RF-rheumatoid factor; Data are expressed as mean ± standard error of the mean

Table 1. Basic characteristics of healthy donors and OA patients

The intensification of OA symptoms at established phase of the disease can be due to calcium-containing crystals. The basic calcium phosphate (BCP) and hydroxyapatite (HA) crystals are often found in joint fluid and tissues of OA patients. The reason for their accumulation is not clear but their contribution to the aggravation of inflammation is obvious (Mebarek et al., 2011; Rosenthal et al., 2011). The elevated ESR might reflect their action on innate immunity cells, inducing inflammatory signals and amplification of already generated. Moreover, the increase of BCP concentration correlates with the severity of the disease (Yavorskyy et al., 2008). To provoke an inhibition of crystal deposition or their degradation represents a novel and tempting approach for application in chronic phase which can limit joint damage.

In our study low percentage of RANKL positive blood neutrophils was detected in healthy donors (0.8 ± 0.4%). After their *in vitro* stimulation with TLR2 agonist, zymosan, they responded with an increased RANKL expression (8.22 ± 0.07%). Significantly higher percentage of RANKL positive blood neutrophils were observed in patients with active OA (14.75 ± 5.07 %; p<0.001 vs healthy) and inactive OA (9.77 ± 2.16%; p<0.01 vs healthy) but only inactive group responded to zymosan stimulation (Fig. 1).

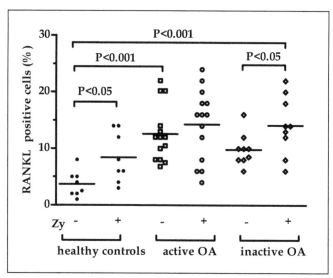

Fig. 1. RANKL expression on neutrophils isolated from healthy controls and patients with active and inactive osteoarthritis (OA). Cells (1x10⁶/ml) were incubated (37⁰C, 2 h) in the absence or presence of 10 µg/ml of zymosan (Zy). After washing neutrophils were stained with rat antibody against human RANKL and isotype control, followed by secondary FITC-conjugated anti-rat antibody. Data represent percentage of RANKL positive cells with the median value in the group (see lines in each group).

Experimental osteoarthritis was induced according to a method described by Blom et al. (Blom, et al. 2007). Mice received two intra-articular injections of collagenase (2 times x1U collagenase) at day 0 and 2. Arthritis onset occurs within 7 days. ZIA was induced by intra-articular injection of 180 µg (10 µl) of zymosan. In both models BALB/c mice 10-12 week old with weight 20-22 g were used. Whole-blood samples were collected in heparin and neutrophils were isolated by dextran sedimentation followed by gradient centrifugation, resuspended at 1x10⁶/ml and stimulated for 2 h with zymosan (10 µg/ml). After washing neutrophils were stained with rat antibody against mouse RANKL and isotype control, followed by secondary FITC-conjugated anti-rat antibody. Data from one representative experiment shows the mean fluorescence intensity and the percentage of RANKL positive cells.

Further, we have investigated RANKL expression on neutrophils in two mouse models: collagenase-induced osteoarthritis and zymosan-induced arthritis. We found low frequencies of RANKL positive neutrophils in blood of CIOA mice and a weak response to *in vitro* zymosan stimulation (Fig. 2). Blood neutrophis from ZIA mice expressed RANKL and responded to TLR2 engagement with increased RANKL expression (Fig. 2).

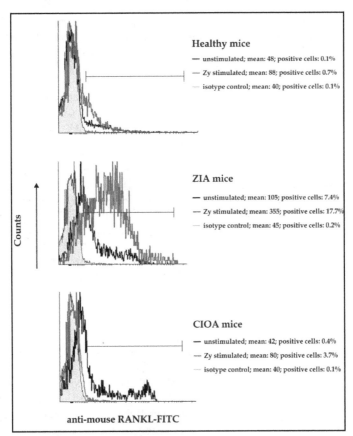

Fig. 2. RANKL expression by blood neutrophils isolated from mice with zymosan-induced arthritis (ZIA) and collagenase-induced osteoarthritis (CIOA) at day 30 of disease.

2.3 MRP8/MRP14 as a potential OA marker related to neutrophil recruitment

The rate of neutrophil and macrophage infiltration at the site of inflammation is associated with myeloid-related proteins (MRP)-8 and -14, belonging to S-100 family of calcium binding proteins. MRP8 and MRP14 are secreted by human monocytes after activation of protein kinase C (PKC) (Rammes et al., 1997). In inflammation they are expressed by infiltrating neutrophils, keratinocytes and monocytes in contrast to resting-tissue macrophages and lymphocytes (Frosch et al., 2000; Kerkhoff et al., 1998). Increased expression of these molecules has been established in various inflammatory disorders including RA (Youssef et al., 1999), psoriasis (Kunz et al., 1992), inflammatory bowel disease (Rugtveit et al., 1994), PsA (Kane et al., 2003). MRP8/MRP14 expression is very low in normal tissues and in RA patients in clinical remission, but high in patients with active disease (Brun et al., 1994). Similar levels of MRP8/MRP14 are found in synovial fluid from patients with psoriatic arthritis, RA and spondyloarthritis without a correlation with disease duration and clinical expression of arthritis activity (Bhardwaj et al., 1992). The proteins enriched more the synovial fluid than the blood circulation as a result of infiltration and activation of neutrophils and macrophages in the joints of RA patients. Very scarce data are available about MRP proteins in OA. It is supposed that the contact of phagocytes with activated endothelium leads to release of MRP8/MRP14, which induces the switch from selectin-mediated reversible adhesion to integrin-dependent tight contact (Frosch et al., 2000).

However, MRP8/MRP14 levels might be reliable prognostic marker for disease activity and for the effectiveness of immunosuppressive therapy. Methotrexate (MTX) treatment resulted in reduced MRP8/MRP14 serum levels (Kane et al., 2003; Ryckman et al., 2003). It is considered that in acute inflammation MRP8/14 and MRP14 are well represented, while MRP8 is associated with chronic inflammatory conditions (Roth et al., 2003). In our study we have included OA patients with or without an active inflammatory process in one or more joints (Toncheva et al., 2009). We observed high MRP8 plasma level in 30% of the patients with active OA (number of patients =37) and in 8% of the patients with inactive OA (number of patients =19). In healthy donors MRP8 level was very low (number of donors =31). Although our data suggest that the severity of OA might correlate with MRP8 plasma level it will be important to continue such investigations in larger groups of patients. The diagnostic value and advantage of MRPs over other disease markers is that they are released immediately upon activation of the particular cell population.

2.4 TLR2 expression by OA neutrophils

The progression of arthritic processes might be supported by the recognition of microbial or host-derived ligands found in arthritic joints. It has been shown that TLR2 and TLR4, but not TLR9, play distinct roles in disease pathogenesis (Abdollahi-Roodsaz et al., 2008). Knockout (IL1rn-/-) mice spontaneously develop T cell-mediated arthritis dependent on TLR activation since germ-free mice fail to develop arthritis. Activation of TLRs on macrophages and dendritic cells leads to the production of proinflammatory cytokines, including TNF-α and IL-1β. The role of the innate immune system in RA and in experimental models of RA has been the object of recent investigations. An increased expression of TLR2 and TLR4 on peripheral blood monocytes and in the synovial tissues from patients with RA has been observed (De Rycke et al., 2005; Iwahashi et al., 2004). Limited data exist on the quantitative TLR2 and TLR4 expression by synovial macrophages, but it is known that their expression was increased in RA compared with osteoarthritis or normal synovial tissue (Radstake et al., 2004). TLRs through NF-κB activation provoke the production of innate immunity mediators, like IL-1, IL-6, IL-8, and TNF-α (Takeuchi et al., 2000; Wang et al., 2001). Consequently, these molecules up-regulate TLR expression, e.g. TNF-α stimulates TLR2 gene expression in contrast to TLR4 (Matsuguchi et al., 2000). The stimulation of cultured RA synovial cells with IL-1β and TNF-α leads to an increase of TLR2 mRNA expression but such increase of TLR4 and TLR9 expression is not detected in the absence or in the presence of stimuli (Seibl et al., 2003). These results are not specific for RA, because cells derived from joints of patients with OA responded similarly to TNF-α stimulation.

Neutrophils express all known human TLRs except TLR3 (Hayashi et al., 2003). TNF-α and IL-6 production in neutrophils can be triggered upon the engagement of TLR2, TLR4, TLR9. In neutrophils the ligation of TLRs results in activation of MAPK and NF-kB but not always involves the adaptor protein MyD88. In respect to TLR4, recently it has been reported that

LPS can induce different response in adherent and in suspended neutrophils. In adherent cells TLR4 ligation triggers Jun activation and the release of the chemokine monocyte chemoattractant protein-1, an activated protein-1-dependent gene product that is important for monocyte recruitment. Adherent neutrophils interact with matrix proteins through sheded CD43. CD43 (leukosialin) is a heavily sialylated molecule that is cleaved by neutrophil elastase near the plasma membrane. In blood CD43 binds albumin that protects it from the elastase action. In inflammatory conditions neutrophils secrete elastase enhancing the spread and rolling of neutrophils. In RA the destruction of cartilage and bone might be associated with the activation of synovial cells through TLR2. The ligands of TLR2 include lipopetides and peptidoglycan (Aliprantis et al., 1999; Schwandner et al., 1999), and zymosan acting in collaboration with TLR6 and CD14 (Ozinsky et al., 2000). While TLR4 is weakly represented on the surface of human neutrophils, TLR2 and CD14 are well expressed (Kurt-Jones et al., 2002).

To investigate the involvement of TLR2 in OA we followed its constitutive and Zy-induced expression in blood neutrophils. Data in Fig. 3 show that the percentage of TLR2 positive neutrophils from OA patients was approximately 4 fold higher compared to healthy donors. Zymosan stimulation resulted in 2 fold enhancement of TLR2 expression on neutrophils from all groups.

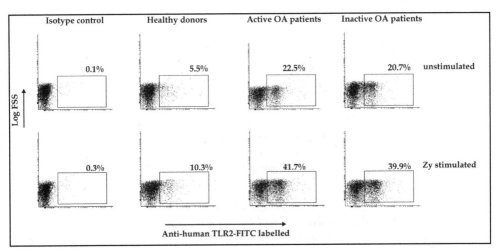

Fig. 3. TLR2 positive neutrophils from healthy donors and patients with active and inactive osteoarthritis (OA). Cells (1×10^6/ml) were incubated (37^0C, 2 h) in the absence or presence of 10 μg/ml of zymosan (Zy). Cells were collected, washed and stained with rat antibodies against human TLR2 (3 μg/ml), followed by secondary FITC-conjugated anti-rat antibody.

Neutrophils isolated from healthy and OA donors were *in vitro* simulated with zymosan and the secretion of TNF-α was determined. Neutrophils from patients with active OA spontaneously release the cytokine in contrast to healthy and inactive OA groups. Zymosan significantly enhanced TNF-α secretion of healthy donors and inactive OA (Fig. 4A). The spontaneous release of TNF-α was higher in ZIA and CIOA groups compared to healthy group. Neutrophils from arthritic mice did not respond significantly to zymosan stimulation, while healthy group showed increased TNF-α production (Figure 4B).

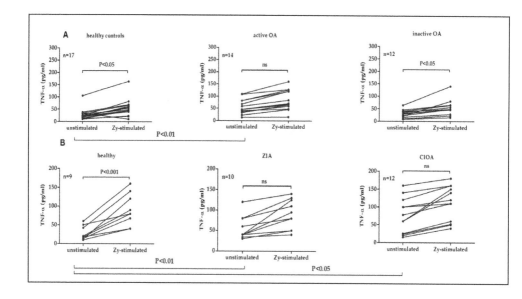

Fig. 4. Spontaneous and zymosan-induced TNF-α production by blood neutrophils. (A) Cells isolated from healthy donors and patients with active and inactive osteoarthritis (1x10⁶/ml) were incubated (37⁰C, 24 h) in the absence or presence of 10 µg/ml of zymosan. (B) Cells isolated from healthy mice and mice with zymosan-induced arthritis (ZIA,) and collagenase-induced osteoarthritis (CIOA) at day 30 of arthritis (1x10⁶/ml) were incubated (37⁰C, 24 h) in the absence or presence of 10 µg/ml of zymosan. TNF-α concentration in the supernatants was determines by ELISA.

The up-regulation of TLR2 corresponds either to a response to an exposure to microbial compounds or is secondary to the inflammatory milieu present in the rheumatoid joints. TNF-α is a key mediator in inflammatory joint diseases. We observed the activation state of neutrophils at least in active OA, which was witnessed by their spontaneous *ex vivo* TNF-α release. Our previous results showed that TLR4 ligand LPS is able to trigger *in vitro* TNF-α release by neutrophils from patients with inactive OA (Toncheva et al., 2009). Zymosan also enhanced TNF-α production of neutrophils from inactive OA patients. Probably in active OA, being in activated state cells has reached a threshold after which they become unresponsive. The results from ZIA and CIOA point on such possibility if we accept that ZIA is relevant to more severe inflammatory condition than CIOA. In synovial explant cultures it has been proved that a monoclonal antibody against TLR2 can inhibit the spontaneous release of TNF-α, IFN-γ, IL-1β and IL-8. Such data are a good base for future investigations on the use of TLR2 antagonists by clinicians, because the effect of anti-TLR2 antibodies is comparable with that of the TNF inhibitor adalimumab (Nic An Ultaigh et al., 2011).

2.5 Activation of monocytes and macrophages during OA

Monocytes and macrophages play an important role in various inflammatory conditions, depending on their stage of activation (Burmester et al., 1997; Tak et al., 1997). Monocytes are subdivided into two different populations with distinct phenotype and functional activity. While classical monocytes are CD14hiCD16- in humans and GR1+ in mouse, non-classical monocytes are CD14lowCD16+ in man and GR1- in mouse. Classical monocytes highly express the CC-chemokine receptor 2 (CCR2), CD62 ligand (CD62L) (Tacke et al., 2007) and vascular cell adhesion molecule 1 (VCAM1 or CD106), and produce low levels of proinflammatory cytokines like TNF-α and IL-1. The latter mediators activate synovial endothelial cells and other leukocytes and initiate inflammatory process. Non-classical monocytes or "resident" monocytes express high level of CX$_3$C-chemokine receptor 1 (CX$_3$CR1) and are potent antigen-presenting cells. It has been shown that monocytes from arthritic patients with active disease have reduced HLA–DR expression and decreased capacity to stimulate T cells *in vitro* than healthy cells (Muller et al., 2009). Moreover, TNF-α inhibits HLA-DR synthesis in arthritic myeloid cells via the expression of class II transactivator (CIITA). In comparison to RA, OA patients showed lower density of HLA-DR expression on peripheral monocytes (Koller et al., 1999) suggesting their intrinsic functional abnormality to act as antigen-presenting cells.

An accumulation of macrophages is found in the synovium of patients with early OA (Benito et al., 2005). These resident tissue cells are CD68 positive. CD68+ macrophages in OA synovium were restricted to the lining layer while in RA patients they were found in the sublining layer and the areas around newly formed micro-vessels. In the study of Bloom et al. macrophages are depleted prior the development of early OA by injection of clodronate liposomes (Blom et al., 2004). The lack of macrophages reduced the size of osteophytes and lining thickness, and inhibits chondrocyte ossification and fibrosis. Macrophage depletion also down-regulates the expression of bone morphogenetic proteins, BMP2 and BMP4 in synovium (van Lent et al., 2004). Both molecules are important regulators of bone remodeling process and their inhibition has good therapeutic potential in OA as we have observed in a model of CIOA (Ivanovska & Dimitrova, 2011).

Under OA conditions, CD68+ macrophages in synovial lining layer are persistently activated via NF-κB, STAT and Pi3K signaling pathways. They are the source of inducible nitric oxide and of proinflammatory cytokines like TNF-α and IL-1β (Benito et al., 2005) driving inflammatory process in OA and causing synovitis and bone erosion. Apart of this role, macrophages can participate directly in cartilage degradation. They are capable to produce enzymes degrading extracellular matrix macromolecules like disintegrin-metalloproteinases with thrombospondin motifs and MMPs like MMP-2, MMP-3 and MMP-9 (Smeets et al., 2003). While MMP-2 activates the expression of other MMPs in chondrocytes, MMP-3 is directly involved in cartilage destruction. Serum level of MMP-3 is associated with joint space narrowing in OA patients (Lohmander et al., 2005). MMP-3-deficient mice show significantly decreased cartilage damage (Blom et al., 2007). In rabbit model of experimental arthritis MMP-3 is initially up-regulated in the synovium contributing to the appearance of cartilage lesions while MMP-3 derived from chondrocyte exacerbate cartilage loss at late phases of OA (Mehraban et al., 1998). Blom et al. showed that at early experimental OA synovial macrophages are responsible for the initial MMP-3 production (Blom et al., 2007). These data are based on the observation that MMP-3 expression in the synovium is strongly reduced in the absence of synovial macrophages.

Secreted by macrophages MMPs are proteases that cleave not only collagen in bone matrix but also can modify other molecules present in the OA synovium. For example MMP-9 cleaves chemokines CXCL1 and CXCL8 increasing their potency to attract neutrophils and to amplify inflammation and bone erosion (Van den Steen et al., 2000).

Synovial macrophages can secrete pro-inflammatory mediators that increase MMP expression by synovial cells or chondrocytes. Macrophages isolated from synovial lining layer of OA patients produce spontaneously IL-1β and TNF-α. In synovial cell co-cultures macrophages stimulate the synovial fibroblasts to produce MMPs and cytokines like IL-6 and IL-8 via a synergistic action of IL-1β and TNF-α (Bondeson et al., 2006). IL-1β synthesis in OA is independent of TNF-α and correlates with OA severity. The biological activity of IL-1β is regulated by the balance between the expression of the active receptor IL-1RI and the inactive or decoy receptor IL-1RII. While the IL-1RI is highly expressed the decoy receptor IL-1RII is little or missing in OA. This receptor imbalance in turn decreases the ability of IL-1RII to neutralize completely and eliminate active IL-1. IL-1 together with TNF-α promotes osteoclast differentiation and bone resoption. It has been shown that IL-1 alone can induce osteoclastogensis but only in osteoclast precursors over-expressing IL-1R1 (Kim et al., 2009). Several *in vitro* studies show that IL-1 inhibition by natural inhibitors such as IL-1 receptor antagonist or soluble receptors decreases MMP expression and cartilage destruction in OA (Jacques et al., 2006).

Macrophages can produce pro-inflammatory cytokine IL-18. The administration of IL-18 at the initial and late phase of arthritis accelerates the development of disease. Despite that IL-18 is detected at low amounts in OA synovium (Gracie et al., 1999) it can stimulate the expression of MMP-3, MMP-13, aggrecanase-2, TIMP-1 in chondrocytes promoting bone destructive process. Recently, it has been shown that IL-21 is a proinflammatory cytokine that increases CXCL8 production by monocyte-derived macrophages. The receptor for IL-21 was detected on monocytes, monocyte-derived macrophages and on synovial macrophages from RA patients (Jungel et al., 2004). IL-21R has limited expression in OA synovium but it is expressed in the areas with enhanced catabolic processes and might participate in destructive process.

Macrophages also release factors that are important for tissue repair and suppression of inflammatory response. Among these factors are vascular endothelial growth factor CD106 (Haywood et al., 2003), prostaglandin E2, IL-10 and TGF-β. TGF-β expression from macrophages can be triggered by lipoxin A4 produced by activated neutrophils. TGF-β inhibits T cell proliferation and inflammatory responses. The anti-inflammatory cytokine IL-10 regulates the synthesis of IL-4, and inhibits IFN-γ production in T cells and TNF-α and IL-1β production in macrophages. The important role of anti-inflammatory cytokines IL-10 and IL-4 in OA has been well described in studies on experimental OA where these cytokine are administrated. The combined treatment with low dosages of IL-4 and IL-10 has potent anti-inflammatory effects and markedly protected against OA cartilage destruction. Improved anti-inflammatory effect was achieved with IL-4/prednisolone treatment (Joosten et al., 1999).

The progression of OA might result in an inappropriate differentiation of resident tissue macrophages, and expression of functionally distinct phenotype (Mantovani et al., 2007; Xu et al., 2005). Macrophage functions are tightly regulated by reversible histone acetylation with acetylases (HAT enzymes) and deacetylation with deacetylases (HDAC enzymes) (Grabiec et al., 2010).

Resident macrophages in different tissues such as lung, liver and synovium express Z39Ig (CRIg) protein (Helmy et al., 2006). The Z39Ig is a receptor for complement fragments C3b and iC3b and is a type 1 transmembrane protein of the immunoglobulin superfamily member. Significant Z39Ig staining is detected in macrophage-enriched areas in the lining and sublining areas of RA synovium (Lee et al., 2006). In OA synovial tissue the number of cells expressing Z39Ig was lower and the positive staining was restricted to the lining-layer macrophages. A significant number of Z39Ig+CD11c+cells observed in some cases of OA and PsA points that Z39Ig+CD11c+cells deserve extended investigations to clarify their functional activity in OA (Tanaka et al., 2008).

It has been shown that prostaglandin E2 secreted by macrophages contributes to pain hypersensitivity by promoting sensory neurons hyperexcitability. Tissue-resident macrophages constitutively express receptor P2X4 and the stimulation via P2X4R triggers calcium influx and p38 MAPK phosphorylation and COX-dependent release of PGE2 (Ulmann et al., 2010). These data suggest that synovial lining macrophages might be important effectors that control pain relieve in OA patients.

Osteoclasts and monocytes are not only derived from a common myeloid progenitor but their activity might be influenced by common mediators (Ross, 2000). Activation of CD40 signaling in monocytes/macrophages results in up-regulation of nitric oxide generation (Tian et al., 1995), and induction of metalloproteinase production (Malik et al., 1996). Recently, it was found that except CD40L, the known activator of monocytes/macrophages, also OPGL can express such function (Andersson et al., 2002). Mice deficient in CD40L expression display a deficiency in T cell-dependent macrophage-mediated immune responses (Stout et al., 1996). The development of osteoclasts is strongly dependent on the interactions between two members of TNF superfamily, OPGL and its receptor RANK (Lacey et al., 1998; Yasuda et al., 1998). One of the pathways for triggering inflammatory processes by OPGL is through p38 MAPK and p42/44 ERK and inducing cytokine and chemokine secretion (Suttles et al., 1996). Results from in vivo application of RANK-Fc in a model of antibody-mediated arthritis showed that it blocked OPGL activity and ameliorated arthritis development (Seshasayee et al., 2004).

3. TLR9 expression in OA

Toll-like receptors are involved not only in pathogen recognition but they can participate in triggering the inflammatory and joint destructive process in arthritis or they can enhance the progression of already established synovitis. TLR-mediated inflammatory response may induce further tissue damage and can provoke a self-sustaining inflammatory loop responsible for chronic progression of arthritis processes. The expression of TLR9 in the joints was assessed in chronic phase (day 30) of ZIA and CIOA. In healthy mice no detectable expression of TLR9 was found in the synovium in contrast to CIOA and ZIA, where synovial lining was extensively stained (Fig. 5A).

We observed stronger TLR9 positive staining in the bone and bone marrow of ZIA than of CIOA, in comparison to healthy mice showing only single positive cells (Fig. 5B). Most intensive accumulation of TLR9 positive cells was established in ZIA mice, especially well exerted in the sites of osteophyte formation (Fig. 5C)

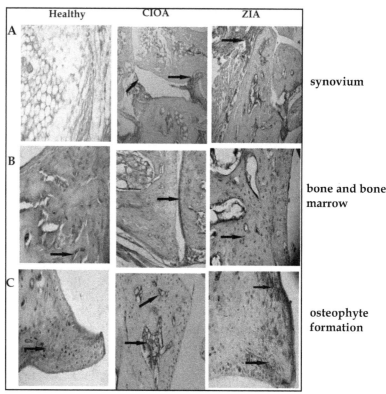

Fig. 5. Histological analyses of TLR9 expression in the joint. Dissected ankle joints were fixed in 10% paraformaldehyde/PBS, decalcified in 5% nitric acid for 1 week, dehydrated and embedded in paraffin. Sections (6 μm thickness) were blocked with 5% bovine serum albumin/PBS for 1 h and the endogenous peroxidase was blocked with 0.3% H_2O_2 in 60% methanol for 10 min. After washing, the sections were incubated for 40 min at room temperature with antibodes against mTLR9 (10 μg/ml). Isotype anti-mouse IgG was used as a background staining control. Then, the joint sections were incubated for 10 min with biotinylated anti-mouse IgGs and streptavidin-peroxidase was added for 10 min. The sections were washed and incubated with DAB solution kit (3',3'diaminobenzididne kit, Abcam) for 10 min and counterstained with Gill's hematoxylin. Arrows show positive TLR9 staining (magnification 40x).

The different TLR9 expression might be due to the difference in both models. Zymosan-induced arthritis is an example for proliferative arthritis, which is restricted to the joint injected with zymosan (Bernotiene et al., 2004). Using this model we found that histologically, joint sections showed cell infiltration into cartilage, capsule, osteoid and surrounding soft tissue and synovial hyperplasia without aggressive pannus formation. Proteoglycan depletion in cartilage, detected by loss of safranin O staining intensity, and changes in joint architecture were observed at late stage of arthritis. Interestingly, we observed the immunoreactivity for TNF-αR and C5aR in cartilage, along with C5aR positive inflammatory cells in the areas of bone and synovium. At the onset of ZIA, TNF-α plays a dominant role in inflammation. In the synovial extracts were found increased levels of IL-6 and C5a that can regulate the expression of C5aR on infiltrating neutrophils (Dimitrova et al., 2010; Dimitrova et al., 2011). CIA was provoked by intraarticular injections of collagenase, leading to acute ligament instability and prolonged inflammatory cartilage erosion over a period of six weeks. The model is relevant to human osteoarthritis pathology. In order to look for correlation between elevated TLR expression and the severity of arthritis we investigated the changes of TLR9 expression by macrophages from different origin in established ZIA. Data showed high presence of TLR9 positive cells in peritoneal exudates and PLNs in arthritic animals, while such elevation was not established for spleens (Fig. 6). These results deserve further experiments on the role of macrophages in the maintenance of inflammation in different organs. The elevation in lymph node population might be due to the fact that PLN is located most closely to the site of zymosan injection in inflamed joint.

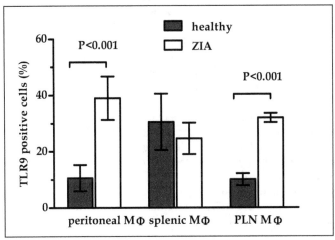

Fig. 6. TLR9 expression in macrophages isolated from different compartments at day 30 of ZIA. Differentiated macrophages isolated from peritoneal exudates (peritoneal Mφ), spleens (splenic Mφ) and popliteal lymph nodes (PLN Mφ) of healthy and ZIA mice (1x10⁶/ml) were stained with antibodies against mouse TLR9 (1 μg/ml), followed by secondary FITC-conjugated anti-mouse antibody and subjected to FACS analysis.

4. Natural killer cells

Natural killer cells are firstly described by their capacity to limit the growth of malignant cells and to eliminate virus-infected cells. They are innate immune effectors that produce immunoregulatory cytokines, such as interferon (IFN)-γ and granulocyte macrophage-colony-stimulating factor GM-CSF (Bancroft, 1993; Feng et al., 2006). Later, it became evident that NK cells can play a critical role in various autoimmune diseases, including rheumatoid arthritis by improving or exacerbating immune responses. They can play dual role in autoimmune diseases, either support or suppress pathogenic processes. In animal models it is established that NK cells are responsible for the induction and progression of K/BxN serum transfer model, being engaged through activation of their FcgIII receptors (Kim et al., 2006) and also being involved in the acceleration and exacerbation of CIA (Chu et al., 2007). The induction of CIA in NK-depleted mice reduces the severity of arthritis and almost completely prevents bone erosion (Soderstrom et al., 2010). In these experiments, also significantly reduced inflammation, pannus formation, and synovitis have been observed. NK cells are enriched within the joints of RA patients but how they contribute to disease pathology is currently not fully elucidated. In RA patients NK cells comprise 20 % of the synovial fluid cells at the early phase of disease (de Matos et al., 2007; Tak et al., 1994). These cells express CD56 and CD94/NKG2A phenotype, but failed to express CD16 similarly to peripheral RA NK cells.

Two distinct subsets of mature NK cells have been recognized, CD56[bright] and CD56[dim]. CD56[bright] subset is the source of IFN-γ, TNF-β, IL-10, IL-13, and GM-CSF, whereas the CD56[dim] NK cell subset produces significantly less of these cytokines in vitro (Cooper et al., 2001). The CD56[bright] NK cells express a chemokine receptor pattern similar to that of monocytes including high-affinity receptors for IL-15 (Carson et al., 1994). This subset has been identified in the joints of patients with early synovitis in RA. Several studies have shown that IL-15 is a critical factor for the development of human and murine NK cells (Kennedy et al., 2000; Mrozek et al., 1996). This might be due to its stimulation of M-CSF and RANKL expression by NK cells. IL-15 alone did not change the ability of monocytes to enhance osteoclast formation, while this process was dramatically supported in the presence of both NK cells and IL-15, indicating that the effect of IL-15 is mediated through NK cells (Soderstrom et al., 2010).

NK cells may be implicated in the initiation, the maintenance or the progression of autoimmune diseases directly or through their interaction with dendritic cells, macrophages or T lymphocytes. Whether neutrophils are capable to regulate and influence the activity of NK cells is not well defined. Generally, data on neutrophils and NK cells concern RA and are focused mainly on cytokines. There are no available investigations in OA in regard to remodeling events and the participation of these cells in OA has been underestimated. The investigations of NK-cell functions in patients with OA will improve our capacity to monitor these cells as possible markers for disease activity and will provide new prospects for NK-cell–directed therapies.

5. Mast cells

Nearly two decades ago available data show that when compared with healthy individuals, patients with OA had elevated numbers of intact and degranulated mast cells in the synovium and synovial fluid of diseased joints. Histological studies confirmed significant numbers of mast cells in both RA and OA synovium (Dean et al., 1993; Kopicky-Burd et al., 1988). Moreover, the numbers of mast cells in OA are comparable with those in RA when clinically active arthritis is envisaged. Prednisone used as anti-rheumatic drug lowered synovial mast cell number (Bridges et al., 1991). Mast cells containing triptase (MCT) expanded in the SF of OA patients (Buckley et al., 1998), while cells containing triptase and chimase (MCTC) expand in RA but not in OA (Gotis-Graham et al., 1998). When mast cell numbers in RA and OA patients are compared without respect to mast cell distribution in the subsynovial layer or the stratum fibrosum, no statistical differences between the diseases could be observed (Fritz et al., 1984). Synovial fluid collected from patients with hand OA expressed elevated number of mast cells in correlation with high content of histamine and elevated levels of tryptase and NO (Renoux et al., 1996). Such data support the hypothesis that in OA the increase of mast cells may participate in the pathological process, at least they can contribute in concert with other inflammatory cells.

6. Adipokines as potential participants in OA

Although leptin has been discovered fifteen years ago, the investigations on adipokines as potential participants in arthritic diseases are now at its beginning. Innate immunity cells appeared to be a source of adipokines as well as an object of their action. Leptin realizes its action as a proinflammatory cytokine through modulation of monocytes, macrophages, neutrophils, basophils, eosinophils, natural killer and dendritic cells (Otero et al., 2005). It seems to play a role in auto immune diseases such as RA and OA, by expressing harmful as well protective action on joint structures in RA (Lago et al., 2007). Leptin has been detected in SF obtained from patients with OA, and it was strongly overexpressed in human OA cartilage and in osteophytes (Dumond et al., 2003). The administration of exogenous leptin in rats increases IGF1 and TGFβ1 production suggesting that high circulating leptin levels might protect cartilage from osteoarthritic erosion but it also can induce osteophyte formation. Although adiponectin was discovered almost at the same time as leptin, its role in obesity-related dis orders has now begun to be investigated. In joint disorders adiponectin might play proinflammatory role beimg involved in matrix degradation. The pathogenic role of adiponectin is largely unknown in concern to RA and OA. Recent data proved that in chronic RA patients adiponectin plasma levels are higher compared to healthy controls, but lower plasma levels than in OA (Laurberg et al., 2009). Another member of this group is resistin (FIZZ3) which is found in adipocytes, macrophages and other cell types. It has been determined in the plasma and the synovial fluid of RA patients. The injection of resistin into mice joints induces an arthritis-like condition, with typical leukocyte infiltration in the synovium and tissue hypertrophy (Bokarewa et al., 2005). There are not enough data to make firm conclusions about the exact role of adipokines in arthritic processes. Their physiological role in RA or OA and their use as disease markers deserve to be a subject of further studies.

7. Conclusions

In the hope of defining novel therapeutic targets in OA much attention has been paid on degenerative processes of cartilage and secondary bone damage. But in recent years, the synovium, and in particular the participation of synovial cells and their mediators are under intensive study. Macrophages, neutrophils and lymphocytes act together with resident fibroblasts in the destructive phases of arthritis through liberation of proinflammatory molecues. Activated macrophages produced chemoattractants such as chemoattractant protein 1, RANTES, MIP-2α and epithelial neutrophil activator (Choy & Panayi, 2001). Many studies have been devoted to investigating various signaling pathways involved in proinflammatory cytokine production from OA synovial macrophages. The promising results of anticytokine therapies in RA prompted that such approach might be used in OA (Bondeson, 2010). Major population of infiltrated cells in synovium are neutrophils. This is valid for the early phase of inflammation as well as for its maintenance. The injection of anti-neutrophil antibodies ameliorated the established disease in collagen-LPS-induced model and K/BxN model (Nandakumar et al., 2003; Tanaka et al., 2006). Instead of macrophage/monocyte or neutrophil depletion which can impair host resistance, neutralizing antibodies blocking their chemotaxis might be used. Promising results in animal models have been obtained with ant-MIP-1α antibodies (Kagari et al., 2003) and pertussis toxin blocking of signals from G protein-coupled receptors (GPCRs) (Becker et al., 1985; Painter et al., 1987; Spangrude et al., 1985).

There is a large unmet need for reliable biochemical markers that will predict the subset of patients who are at risk of the disease progression and will be used to find molecular targets in future therapies. Elevated RANKL levels in synovium and circulation, and particularly increased RANKL expression by neutrophils in OA, makes it a suitable candidate for disease prognosis.

The ability of known TLR agonists to activate neutrophil functions supports the notion that TLRs are an important pattern recognition receptors in the function of these cells. Consequently, while producing chemokines they trigger migration of other immune cells, such as more neutrophils, monocytes, macrophages, NK cells, and immature dendritic cells. These results prompt a possible correlation between the increase of TLR2 positive blood cells, including neutrophils and existing OA condition and strongly support the idea that OA inflammation might be influenced through TLR2. Also, elevated TLR9 expression is detected in the joints of arthritic mice. Whether TLRs involvement is similar for both inactive and active OA is a question to be resolved. TLR-dependent mechanisms may contribute to the activation of synovial cells, possibly leading to the destruction of cartilage and bone in the pathogenesis of RA and OA.

8. Acknowledgments

This work has been supported by the project BG051PO001/3.3-05-001 „Science and Business, financed by Operating Program "Development of human resources" to European Social Fund.

9. Abbreviations

CIOA – collagenase-induced osteoarthritis; ERK – extracellular signal-regulated kinase; FITC - fluorescein isothiocianate; GM-CSF - granulocyte-macrophage colony-stimulating factor; IFN-γ - interferon gamma; IL – interleukine; MAPK-mitogen-activated protein kinase; MIP-2 - macrophage inflammatory protein; MMP - matrix metalloproteinase; MRPs – myeloid-related proteins; NF-kB – nuclear factor-kappa B; NK cells – natural killer cells; OA – osteoarthritis; OPG - osteoprotegerin ; Pi3K - phosphatidylinositol 3-kinases; RA – rheumatoid arthritis; RANK – receptor activator of nuclear factor-kappa B; RANKL - receptor activator of nuclear factor-kappa B ligand; RANTES - Regulated upon Activation, Normal T-cell Expressed, and Secreted; STAT - Signal Transducer and Activator of Transcription; TGF-β – transforming growth factor beta; TIMP-1 - TIMP metallopeptidase inhibitor 1; TLR – Toll-like receptor; TNF - tumor necrosis factor; Z39Ig - Immunoglobulin superfamily protein Z39IG; ZIA – zymosan-induced arthritis

10. References

Abdollahi-Roodsaz, S., Joosten, L.A., Koenders, M.I., Devesa, I., Roelofs, M.F., et al. (2008). Stimulation of TLR2 and TLR4 differentially skews the balance of T cells in a mouse model of arthritis. *Journal of Clinical Investigation*, Vol.118, No1, pp. 205-216, ISSN 0021-9738

Aliprantis, A.O., Yang, R.B., Mark, M.R., Suggett, S., Devaux, B., et al. (1999). Cell activation and apoptosis by bacterial lipoproteins through toll-like receptor-2. *Science*, Vol.285, No5428, pp. 736-739.

Andersson, U., Erlandsson-Harris, H., Yang, H. & Tracey, K.J. (2002). HMGB1 as a DNA-binding cytokine. *Journal of Leukocyte Biology*, Vol.72, No6, pp. 1084-1091, ISSN 0741-5400

Bancroft, G.J. (1993). The role of natural killer cells in innate resistance to infection. *Current Opinion in Immunology*, Vol.5, No4, pp. 503-510, ISSN 0952-7915

Becker, E.L., Kermode, J.C., Naccache, P.H., Yassin, R., Marsh, M.L., et al. (1985). The inhibition of neutrophil granule enzyme secretion and chemotaxis by pertussis toxin. *Journal of Cell Biology*, Vol.100, No5, pp. 1641-1646, ISSN 0021-9525

Bell, A.L., Magill, M.K., McKane, R. & Irvine, A.E. (1995). Human blood and synovial fluid neutrophils cultured in vitro undergo programmed cell death which is promoted by the addition of synovial fluid. *Annals of the Rheumatic Diseases*, Vol.54, No11, pp. 910-915, ISSN 0003-4967

Benito, M.J., Veale, D.J., FitzGerald, O., van den Berg, W.B. & Bresnihan, B. (2005). Synovial tissue inflammation in early and late osteoarthritis. *Annals of the Rheumatic Diseases*, Vol.64, No9, pp. 1263-1267.

Bernotiene, E., Palmer, G., Talabot-Ayer, D., Szalay-Quinodoz, I., Aubert, M.L., et al. (2004). Delayed resolution of acute inflammation during zymosan-induced arthritis in leptin-deficient mice. *Arthritis Research and Therapy*, Vol.6, No3, pp. R256-263, ISSN 1478-6362

Bhardwaj, R.S., Zotz, C., Zwadlo-Klarwasser, G., Roth, J., Goebeler, M., et al. (1992). The calcium-binding proteins MRP8 and MRP14 form a membrane-associated heterodimer in a subset of monocytes/macrophages present in acute but absent in chronic inflammatory lesions. *European Journal of Immunology*, Vol.22, No7, pp. 1891-1897, ISSN 0014-2980

Blom, A.B., van Lent, P.L., Holthuysen, A.E., van der Kraan, P.M., Roth, J., et al. (2004). Synovial lining macrophages mediate osteophyte formation during experimental osteoarthritis. *Osteoarthritis and Cartilage*, Vol.12, No8, pp. 627-635, ISSN 1063-4584

Blom, A.B., van Lent, P.L., Libregts, S., Holthuysen, A.E., van der Kraan, P.M., et al. (2007). Crucial role of macrophages in matrix metalloproteinase-mediated cartilage destruction during experimental osteoarthritis: involvement of matrix metalloproteinase 3. *Arthritis and Rheumatism*, Vol.56, No1, pp. 147-157, ISSN 0004-3591

Bokarewa, M., Nagaev, I., Dahlberg, L., Smith, U. & Tarkowski, A. (2005). Resistin, an adipokine with potent proinflammatory properties. *Journal of Immunology*, Vol.174, No9, pp. 5789-95, SSN 0022-1767

Bondeson, J. (2010). Activated synovial macrophages as targets for osteoarthritis drug therapy. *Curr Drug Targets*, Vol.11, No5, pp. 576-585, ISSN 1873-5592

Bondeson, J., Wainwright, S.D., Lauder, S., Amos, N. & Hughes, C.E. (2006). The role of synovial macrophages and macrophage-produced cytokines in driving aggrecanases, matrix metalloproteinases, and other destructive and inflammatory responses in osteoarthritis. *Arthritis Research and Therapy*, Vol.8, No6, pp. R187, ISSN 1478-6362

Brach, M.A., deVos, S., Gruss, H.J. & Herrmann, F. (1992). Prolongation of survival of human polymorphonuclear neutrophils by granulocyte-macrophage colony-stimulating factor is caused by inhibition of programmed cell death. *Blood*, Vol.80, No11, pp. 2920-2924, ISSN 0006-4971

Bridges, A.J., Malone, D.G., Jicinsky, J., Chen, M., Ory, P., et al. (1991). Human synovial mast cell involvement in rheumatoid arthritis and osteoarthritis. Relationship to disease type, clinical activity, and antirheumatic therapy. *Arthritis and Rheumatism*, Vol.34, No9, pp. 1116-1124, ISSN 0004-3591

Brun, J.G., Jonsson, R. & Haga, H.J. (1994). Measurement of plasma calprotectin as an indicator of arthritis and disease activity in patients with inflammatory rheumatic diseases. *Journal of Rheumatology*, Vol.21, No4, pp. 733-738, ISSN 0315-162X

Buckley, M.G., Gallagher, P.J. & Walls, A.F. (1998). Mast cell subpopulations in the synovial tissue of patients with osteoarthritis: selective increase in numbers of tryptase-positive, chymase-negative mast cells. *Journal of Pathology*, Vol.186, No1, pp. 67-74, ISSN 0022-3417

Burmester, G.R., Stuhlmuller, B., Keyszer, G. & Kinne, R.W. (1997). Mononuclear phagocytes and rheumatoid synovitis. Mastermind or workhorse in arthritis? *Arthritis and Rheumatism*, Vol.40, No1, pp. 5-18, ISSN 0004-3591

Carson, W.E., Giri, J.G., Lindemann, M.J., Linett, M.L., Ahdieh, M., et al. (1994). Interleukin (IL) 15 is a novel cytokine that activates human natural killer cells via components of the IL-2 receptor. *Journal of Experimental Medicine*, Vol.180, No4, pp. 1395-1403, ISSN 0022-1007

Chakrabarti, S. & Patel, K.D. (2005). Regulation of matrix metalloproteinase-9 release from IL-8-stimulated human neutrophils. *Journal of Leukocyte Biology*, Vol.78, No1, pp. 279-288,

Chakravarti, A., Rusu, D., Flamand, N., Borgeat, P. & Poubelle, P.E. (2009). Reprogramming of a subpopulation of human blood neutrophils by prolonged exposure to cytokines. *Laboratory Investigation*, Vol.89, No10, pp. 1084-1099, ISSN 1530-0307

Choy, E.H. & Panayi, G.S. (2001). Cytokine pathways and joint inflammation in rheumatoid arthritis. *New England Journal of Medicine*, Vol.344, No12, pp. 907-916, ISSN 0028-4793

Chu, C.Q., Swart, D., Alcorn, D., Tocker, J. & Elkon, K.B. (2007). Interferon-gamma regulates susceptibility to collagen-induced arthritis through suppression of interleukin-17. *Arthritis and Rheumatism*, Vol.56, No4, pp. 1145-1151, ISS N0004-3591

Cooper, M.A., Fehniger, T.A., Turner, S.C., Chen, K.S., Ghaheri, B.A., et al. (2001). Human natural killer cells: a unique innate immunoregulatory role for the CD56(bright) subset. *Blood*, Vol.97, No10, pp. 3146-3151, ISSN 0006-4971

Cross, A., Bucknall, R.C., Cassatella, M.A., Edwards, S.W. & Moots, R.J. (2003). Synovial fluid neutrophils transcribe and express class II major histocompatibility complex molecules in rheumatoid arthritis. *Arthritis and Rheumatism*, Vol.48, No10, pp. 2796-2806.

Crotti, T.N., Smith, M.D., Weedon, H., Ahern, M.J., Findlay, D.M., et al. (2002). Receptor activator NF-kappaB ligand (RANKL) expression in synovial tissue from patients with rheumatoid arthritis, spondyloarthropathy, osteoarthritis, and from normal patients: semiquantitative and quantitative analysis. *Annals of the Rheumatic Diseases*, Vol.61, No12, pp. 1047-1054.

De Matos, C.T., Berg, L., Michaelsson, J., Fellander-Tsai, L., Karre, K., et al. (2007). Activating and inhibitory receptors on synovial fluid natural killer cells of arthritis patients: role of CD94/NKG2A in control of cytokine secretion. *Immunology*, Vol.122, No2, pp. 291-301.

De Rycke, L., Vandooren, B., Kruithof, E., De Keyser, F., Veys, E.M., et al. (2005). Tumor necrosis factor alpha blockade treatment down-modulates the increased systemic and local expression of Toll-like receptor 2 and Toll-like receptor 4 in spondylarthropathy. *Arthritis and Rheumatism*, Vol.52, No7, pp. 2146-2158, ISSN0004-3591

Dean, G., Hoyland, J.A., Denton, J., Donn, R.P. & Freemont, A.J. (1993). Mast cells in the synovium and synovial fluid in osteoarthritis. *British Journal of Rheumatology*, Vol.32, No8, pp. 671-675, ISSN 0263-7103

Dimitrova, P., Ivanovska, N., Schwaeble, W., Gyurkovska, V. & Stover, C. (2010). The role of properdin in murine zymosan-induced arthritis. *Molecular Immunology*, Vol.47, No7-8, pp. 1458-1466, ISSN0161-5890

Dimitrova, P., Toncheva, A., Gyurkovska, V. & Ivanovska, N. (2011). Involvement of soluble receptor activator of nuclear factor-kappaB ligand (sRANKL) in collagenase-induced murine osteoarthritis and human osteoarthritis. *Rheumatology International*, published online February 03 2011, DOI:10.1007/s00296-010-1723-8, ISSN0172-8172

Duan, H., Koga, T., Kohda, F., Hara, H., Urabe, K., et al. (2001). Interleukin-8-positive neutrophils in psoriasis. *Journal of Dermatological Science*, Vol.26, No2, pp. 119-124, ISSN0923-1811

Dumond, H., Presle, N., Terlain, B., Mainard, D., Loeuille, D. et al. (2003). Evidence for a key role of leptin in osteoarthritis. *Arthritis and Rheumatism*, Vol.48, No11, pp. 3118-29, ISSN0004-3591

Edwards, S.W. & Hallett, M.B. (1997). Seeing the wood for the trees: the forgotten role of neutrophils in rheumatoid arthritis. *Immunology Today*, Vol.18, No7, pp. 320-324, ISSN0167-5699

Felzmann, T., Gadd, S., Majdic, O., Maurer, D., Petera, P., et al. (1991). Analysis of function-associated receptor molecules on peripheral blood and synovial fluid granulocytes from patients with rheumatoid and reactive arthritis. *Journal of Clinical Immunology*, Vol.11, No4, pp. 205-212.

Feng, C.G., Kaviratne, M., Rothfuchs, A.G., Cheever, A., Hieny, S., et al. (2006). NK cell-derived IFN-gamma differentially regulates innate resistance and neutrophil response in T cell-deficient hosts infected with Mycobacterium tuberculosis. *Journal of Immunology*, Vol.177, No10, pp. 7086-7093, ISSN 0022-1767

Fritz, P., Muller, J., Reiser, H., Saal, J.G., Hadam, M., et al. (1984). Distribution of mast cells in human synovial tissue of patients with osteoarthritis and rheumatoid arthritis. *Zeitschrift fur Rheumatologie*, Vol.43, No6, pp. 294-298, ISSN 0340-1855

Frosch, M., Strey, A., Vogl, T., Wulffraat, N.M., Kuis, W., et al. (2000). Myeloid-related proteins 8 and 14 are specifically secreted during interaction of phagocytes and activated endothelium and are useful markers for monitoring disease activity in pauciarticular-onset juvenile rheumatoid arthritis. *Arthritis and Rheumatism*, Vol.43, No3, pp. 628-637, ISSN 0004-3591

Gotis-Graham, I., Smith, M.D., Parker, A. & McNeil, H.P. (1998). Synovial mast cell responses during clinical improvement in early rheumatoid arthritis. *Annals of the Rheumatic Diseases*, Vol.57, No11, pp. 664-671, ISSN 0003-4967

Grabiec, A.M., Krausz, S., de Jager, W., Burakowski, T., Groot, D., et al. (2010). Histone deacetylase inhibitors suppress inflammatory activation of rheumatoid arthritis patient synovial macrophages and tissue. *Journal of Immunology*, Vol.184, No5, pp. 2718-2728, ISSN 0022-1767

Gracie, J.A., Forsey, R.J., Chan, W.L., Gilmour, A., Leung, B.P., et al. (1999). A proinflammatory role for IL-18 in rheumatoid arthritis. *Journal of Clinical Investigation*, Vol.104, No10, pp. 1393-1401, ISSN 0021-9738

Hayashi, F., Means, T.K. & Luster, A.D. (2003). Toll-like receptors stimulate human neutrophil function. *Blood*, Vol.102, No7, pp. 2660-2669, ISSN 0006-4971

Haywood, L., McWilliams, D.F., Pearson, C.I., Gill, S.E., Ganesan, A., et al. (2003). Inflammation and angiogenesis in osteoarthritis. *Arthritis and Rheumatism*, Vol.48, No8, pp. 2173-2177, ISSN 0004-3591

Hedbom, E. & Hauselmann, H.J. (2002). Molecular aspects of pathogenesis in osteoarthritis: the role of inflammation. *Cellular and Molecular Life Sciences*, Vol.59, No1, pp. 45-53.

Helmy, K.Y., Katschke, K.J., Jr., Gorgani, N.N., Kljavin, N.M., Elliott, J.M., et al. (2006). CRIg: a macrophage complement receptor required for phagocytosis of circulating pathogens. *Cell*, Vol.124, No5, pp. 915-927, ISSN 0092-8674

Ivanovska, N. & Dimitrova, P. (2011). Bone resorption and remodeling in murine collagenase-induced osteoarthritis after administration of glucosamine. *Arthritis Research and Therapy*, Vol.13, No2, pp. R44, ISSN 1478-6354

Iwahashi, M., Yamamura, M., Aita, T., Okamoto, A., Ueno, A., et al. (2004). Expression of Toll-like receptor 2 on CD16+ blood monocytes and synovial tissue macrophages in rheumatoid arthritis. *Arthritis and Rheumatism*, Vol.50, No5, pp. 1457-1467, ISSN 0004-3591

Jacques, C., Gosset, M., Berenbaum, F. & Gabay, C. (2006). The role of IL-1 and IL-1Ra in joint inflammation and cartilage degradation. *Vitamins and Hormones*, Vol.74pp. 371-403, ISSN 0083-6729

Ji, H., Pettit, A., Ohmura, K., Ortiz-Lopez, A., Duchatelle, V., et al. (2002). Critical roles for interleukin 1 and tumor necrosis factor alpha in antibody-induced arthritis. *Journal of Experimental Medicine*, Vol.196, No1, pp. 77-85

Joosten, L.A., Lubberts, E., Helsen, M.M., Saxne, T., Coenen-de Roo, C.J., et al. (1999). Protection against cartilage and bone destruction by systemic interleukin-4 treatment in established murine type II collagen-induced arthritis. *Arthritis Research and Therapy*, Vol.1, No1, pp. 81-91, ISSN 1465-9905

Jungel, A., Distler, J.H., Kurowska-Stolarska, M., Seemayer, C.A., Seibl, R., et al. (2004). Expression of interleukin-21 receptor, but not interleukin-21, in synovial fibroblasts and synovial macrophages of patients with rheumatoid arthritis. *Arthritis and Rheumatism*, Vol.50, No5, pp. 1468-1476, ISSN 0004-3591

Kagari, T., Tanaka, D., Doi, H. & Shimozato, T. (2003). Essential role of Fc gamma receptors in anti-type II collagen antibody-induced arthritis. *Journal of Immunology*, Vol.170, No8, pp. 4318-4324, ISSN 0022-1767

Kamijo, S., Nakajima, A., Ikeda, K., Aoki, K., Ohya, K., et al. (2006). Amelioration of bone loss in collagen-induced arthritis by neutralizing anti-RANKL monoclonal antibody. *Biochemical and Biophysical Research Communications*, Vol.347, No1, pp. 124-132.

Kane, D., Roth, J., Frosch, M., Vogl, T., Bresnihan, B., et al. (2003). Increased perivascular synovial membrane expression of myeloid-related proteins in psoriatic arthritis. *Arthritis and Rheumatism*, Vol.48, No6, pp. 1676-1685, ISSN 0004-3591

Keffer, J., Probert, L., Cazlaris, H., Georgopoulos, S., Kaslaris, E., et al. (1991). Transgenic mice expressing human tumour necrosis factor: a predictive genetic model of arthritis. *EMBO Journal*, Vol.10, No13, pp. 4025-4031.

Kennedy, M.K., Glaccum, M., Brown, S.N., Butz, E.A., Viney, J.L., et al. (2000). Reversible defects in natural killer and memory CD8 T cell lineages in interleukin 15-deficient mice. *Journal of Experimental Medicine*, Vol.191, No5, pp. 771-780, ISSN 0022-1007

Kerkhoff, C., Klempt, M. & Sorg, C. (1998). Novel insights into structure and function of MRP8 (S100A8) and MRP14 (S100A9). *Biochimica et Biophysica Acta*, Vol.1448, No2, pp. 200-211, ISSN 0006-3002

Kilpatrick, L.E., Sun, S., Mackie, D., Baik, F., Li, H., et al. (2006). Regulation of TNF mediated antiapoptotic signaling in human neutrophils: role of delta-PKC and ERK1/2. *Journal of Leukocyte Biology*, Vol.80, No6, pp. 1512-1521, ISSN 0741-5400

Kim, H.Y., Kim, S. & Chung, D.H. (2006). FcgammaRIII engagement provides activating signals to NKT cells in antibody-induced joint inflammation. *Journal of Clinical Investigation*, Vol.116, No9, pp. 2484-2492, ISSN 0021-9738

Kim, J.H., Jin, H.M., Kim, K., Song, I., Youn, B.U., et al. (2009). The mechanism of osteoclast differentiation induced by IL-1. *Journal of Immunology*, Vol.183, No3, pp. 1862-1870, ISSN 1550-6606

Koller, M., Aringer, M., Kiener, H., Erlacher, L., Machold, K., et al. (1999). Expression of adhesion molecules on synovial fluid and peripheral blood monocytes in patients with inflammatory joint disease and osteoarthritis. *Annals of the Rheumatic Diseases*, Vol.58, No11, pp. 709-712, ISSN 0003-4967

Kopicky-Burd, J.A., Kagey-Sobotka, A., Peters, S.P., Dvorak, A.M., Lennox, D.W., et al. (1988). Characterization of human synovial mast cells. *Journal of Rheumatology*, Vol.15, No9, pp. 1326-1333, ISSN 0315-162X

Kragstrup, T.W., Otkjaer, K., Holm, C., Jorgensen, A., Hokland, M., et al. (2008). The expression of IL-20 and IL-24 and their shared receptors are increased in rheumatoid arthritis and spondyloarthropathy. *Cytokine*, Vol.41, No1, pp. 16-23.

Kunz, M., Roth, J., Sorg, C. & Kolde, G. (1992). Epidermal expression of the calcium binding surface antigen 27E10 in inflammatory skin diseases. *Archives of Dermatological Research*, Vol.284, No7, pp. 386-390, ISSN 0340-3696

Kurt-Jones, E.A., Mandell, L., Whitney, C., Padgett, A., Gosselin, K., et al. (2002). Role of toll-like receptor 2 (TLR2) in neutrophil activation: GM-CSF enhances TLR2 expression and TLR2-mediated interleukin 8 responses in neutrophils. *Blood*, Vol.100, No5, pp. 1860-1868.

Lacey, D.L., Timms, E., Tan, H.L., Kelley, M.J., Dunstan, C.R., et al. (1998). Osteoprotegerin ligand is a cytokine that regulates osteoclast differentiation and activation. *Cell*, Vol.93, No2, pp. 165-176, ISSN 0092-8674

Lago, F., Dieguez, C., Gomez-Reino, J., Gualillo, O. (2007). Adipokines as emerging mediators of immune response and inflammation. *Nature Clinical Practical Rheumatology*, Vol.3, No12, pp.716-24, ISSN 1745-8382

Laurberg, T.B., Frystyk, J., Ellingsen, T., Hansen, I.T., Jorgensen, A. (2009). Plasma adiponectin in patients with active, early, and chronic rheumatoid arthritis who are steroid- and disease-modifying antirheumatic drug-naive compared with patients with osteoarthritis and controls. *Journal of Rheumatology*, Vol.36, No9, pp.1885-1891, ISSN 0315-162X

Lee, M.Y., Kim, W.J., Kang, Y.J., Jung, Y.M., Kang, Y.M., et al. (2006). Z39Ig is expressed on macrophages and may mediate inflammatory reactions in arthritis and atherosclerosis. *Journal of Leukocyte Biology*, Vol.80, No4, pp. 922-928, ISSN 0741-5400

Lohmander, L.S., Brandt, K.D., Mazzuca, S.A., Katz, B.P., Larsson, S., et al. (2005). Use of the plasma stromelysin (matrix metalloproteinase 3) concentration to predict joint space narrowing in knee osteoarthritis. *Arthritis and Rheumatism*, Vol.52, No10, pp. 3160-3167, ISSN 0004-3591

Malik, N., Greenfield, B.W., Wahl, A.F. & Kiener, P.A. (1996). Activation of human monocytes through CD40 induces matrix metalloproteinases. *Journal of Immunology*, Vol.156, No10, pp. 3952-3960, ISSN 0022-1767

Mantovani, A., Sica, A. & Locati, M. (2007). New vistas on macrophage differentiation and activation. *European Journal of Immunology*, Vol.37, No1, pp. 14-16, ISSN 0014-2980

Marshall, J.C., Malam, Z. & Jia, S. (2007). Modulating neutrophil apoptosis. *Novartis Foundation Symposium*, Vol.280, pp. 53-66; discussion 67-72, 160-164, ISSN 1528-2511

Matsuguchi, T., Musikacharoen, T., Ogawa, T. & Yoshikai, Y. (2000). Gene expressions of Toll-like receptor 2, but not Toll-like receptor 4, is induced by LPS and inflammatory cytokines in mouse macrophages. *Journal of Immunology*, Vol.165, No10, pp. 5767-5772, ISSN 0022-1767

Mebarek, S., Hamade, E., Thouverey, C., Bandorowicz-Pikula, J., Pikula, S., et al. (2011). Ankylosing spondylitis, late osteoarthritis, vascular calcification, chondrocalcinosis and pseudo gout: toward a possible drug therapy. *Current Medicinal Chemistry*, Vol.18, No14, pp. 2196-2203, ISSN 0929-8673

Mehraban, F., Lark, M.W., Ahmed, F.N., Xu, F. & Moskowitz, R.W. (1998). Increased secretion and activity of matrix metalloproteinase-3 in synovial tissues and chondrocytes from experimental osteoarthritis. *Osteoarthritis and Cartilage*, Vol.6, No4, pp. 286-294, ISSN 1063-4584

Mitsuyama, K., Toyonaga, A., Sasaki, E., Watanabe, K., Tateishi, H., et al. (1994). IL-8 as an important chemoattractant for neutrophils in ulcerative colitis and Crohn's disease. *Clinical and Experimental Immunology*, Vol.96, No3, pp. 432-436, ISSN 0009-9104

Mrozek, E., Anderson, P. & Caligiuri, M.A. (1996). Role of interleukin-15 in the development of human CD56+ natural killer cells from CD34+ hematopoietic progenitor cells. *Blood*, Vol.87, No7, pp. 2632-2640, ISSN 0006-4971

Muller, I., Munder, M., Kropf, P. & Hansch, G.M. (2009). Polymorphonuclear neutrophils and T lymphocytes: strange bedfellows or brothers in arms? *Trends Immunol*, Vol.30, No11, pp. 522-530, ISSN 1471-4981

Nandakumar, K.S., Svensson, L. & Holmdahl, R. (2003). Collagen type II-specific monoclonal antibody-induced arthritis in mice: description of the disease and the influence of age, sex, and genes. *American Journal of Pathology*, Vol.163, No5, pp. 1827-1837, ISSN 0002-9440

Nic An Ultaigh, S., Saber, T.P., McCormick, J., Connolly, M., Dellacasagrande, J., et al. (2011). Blockade of Toll-like receptor 2 prevents spontaneous cytokine release from rheumatoid arthritis ex vivo synovial explant cultures. *Arthritis Research and Therapy*, Vol.13, No1, pp. R33, ISSN 1478-6354

Otero, M., Lago, R., Lago, F., Casanueva, F.F., Dieguez. C. et al. Leptin, from fat to inflammation: old questions and new insights. (2005). *FEBS Letters*, Vol.579, No2, pp.295-301, ISSN 0014-5793

Ottonello, L., Cutolo, M., Frumento, G., Arduino, N., Bertolotto, M., et al. (2002). Synovial fluid from patients with rheumatoid arthritis inhibits neutrophil apoptosis: role of adenosine and proinflammatory cytokines. *Rheumatology*, Vol.41, No11, pp. 1249-1260, ISSN 1462-0324

Ozinsky, A., Underhill, D.M., Fontenot, J.D., Hajjar, A.M., Smith, K.D., et al. (2000). The repertoire for pattern recognition of pathogens by the innate immune system is defined by cooperation between toll-like receptors. *Proceedings of the National Academy of Sciences of the United States of America*, Vol.97, No25, pp. 13766-13771.

Painter, R.G., Zahler-Bentz, K. & Dukes, R.E. (1987). Regulation of the affinity state of the N-formylated peptide receptor of neutrophils: role of guanine nucleotide-binding proteins and the cytoskeleton. *Journal of Cell Biology*, Vol.105, No6 Pt 2, pp. 2959-2971, ISSN 0021-9525

Poubelle, P.E., Chakravarti, A., Fernandes, M.J., Doiron, K. & Marceau, A.A. (2007). Differential expression of RANK, RANK-L, and osteoprotegerin by synovial fluid neutrophils from patients with rheumatoid arthritis and by healthy human blood neutrophils. *Arthritis Research and Therapy*, Vol.9, No2, pp. R25.

Pronai, L., Ichikawa, Y., Ichimori, K., Nakazawa, H. & Arimori, S. (1991). Association of enhanced superoxide generation by neutrophils with low superoxide scavenging activity of the peripheral blood, joint fluid, and their leukocyte components in rheumatoid arthritis: effects of slow-acting anti-rheumatic drugs and disease activity. *Clinical and Experimental Rheumatology*, Vol.9, No2, pp. 149-155.

Radstake, T.R., Roelofs, M.F., Jenniskens, Y.M., Oppers-Walgreen, B., van Riel, P.L., et al. (2004). Expression of toll-like receptors 2 and 4 in rheumatoid synovial tissue and regulation by proinflammatory cytokines interleukin-12 and interleukin-18 via interferon-gamma. *Arthritis and Rheumatism*, Vol.50, No12, pp. 3856-3865, ISSN 0004-3591

Rammes, A., Roth, J., Goebeler, M., Klempt, M., Hartmann, M., et al. (1997). Myeloid-related protein (MRP) 8 and MRP14, calcium-binding proteins of the S100 family, are secreted by activated monocytes via a novel, tubulin-dependent pathway. *Journal of Biological Chemistry*, Vol.272, No14, pp. 9496-9502, ISSN 0021-9258

Raza, K., Scheel-Toellner, D., Lee, C.Y., Pilling, D., Curnow, S.J., et al. (2006). Synovial fluid leukocyte apoptosis is inhibited in patients with very early rheumatoid arthritis. *Arthritis Res earch and Therapy*, Vol.8, No4, pp. R120, ISSN 1478-6362

Renoux, M., Hilliquin, P., Galoppin, L., Florentin, I. & Menkes, C.J. (1996). Release of mast cell mediators and nitrites into knee joint fluid in osteoarthritis--comparison with articular chondrocalcinosis and rheumatoid arthritis. *Osteoarthritis and Cartilage*, Vol.4, No3, pp. 175-179, ISSN 1063-4584

Rosenthal, A.K. (2011). Crystals, inflammation, and osteoarthritis. *Current Opinion in Rheumatology*, Vol.23, No2, pp. 170-173, ISSN 1040-8711

Ross, F.P. (2000). RANKing the importance of measles virus in Paget's disease. *Journal of Clinical Investigation*, Vol.105, No5, pp. 555-558, ISSN 0021-9738

Roth, J., Vogl, T., Sorg, C. & Sunderkotter, C. (2003). Phagocyte-specific S100 proteins: a novel group of proinflammatory molecules. *Trends Immunology*, Vol.24, No4, pp. 155-158, ISSN 1471-4906

Rugtveit, J., Brandtzaeg, P., Halstensen, T.S., Fausa, O. & Scott, H. (1994). Increased macrophage subset in inflammatory bowel disease: apparent recruitment from peripheral blood monocytes. *Gut*, Vol.35, No5, pp. 669-674, ISSN 0017-5749

Ryckman, C., Vandal, K., Rouleau, P., Talbot, M. & Tessier, P.A. (2003). Proinflammatory activities of S100: proteins S100A8, S100A9, and S100A8/A9 induce neutrophil chemotaxis and adhesion. *Journal of Immunology*, Vol.170, No6, pp. 3233-3242, ISSN 0022-1767

Santos, L.L., Morand, E.F., Hutchinson, P., Boyce, N.W. & Holdsworth, S.R. (1997). Anti-neutrophil monoclonal antibody therapy inhibits the development of adjuvant arthritis. *Clinical and Experimental Immunology*, Vol.107, No2, pp. 248-253.

Schwandner, R., Dziarski, R., Wesche, H., Rothe, M. & Kirschning, C.J. (1999). Peptidoglycan- and lipoteichoic acid-induced cell activation is mediated by toll-like receptor 2. *Journal of Biological Chemistry*, Vol.274, No25, pp. 17406-17409.

Seibl, R., Birchler, T., Loeliger, S., Hossle, J.P., Gay, R.E., et al. (2003). Expression and regulation of Toll-like receptor 2 in rheumatoid arthritis synovium. *American Journal of Pathology*, Vol.162, No4, pp. 1221-1227, ISSN 0002-9440

Seshasayee, D., Wang, H., Lee, W.P., Gribling, P., Ross, J., et al. (2004). A novel in vivo role for osteoprotegerin ligand in activation of monocyte effector function and inflammatory response. *Journal of Biological Chemistry*, Vol.279, No29, pp. 30202-30209, ISSN 0021-9258

Shen, F., Ruddy, M.J., Plamondon, P. & Gaffen, S.L. (2005). Cytokines link osteoblasts and inflammation: microarray analysis of interleukin-17- and TNF-alpha-induced genes in bone cells. *Journal of Leukocyte Biology*, Vol.77, No3, pp. 388-399.

Simon, T., Opelz, G., Weimer, R., Wiesel, M., Feustel, A., et al. (2003). The effect of ATG on cytokine and cytotoxic T-lymphocyte gene expression in renal allograft recipients during the early post-transplant period. *Clinical Transplantation*, Vol.17, No3, pp. 217-224, ISSN 0902-0063

Smeets, T.J., Barg, E.C., Kraan, M.C., Smith, M.D., Breedveld, F.C., et al. (2003). Analysis of the cell infiltrate and expression of proinflammatory cytokines and matrix metalloproteinases in arthroscopic synovial biopsies: comparison with synovial samples from patients with end stage, destructive rheumatoid arthritis. *Annals of the Rheumatic Diseases*, Vol.62, No7, pp. 635-638, ISSN 0003-4967

Soderstrom, K., Stein, E., Colmenero, P., Purath, U., Muller-Ladner, U., et al. (2010). Natural killer cells trigger osteoclastogenesis and bone destruction in arthritis. *Proceedings of the National Academy of Sciences of the United States of America*, Vol.107, No29, pp. 13028-13033, ISSN 0027-8424

Spangrude, G.J., Sacchi, F., Hill, H.R., Van Epps, D.E. & Daynes, R.A. (1985). Inhibition of lymphocyte and neutrophil chemotaxis by pertussis toxin. *Journal of Immunology*, Vol.135, No6, pp. 4135-4143, ISSN 0022-1767

Stout, R.D., Suttles, J., Xu, J., Grewal, I.S. & Flavell, R.A. (1996). Impaired T cell-mediated macrophage activation in CD40 ligand-deficient mice. *Journal of Immunology*, Vol.156, No1, pp. 8-11, ISSN 0022-1767

Suttles, J., Evans, M., Miller, R.W., Poe, J.C., Stout, R.D., et al. (1996). T cell rescue of monocytes from apoptosis: role of the CD40-CD40L interaction and requirement for CD40-mediated induction of protein tyrosine kinase activity. *Journal of Leukocyte Biology*, Vol.60, No5, pp. 651-657, ISSN 0741-5400

Tacke, F., Alvarez, D., Kaplan, T.J., Jakubzick, C., Spanbroek, R., et al. (2007). Monocyte subsets differentially employ CCR2, CCR5, and CX3CR1 to accumulate within atherosclerotic plaques. *Journal of Clinical Investigation*, Vol.117, No1, pp. 185-194, ISSN 0021-9738

Tak, P.P., Kummer, J.A., Hack, C.E., Daha, M.R., Smeets, T.J., et al. (1994). Granzyme-positive cytotoxic cells are specifically increased in early rheumatoid synovial tissue. *Arthritis and Rheumatism*, Vol.37, No12, pp. 1735-1743

Tak, P.P., Smeets, T.J., Daha, M.R., Kluin, P.M., Meijers, K.A., et al. (1997). Analysis of the synovial cell infiltrate in early rheumatoid synovial tissue in relation to local disease activity. *Arthritis and Rheumatism*, Vol.40, No2, pp. 217-225, ISSN 0004-3591

Takeuchi, O., Hoshino, K. & Akira, S. (2000). Cutting edge: TLR2-deficient and MyD88-deficient mice are highly susceptible to Staphylococcus aureus infection. *Journal of Immunology*, Vol.165, No10, pp. 5392-5396, ISSN 0022-1767

Tanaka, D., Kagari, T., Doi, H. & Shimozato, T. (2006). Essential role of neutrophils in anti-type II collagen antibody and lipopolysaccharide-induced arthritis. *Immunology*, Vol.119, No2, pp. 195-202, ISSN 0019-2805

Tanaka, M., Nagai, T., Tsuneyoshi, Y., Sunahara, N., Matsuda, T., et al. (2008). Expansion of a unique macrophage subset in rheumatoid arthritis synovial lining layer. *Clinical and Experimental Immunology*, Vol.154, No1, pp. 38-47, ISSN 0009-9104

Teitelbaum, S.L. (2000). Bone resorption by osteoclasts. *Science*, Vol.289, No5484, pp. 1504-1508.

Tian, L., Noelle, R.J. & Lawrence, D.A. (1995). Activated T cells enhance nitric oxide production by murine splenic macrophages through gp39 and LFA-1. *European Journal of Immunology*, Vol.25, No1, pp. 306-309, ISSN 0014-2980

Toncheva, A., Remichkova, M., Ikonomova, K., Dimitrova, P. & Ivanovska, N. (2009). Inflammatory response in patients with active and inactive osteoarthritis. *Rheumatology International*, Vol.29, No10, pp. 1197-1203.

Ulmann, L., Hirbec, H. & Rassendren, F. (2010). P2X4 receptors mediate PGE2 release by tissue-resident macrophages and initiate inflammatory pain. *EMBO Journal*, Vol.29, No14, pp. 2290-2300, ISSN 1460-2075

Van den Steen, P.E., Proost, P., Wuyts, A., Van Damme, J. & Opdenakker, G. (2000). Neutrophil gelatinase B potentiates interleukin-8 tenfold by aminoterminal processing, whereas it degrades CTAP-III, PF-4, and GRO-alpha and leaves RANTES and MCP-2 intact. *Blood*, Vol.96, No8, pp. 2673-2681, ISSN 0006-4971

van Lent, P.L., Blom, A.B., van der Kraan, P., Holthuysen, A.E., Vitters, E., et al. (2004). Crucial role of synovial lining macrophages in the promotion of transforming growth factor beta-mediated osteophyte formation. *Arthritis and Rheumatism*, Vol.50, No1, pp. 103-111, ISSN 0004-3591

Wang, J.E., Warris, A., Ellingsen, E.A., Jorgensen, P.F., Flo, T.H., et al. (2001). Involvement of CD14 and toll-like receptors in activation of human monocytes by Aspergillus fumigatus hyphae. *Infection and Immunity*, Vol.69, No4, pp. 2402-2406, ISSN 0019-9567

Xu, H., Manivannan, A., Dawson, R., Crane, I.J., Mack, M., et al. (2005). Differentiation to the CCR2+ inflammatory phenotype in vivo is a constitutive, time-limited property of blood monocytes and is independent of local inflammatory mediators. *Journal of Immunology*, Vol.175, No10, pp. 6915-6923, ISSN 0022-1767

Yasuda, H., Shima, N., Nakagawa, N., Yamaguchi, K., Kinosaki, M., et al. (1998). Osteoclast differentiation factor is a ligand for osteoprotegerin/osteoclastogenesis-inhibitory factor and is identical to TRANCE/RANKL. *Proceedings of the National Academy of Sciences of the United States of America*, Vol.95, No7, pp. 3597-3602.

Yavorskyy, A., Hernandez-Santana, A., McCarthy, G. & McMahon, G. (2008). Detection of calcium phosphate crystals in the joint fluid of patients with osteoarthritis - analytical approaches and challenges. *Analyst*, Vol.133, No3, pp. 302-318, ISSN 0003-2654

Youssef, P., Roth, J., Frosch, M., Costello, P., Fitzgerald, O., et al. (1999). Expression of myeloid related proteins (MRP) 8 and 14 and the MRP8/14 heterodimer in rheumatoid arthritis synovial membrane. *Journal of Rheumatology*, Vol.26, No12, pp. 2523-2528, ISSN 0315-162X

11

Cellular Physiology of Articular Cartilage in Health and Disease

Peter I. Milner, Robert J. Wilkins and John S. Gibson
University of Liverpool, University of Oxford & University of Cambridge
United Kingdom

1. Introduction

Articular chondrocytes live in an unusual and constantly changing physicochemical environment. Due to the structure of the extracellular matrix, adult cartilage is avascular, relatively hypoxic and acidic compared to other tissues (Wilkins et al., 2000). In this challenging environment the maintenance and regulation of extracellular matrix by chondrocytes is dependent on signals received through this milieu (Lai et al., 2002). In joint disease, such as osteoarthritis, the extracellular environment is altered and the cellular physiology of the chondrocyte will change to reflect this, leading to alterations in its key role of regulating matrix turnover and hence contributing to the pathophysiology of joint disease (Goldring 2006).

This chapter will discuss the challenges to the chondrocyte and how cellular physiology is affected in both health and disease. We will discuss how the structure of the matrix confers its biomechanical properties to cartilage and how this translates to physiological sensing by the cartilage during static and dynamic loading with particular emphasis on effects on membrane transporters and cell signalling pathways. We will also consider how other features of cartilage in the adult influence the chondrocyte, such as oxygen tension, osmolarity and pH. Finally we will consider the changes that occur in osteoarthritis and how these translate to alterations in cellular physiology and hence matrix integrity, the loss of the which is the key feature of osteoarthritis, and how these events may be new targets for treatment of this condition.

2. Structure of articular cartilage

Articular cartilage is a highly specialised tissue that provides a resilient, smooth, almost frictionless surface for joints to function efficiently and pain-free (Morris et al., 2002). In the adult, articular cartilage is avascular and predominately composed of extracellular matrix with a low density of resident cells, articular chondrocytes, which are responsible for the maintenance of the matrix in the healthy joint (Palmer & Bertone, 1994). Chondrocytes are embedded within a structurally organised matrix consisting of water, collagens, proteoglycans, glycosaminoglycans and non-collagenous proteins (Huber et al., 2000). The biochemical composition and structural alignment of these components within cartilage is responsible for the mechanical properties of this tissue and the cellular responses of the chondrocyte (Jeffery et al., 1991; Kuettner et al., 1991).

2.1 Articular chondrocytes and zonal organisation

Articular cartilage is organised to allow its main role to occur, that is, providing a smooth almost frictionless surface for pain-free mobility but also as a biomaterial that can also withstand compressive and shear forces. As well as the actual biochemical content of articular cartilage, the biomechanical properties rely on the structural organisation of the extracellular matrix and the cells embedded within them. The structure and organisation of articular cartilage not only varies with depth from the articular surface (divided into zones) but also the location within the joint (for example, weightbearing versus non-weightbearing surfaces).

Articular chondrocytes occupy 2-5% of the tissue volume and are sometimes considered relatively inactive metabolically due to an absence of a vascular supply but are responsible for maintaining the integrity of the extracellular matrix and can respond to mechanical stimuli, growth factors and cytokines. Articular cartilage has four distinct histological and biochemical zones (I-IV): superficial (tangential), intermediate (transitional), deep (radial) and calcified. The superficial zone is the thinnest along the articular surface and merges with the perichondrium at the articular margin. Type II collagen in the superficial zone is orientated tangentially to the articular surface to provide resistance to tensile forces. Proteoglycan composition in this zone acts as a non-selective barrier to diffusion of oxygen and water and a selective barrier to the diffusion of nutrients and hormones. This is largely due to the large amount of negatively charged anionic groups on the sulphated side chains on proteoglycans which allows smaller, non-ionic molecules through the matrix more readily than larger charged molecules. The pericellular matrix in the chondron (the chondrocyte and its pericellular microenvironment) consists of high levels of collagen type VI and aggregating proteoglycans and defines the physiochemical environment of the chondrocyte (Wang et al, 2008) and biochemical or mechanical signals perceived by the chondrocyte are therefore influenced by the structural and functional composition of the chondron (Guilak et al., 2006). Proteoglycans in the pericellular zone are thought to have a role in binding the chondrocyte to the matrix rather that the direct biomechanical role seen in the interterritorial matrix. Within the matrix surrounding the chondrocytes (territorial matrix) are thin type II and VI collagen fibrils, organised in a "basket-weave" formation and these fibrils extend out in a parallel arrangement to bind with larger type II collagen fibrils in the interterritorial matrix. In the intermediate zone the chondron structure is more typical. In this zone the collagen fibrils appears more widely spaced and their orientation is more random and there are increased amounts of proteoglycan compared to the superficial zone. In the deep zone the chondrocytes start to align themselves in columns perpendicularly to the joint surface along with thicker collagen fibrils. The collagen fibrils are orientated radially between these chondrocytic columns. The abundant proteoglycan within the interterritorial matrix with higher amounts of keratin sulphate side chains increases the permeability of the matrix in the deep zone and may be important in allowing diffusion of nutrients to the deeper layers of cartilage. Between the deep and calcified zones, there is a demarcation consisting of mineral associated with matrix vesicles within the interterritorial matrix and this is known as the tidemark.

2.2 The extracellular matrix

The extracellular matrix is a mechanically resilient structure comprising of collagens, proteoglycans and other non-collagenous proteins (Wilkins et al., 2000). Hydrated proteoglycans confer resistance to compression and are constrained by the collagen fibrillar meshwork (thought of as a "string-and-balloon" model). Proteoglycans, with highly sulphated glycosaminoglycan (GAG) side chains and fixed negative charges, attract free cations and osmotically obliged water, leading to a hydrated matrix of raised osmolarity and lowered pH. Avascularity of matrix means that movement of hormones, cytokines, nutrients and metabolites occurs over relatively large distances along steep gradients. The low partial pressures of oxygen denote that cells undergo predominately anaerobic glycolysis and must endure high concentrations of lactic acid. Added to these challenges, normal mechanical loading causes profound fluctuations in the physiochemical environment.

2.2.1 Collagen

There are a number of collagen types recognised in articular cartilage, but type II collagen is the primary collagen of articular cartilage, comprising 80-90% of the total collagen content (Becerra et al., 2010). Type II collagen acts primarily to provide tensile stiffness in cartilage (Kaab et al., 1998). Other collagens are formed due to different gene expression, translational splicing and post-translational modification and many have important regulatory and structural roles and may be associated with type II collagen (e.g. functional binding) or other components of the matrix (for example binding and interactions with proteoglycans and the chondrocyte).

Collagen fibrils extend out from the pericellular envelope into the territorial matrix (Morris et al., 2002). Further collagen fibrils extend out into the interterritorial matrix, intimately involved with proteoglycans. Numerous contacts are present between the plasma membrane, collagens and proteoglycans through the extracellular matrix. Pericellular matrix contains little or no fibrillar collagen but type VI collagen microfibrils that interact with hyaluronic acid (HA), small proteoglycans and cell surface molecules. Type IX collagen is found throughout cartilage matrix and type XI collagen is mainly localised to the territorial matrix interacting with type II collagen, adding to tensile strength. Type IX collagen appears to localise with type II collagen fibrils in particular regions and covalent cross-linking may alter size and stability and hence mechanical properties of the type II collagen fibrils.

2.2.2 Proteoglycans

Proteoglycans and glycosaminoglycans contribute compressive stiffness to articular cartilage (Hardingham & Forsang, 1992). There are a number of different types of these macromolecules present throughout cartilage and they can also function as regulatory proteins and binding sites for other matrix components. Aggrecan, one of the most common proteoglycans in cartilage, is a high molecular weight proteoglycan ($1\text{-}2 \times 10^6$ kDa) that binds HA in the matrix. Proteoglycans and proteoglycan link proteins are present throughout the extracellular matrix including the pericellular matrix and have structural relationships with collagens. Proteoglycans act as a selective permeability barrier and the structure of the matrix will dampen kinetic responses as diffusion through the matrix is slow. As well as contributing important mechanical properties to cartilage, proteoglycans are also important modulators of cell signalling and function.

2.2.3 Glycosaminoglycans

Glycosaminoglycans contain highly negatively charged polyanionic sulphate groups. It is this, as well as the large molecular weight of the proteoglycan aggrecan, that attracts cations, such as Na^+ and thereby water into the cartilage matrix and thus increasing tissue osmotic pressure (Wilkins et al., 2000). The resistance of the collagen fibrillar network to expansion therefore provides cartilage with an ability to resist compressive forces.   The main glycosaminoglycans identified in articular cartilage are chondroitin-4-sulphate, chondroitin-6-sulpate, keratin sulphate and hyaluronic acid (Morris et al., 2002).

In a typical aggrecan molecule there can be up to 100 chondroitin sulphate side chains attached to the core protein (via xyulose-serine bond), each with up to 1000 repeating disaccharide units.   Keratan sulphate is a smaller polysaccharide and there are usually around 50 keratin sulphate side chains linked to the aggrecan core protein (via a galactose-N-acetyl-threonine or –serine bond).   Hyaluronic acid ($1x10^4$ kDa) is also classified as a glycosaminoglycan although it lacks the sulphated groups on its D-glucosamine and D-glucuronic acid disaccharide chains.   Each HA can bind up to 100 aggrecan proteins. Early release of HA of the cell during synthesis may be important in articular cartilage structure since the length of HA influences proteoglycan binding and may affect proteoglycan aggregation and function (Palmer & Bertone 1994).

2.2.4 Water and water flow in cartilage

Water makes up approximately 70% of cartilage weight. Negatively charged proteoglycans attract cations and water follows leading to swelling of proteoglycans, resisting tension and shear forces.   Since the macromolecular composition of extracellular matrix of cartilage determines matrix hydration and tissue volume it therefore determines the space for molecular transport and offers compressive resistance (as water is essentially incompressible).   The hydrodynamic processes controlling the water content include osmosis, filtration, swelling and diffusion.

Osmotic flow of water occurs up gradients of osmotic pressure and cartilage can be thought of as a gel consisting of cross-linked non-ideal macromolecules (i.e. yield parameters which vary nonlinearly with concentration, a feature of a number of biological systems).   It is thought that within the proteoglycan network, an ensemble of segments interacting with each other may form "pores" through which the flow resistance for water is lowered (Comper 1996).

3. Cellular physiology of articular chondrocytes

The unusual biochemical structure of articular cartilage results in particular biomechanical properties that strongly influence the cellular physiology of the articular chondrocyte (Hall et al., 1996a). Due to the presence of fixed, highly negatively-charged polysulphated proteoglycans, there is an increase in cation (Na^+, K^+ and H^+) concentration in articular cartilage, compared to other tissues (e.g. plasma) leading to cartilage having raised osmolality (350-450mOsm.kg^{-1}) compared to synovial fluid (around 300mOsm.kg $^{-1}$). Under load, the physical and ionic environment of cartilage alters. Dynamic load leads to increased hydrostatic pressure causing cartilage deformation/ membrane stretch and fluid flows (Urban, 1994). On removal of load the matrix regains its steady-state conformation. If loading continues, though, these dynamic components are followed by slower osmotic consequences. Under static loading conditions, fluid expression results in changes to the extracellular environment, raising fixed negative charge of glycosaminoglycans and hence increases osmotic pressure.   These dynamic changes result in direct effects on articular chondrocyte function since not only does the extracellular environment change, intracellular cation concentrations fluctuate with load and altered membrane transport activities occur due to mechanical deformation of membranes and changes in pressure, osmolarity and pH. Additionally, this environment is altered in joint disease such as osteoarthritis since biochemical and biomechanical changes occur which will directly influence the chondrocyte.

3.1 Membrane transport in articular chondrocytes
Chondrocytes possess many of the membrane transport systems found in other cell types (Wilkins et al., 2000). Active membrane transport systems exchange cations whose intracellular concentrations fluctuate with load not only to maintain cellular homeostasis but these mechanisms can be linked to solute transport and intracellular signalling events and mechanotransduction events, important in the articular chondrocyte to maintain cartilage integrity through extracellular matrix synthesis.

3.1.1 Electrophysiology of articular chondrocytes
The resting membrane potential of articular chondrocytes is thought to be between -15mV and -44mV, maintained by Na^+/K^+ ATPase and is influenced by cyclical pressure (Clarke et al., 2010; Funabashi et al., 2010; Hall et al., 1996a). Potassium channels are integral membrane proteins, participating in cell membrane potential and belong to a large superfamily including voltage-activated potassium channels (K_v), Ca^{2+}-activated potassium channels (K_{Ca}) and inward rectifier potassium channels (Kir). Using whole cell-patch clamp techniques, a voltage-dependent, Ca^{2+}-independent K^+ current with rapid activation and very slow inactivation has been described in isolated canine articular chondrocytes (Wilson et al., 2004). ATP-sensitive K_{ATP} channels have also been demonstrated in articular cartilage (Mobasheri et al., 2007). K_{ATP} channels may couple metabolic events (i.e. intracellular ATP levels) to membrane electrical activity and potentially their activity may be may be important in low oxygen conditions since hypoxia is known to lead to activation of K_{ATP} channels in other systems (Miki & Seino, 2005). Additionally, electrophysiological responses of chondrocytes from osteoarthritic cartilage appears to differ from healthy cartilage (Sanchez & Lopez-Zapata 2010).

3.1.2 Volume regulation
The maintenance of cell volume in the face of alterations in the extracellular environment is an important cellular function (Hoffmann et al., 2009). Chondrocyte cell volume, as with other cell types, is determined by a pump-leak model where a double Donnan equilibrium exists between intracellular compartments and the matrix (Wilkins et al., 2000). Exclusion of Na^+ ions from the cell is maintained by Na^+-K^+ ATPase and cell volume is maintained by altered balance of leaks and pumps to hold cell water constant.

In articular chondrocytes, hypertonicity leads to regulatory volume increase (RVI) and raises intracellular potassium ($[K^+]_i$) via $Na^+/K^+/2Cl^-$ co-transporter (Hall et al., 1996b). Na^+/H^+ exchange (NHE), unlike in other cell systems in the body, does not appear to play a role in volume regulation in cartilage due to the lack of $Cl^- - HCO_3^-$ exchange activity which is required for RVI. During RVI, $[Na^+]_i$ is increased and the Na^+/K^+ pump is stimulated to keep $[K^+]_i:[Na^+]_i$ ratio optimal for protein and enzyme function. Removal of static load in cartilage results in cell swelling and the activation of regulatory volume decrease (RVD) processes. Cell swelling following hypotonic challenge leads to RVD in many cells via Cl^- -

dependent K^+ transporter, Ca^{2+}-activated K^+ (with associated Cl^- ions) channel or an "osmolyte" channel (e.g. taurine, sorbitol and myo-inositol) (Hoffmann et al., 2009). In chondrocytes, loss of osmolytes appears to occur via "osmolyte" channel and volume activated K^+ transport may also occur by this route (Hall & Bush 2001). Hypotonic challenge also leads to depolarisation via Na^+ influx through stretch activated cation channels (SACC) (Sanchez et al., 2003).

In cartilage, cells lysis is prevented by the ECM (akin to plant cells and cell wall) and thus avoiding the effects extremes of hyposmolarity (although static loading in normal joints only leads to fluid losses and decrease in cartilage hydration of only around 5% per day and these losses are restored when load is removed). However, in osteoarthritis (OA), proteoglycans are lost and reduced Na^+ and water content affects joint function. This increase in cartilage hydration under load is an early event in OA and could lead to changes in chondrocyte volume regulation (Bush & Hall 2005). Indeed the first changes in osteoarthritis are cell swelling suggesting the mechanisms for regulating cell volume are either lost or impaired.

3.1.3 Intracellular pH (pH$_i$) regulation

The acidic extracellular environment (pH 6.8) promotes inward leak of H^+ ions so chondrocytes are subjected to chronic acid loading. With low O_2 and anaerobic glycolysis as the primary source of metabolism resulting in lactate production, additional intracellular loading is also encountered. Articular chondrocytes have resting pH$_i$ of around 7.1 and a relatively high intracellular buffering capacity of around 30mmol.l^{-1} (pH$_i$) (Wilkins & Hall 1992). Intracellular pH (pH$_i$) regulation in chondrocytes predominately occurs through the amiloride-sensitive sodium-dependent Na^+/H^+ exchanger (NHE). As discussed previously the extracellular matrix is rich in Na^+ but poor in anions and therefore it appears that anion-dependent pH regulation been sacrificed in favour of SO_4^- uptake; an essential precursor for proteoglycan synthesis.

Extracellular acidity is an important regulator of cartilage matrix metabolism and activity of degradative enzymes. Changes in extra-and intracellular pH both elicit a bi-modal response of matrix synthesis (Wilkins & Hall, 1995). Small changes in extracellular pH (pH$_o$) quickly and significantly (up to 50%) inhibit synthesis rates (particularly below pH 6.9). It is possible, in normal cartilage, that matrix acidification could provide a means of regulating proteoglycan synthesis by a negative feedback system such that increased proteoglycan content raises H^+, thereby inhibiting synthesis.

There are a number of NHE isoforms characterised but the main "housekeeping" form is NHE-1 (Pedersen & Cala, 2004). Static loading leads to hyperosmolarity and hyperosmosis results in increased acid efflux in chondrocytes through the activation of NHE (Yamazaki et al., 2000). Enhanced H^+ extrusion under conditions of loading may allow a defence versus cellular acidosis and a mechanism whereby effects of this loading can be transduced into changes in cartilage turnover. Hypotonic shock, however, leads to an increase in pH$_i$ (alkalosis) via the opening of voltage-activated H^+ channels (VAHC) (Sanchez & Wilkins, 2003).

Serum leads to increased acid extrusion on response to intracellular acidosis. NHE3 is expressed following exposure to serum and cytokines (Tattersall et al., 2003), particularly IGF-1 (Tattersall et al., 2008). In contrast to NHE1, NHE3 is inhibited by hypertonicity and by PKA pathways but activated by hypotonicity. Exposure to serum factors occurring in osteoarthritic cartilage (damaged tissue more likely to be exposed to serum factors and IGF-1 is elevated in arthritic cartilage - van der Kraan & van den Berg, 2000) could therefore result in a differential response of NHE1 and 3 to hyperosmotic shock. Additionally this may have consequences for matrix synthesis which are dictated by pH. In addition to IGF-1, EGF has been shown to stimulate proton efflux by increasing activity of NHE involving PI3-kinase pathway (Lui et al., 2002).

Despite the chondrocyte already residing in an acidic extracellular matrix, further acidosis occurs in joint disease due to hypoxia and production of inflammatory cytokines altering blood flow. Since extracellular pH has a potent influence on cellular function (Das et al., 2010) any effect on the ability of the cell to regulate intracellular pH is likely to result in alteration in chondrocyte function, including matrix synthesis. Very low levels of oxygen, likely to be experienced in joint disease, reduce the activity of NHE resulting in intracellular acidosis in articular chondrocytes (Milner et al., 2006).

3.1.4 Intracellular calcium regulation

Intracellular calcium $[Ca^{2+}]_i$ in chondrocytes, as in many other cells has numerous physiological functions (Berridge et al., 1998). In articular chondrocytes, $[Ca^{2+}]_i$ is maintained at low levels (around 80nM) and Ca^{2+}-ATPase and Na^+-Ca^{2+} exchanger appear to be the dominant mediators of calcium homeostasis in these cells (Sanchez et al., 2003). The maintenance of calcium is a balance between Ca^{2+} extrusion, influx via membrane channels and Ca^{2+} release from intracellular stores, such as endoplasmic reticulum and mitochondria (Duchen, 2004; Sanchez et al., 2006).

Alterations in intracellular calcium can affect matrix synthesis (Wilkins et al., 2000) and calcium signaling has been implicated in mechanotransduction in articular chondrocytes (Guilak et al., 1999;). There are a number of studies showing that intracellular calcium in chondrocytes can be altered by hydrostatic pressure, osmotic stress and fluid flow (Kerrigan & Hall, 2008; Yellowley et al., 2002). Increased pressure and cell swelling induces a Gd^{3+}-sensitive $[Ca^{2+}]_i$ increase (Wilkins et al., 2003) and it has been shown that intracellular Ca^{2+} levels can also be modulated by pH (Sanchez and Wilkins, 2003).

3.1.5 Metabolite transport

Transport of metabolites across the plasma membrane has an important role in maintaining chondrocytic biosynthetic output and matrix integrity. The uptake of sulphate (SO_4^{2-}) is an important step in the synthesis of glycosaminoglycans and appears to occur in articular chondrocytes via a carrier-mediated mechanism that is Na^+-independent and sensitive to transmembrane H^+ gradient (stimulated by acidic extracellular pH) (Meredith et al., 2007). Probable candidates include SO_4^{2-} x Cl^- and SO_4^{2-} x OH^- exchanger (anion exchanger). Amino acid uptake occurs via Na^+-dependent (proline, glycine and glutamine) and independent (leucine) transporters (Wilkins et al., 2000).

Inorganic phosphate (P_i) uptake in chondrocytes appears to have both Na^+-dependent and – independent components and shows pH- sensitivity (Solomon et al., 2007). Transport of P_i across the cell membrane is an important component of the calcification process, particularly in the growth plate and the inappropriate formation of calcium-phosphate (hydroxyapatite) crystals in osteoarthritis could involve dysfunction of P_i-transporters.

Glucose provides energy source and is an essential precursor for glycosaminoglycan synthesis. GLUT transporters (e.g. IGF-1 modulated GLUT4) are mainly responsible for glucose uptake (Shikhman et al., 2004; Windhaber et al., 2003) whereas lactic acid transport appears via monocarboxylate family of transporters (MCT) including MCT1 ("housekeeper") and MCT4 (Meredith et al., 2002). MCT4 appears to be the main isoform in articular chondrocytes whose kinetics favour lactate export thereby allowing pyruvate conversion back to lactate to assist in NAD^+ regeneration and continued glycolysis.

4. Mechanotransduction in articular cartilage

The main functions of articular cartilage are concerned with load-bearing (Urban, 1994). During normal activity, pressures within cartilage may rise to 100-200 atmospheres (10-20 MPa) within milliseconds. The mechanical failure of extracellular matrix is a key event in the progression of degenerative joint disease since not only direct loss of function of the tissue occurs but detrimental effects on cellular activity and the potential repair process ensues. The ability of the chondrocyte to sense and respond appropriately to mechanical signals (mechanotransduction) is vital in maintaining cartilage integrity.

4.1 Mechano-electrochemical properties of cartilage and signal transduction

Physical environmental factors such as shear stress, fluid flow and electrical field alterations are known to be strong biologic factors in regulating cellular activities (Lai et al., 2002; Mow et al., 1999). During loading, a number of changes occur within cartilage, including increased hydrostatic pressure, cartilage/chondrocyte cell deformation, fluid flow and streaming potentials, changes in chondrocyte cell membrane and fluid loss resulting in changes to interstitial fluid osmolality/ionic content (Urban, 2000). Transducers of mechanotransduction in cells include activation of stretch activated channels allowing ingress of external Ca^{2+}, alteration of membrane transporter activity (eg Na^+/H^+ exchange) and activation of mechanosensitive ion channels and transporters such as transient receptor potential (TRP) channels and purinergic receptors. The ECM is directly linked to the cytoskeleton and nucleus of the cell via integrins. Integrins are central to many mechanotransduction pathways since they integrate a number of important intracellular signalling pathways, for example, focal adhesion kinase signaling via integrin-ECM (involving G-protein signaling) and other pathways (involving, for example MAPK and PI-3 kinases) (Loeser, 2002).

4.1.1 Streaming potential and diffusion potential

Streaming potentials and diffusion potentials can be used to describe the electrical forces generated during ionic species movement and these are thought to be important in mechanical signal transduction in cartilage. The potential induced by convection current (mechano-chemical force generated by cation and anion movement) in the presence of a pressure gradient gives the streaming potential of cartilage, whereas the potential induced by the diffusion in the presence concentration gradient is the diffusion potential and have been shown to be important modulators of chondrocyte metabolism (Kim et al., 1995).

4.1.2 Effects of mechanical load on chondrocyte function and matrix synthesis

Mechanical load is required to maintain cartilage integrity (Hasler et al., 1999). Matrix proteoglycan is lost from cartilage in immobilised joints and there is variation within a normal joint between unloaded and loaded regions. Regions subjected to load are often thicker and have higher proteoglycan content and therefore likely to be mechanically stronger. Dynamic or cyclic loading stimulates proteoglycan and protein synthesis whereas static loading is associated with decreased synthesis and in addition, load-induced solute movement can also influence rates at which growth factors or cytokines reach the cells and alter cellular metabolism.

When load is applied there is an increase in hydrostatic pressure, extracellular pH decreases and there is an increase in extracellular free cation concentration and osmolality. Alterations in the osmotic balance occurs as fluid is expressed to try to restore the hydrostatic equilibrium and this increases the concentrations of proteoglycans and hence cations, resulting in osmotic consequences. The changes in hydrostatic pressure and osmotic alteration lead to cellular deformation and change in volume resulting in changes in $[Na^+]_i$, $[K^+]_i$, pH_i and $[Ca^{2+}]_i$ due to altered transporter activity and therefore this can result in alterations in macromolecular synthesis.

During loading, cartilage from osteoarthritic joints will deform more than cartilage from non-diseased joints, since both the rate and amount of fluid loss are sensitive to proteoglycan concentrations. Therefore cartilage from degenerate joints will lose fluid faster than healthy cartilage and this is likely to alter the stimulus and hence the response of the chondrocyte in diseased tissue.

4.1.3 Hydrostatic pressure

During normal walking, articular cartilage cycles between a resting hydrostatic pressure of 0.2MPa and pressures of 4-5 MPa (2-50atm). It is known that pressures in the 5-50MPa range can alter cellular morphology, reduce exocytosis, dissociate cytoskeletal elements, reduce protein synthesis and inhibit membrane transport. The timing of the cycles is also important – application of cyclical pressures (>0.5Hz) have stimulatory effects on cartilage matrix synthesis. It also appears that isolated chondrocytes are more sensitive to pressure than *in situ* within the matrix and that the cytoskeleton and Golgi apparatus are involved in this response.

Physiological levels of hydrostatic pressure can affect membrane permeability to ions and amino acids and thus affect intracellular solute concentrations. Increase in hydrostatic pressure leads to increased rate of synthesis of matrix components and this may be exerted via alteration in intracellular pH. Browning et al., (1999) showed that application of 20-300atm to isolated cells led to NHE stimulation via phosphorylation-dependent processes. Additionally, hydrostatic pressure has been shown to inhibit membrane transport pathways (such as Na^+/K^+-pump, $Na^+/K^+/2Cl^-$ cotransporter) (Hall et al., 1999). Conformational alterations by cell deformation may be responsible for change in membrane transport activity as well as changes in their phosphorylation status. For example, pressure may uncouple ATP hydrolysis or alter lipid environment as to retard Na^+ binding or constrain conformational changes leading to altered activity of the Na^+/K^+ pump. Alteration in ion channel activity is therefore likely to be intimately linked to matrix synthesis.

4.1.4 Osmotic sensitivity of chondrocytes

Static loading leads to fluid expression and increased interstitial fluid osmolarity. The link between ECM hydration and chondrocyte metabolism appears to be via volume regulation. Cells respond to unequal tonicity by water movement across plasma membrane and this is usually rapid leading to cell volume changes within seconds. The osmometric behaviour of chondrocytes in situ and isolated from matrix appears to be similar although some differences in layers occur in situ (Bush & Hall, 2001). Superficial zone chondrocytes appear to swell more than middle or deeper zone cells and this may reflect less proteoglycan present in this zone. Additionally deeper zone chondrocytes may take longer to respond to water changes in cartilage so the response may depend on zone and local osmotic environment. Potentially, zone-specific alterations in physico-chemical signals may lead to differences in chondrocyte matrix biosynthesis.

Water can flux through membranes via aquaporins. Aquaporins (AQP) are water channel proteins that allow water to move in the direction of osmotic gradient and may also allow small solutes to pass, for example glycerol and urea. A role in cell volume regulation and mechanotransduction in chondrocytes has been proposed (Mobasheri et al., 2004). AQP1 and AQP3 are expressed in cartilage resulting in water permeability and may respond to environment changes since changes in aquaporin expression may be important in pathology.

Hyperosmotic stress induces a transient alteration in cellular volume and $[Ca^{2+}]_i$ (Erickson et al., 2001) but a latency appears to exist between minimum cell volume reached and peak Ca^{2+} levels. This may be explained by Na^+ entering the cell (possibly via voltage-gated sodium channels, VGSC, or epithelial sodium channels, ENaC), leading to depolarisation and subsequent increase in intracellular calcium levels. This then results in membrane hyperpolarisation and Ca^{2+} activated K^+ channels open causing K^+ efflux. Hypotonic shock also results in increased intracellular Ca^{2+} levels (Wilkins et al., 2003). Mechanosensitive Ca^{2+} channels appear to open in response to hypotonicity as well as calcium release from intracellular stores. Prolonged increase of intracellular calcium, however, is detrimental to the cell so mechanisms such as Na^+/Ca^{2+} exchanger are in operation to regulate this Ca^{2+} rise.

These stretch-activated ion channels may act as putative mechanical signal transducers since they lead to fluctuations in intracellular calcium levels that may affect gene expression. Potential mechanosensitive ion channels in chondrocytes could include VGSC, ENaC and N/L-type voltage gated calcium channels (VGCC). In epithelial cells, ENaC is linked to the actin cytoskeleton and integrin. In osteoarthritic cartilage, ENaC is absent and the lack of ENaC means that chondrocytes may have lost the ability to transduce mechanical signals effectively.

4.1.5 Integrins

Integrins play a key role in the interactions between the cell and the extracellular matrix including cell anchorage, growth, differentiation, migration and matrix synthesis and degradation (Loeser, 1993). Integrins are cell surface receptors that recognise and bind to an Arg-Gly-Asp sequence on ECM proteins and are heterodimeric (one α and one β subunit) transmembrane glycoproteins (Loeser, 2000). The importance of integrins, as well as being cell adhesion molecules, is that they may function as transmitters of information and be able to mediate intracellular responses to extracellular stimuli. The pericellular matrix and chondrocytes in the chondron contain collagen types II, VI and IV, aggrecan and fibronectin and integrins are known to interact with these proteins found in pericellular matrix. Immunoprecipitation and immunofluorescence experiments show co-localisation and association of integrin with ENaC and VGCC and therefore integrins may functionally activate ion transporters following deformation of the pericellular matrix.

Extracellular protein binding to the cell leads to receptor clustering and activates integrin. Integrins however, have no inherent kinase activity but will often complex with Shc, Crk, paxillin, vinculin, caveolin and/or FAK. Many of these proteins in the complex are activated by tyrosine phosphorylation which then leads to activation of other kinases such as Src, RhoA, Rac1, Ras, Raf1, Sos, Grb2, MEK kinase and member of the MAP kinase family (including ERK1/2, JNK and p38). This then leads to downstream signalling that regulate gene expression, for example MAP kinase, that lead to activation of transcription factors such as AP-1 and NF-κB.

The regulation of chondrocyte integrin function is important in the homeostasis of cartilage as well as in disease states in which interactions between chondrocytes and their ECM are altered. Factors that modulate chondrocyte ECM synthesis, such as IGF-1 and TGF-β, also appear to modulate integrin-mediated attachment of chondrocytes to ECM proteins (Loeser 1994, 1997). The effects of IGF-1 and TGF-β on chondrocyte integrin expression and function, however, in vivo may depend on the relative levels of each growth factor present and thereby providing a means for sophisticated control of cell-matrix interactions in cartilage. Growth factor receptor phosphorylation leads to increased integrin aggregation, possibly via MAP kinase activation. There appears to be co-localisation of IGF-1 receptor and β_1 integrin subunit in chondrocytes. Cross-talk exists between integrins and growth factors/cytokines and as well as integrin activity being affected by growth factors, growth factor activity itself is dependent on integrin binding. Therefore a two-way signalling process occurs with integrin occupying a central role in this system. Increased expression of IGF-1 has been noted in osteoarthritic cartilage and could act in an autocrine manner to increased $\alpha_1\beta_1$ possibly as part of a repair response mediating signals important for cell survival/proliferation.

Integrins have a central role in cell survival and inhibition of integrin function results in apoptosis (Loeser, 2002; Mobasheri et al., 2002). The Ras-MAPK pathway is important to chondrocyte survival and integrins are linked to Ras-MAPK pathway by downstream signaling factors including the docking protein Shc. Interruption of the Ras-MAPK pathway produces apoptosis (via increased expression of pro-apoptotic proteins or repression of anti-apoptotic proteins). Therefore disruption of the interactions between chondrocytes and the ECM (via integrins) may induce apoptotic cell death and may contribute to pathogenesis of osteoarthritis.

4.1.6 Purinergic signaling

The potential role of purinergic signalling in mechanotransduction in cartilage was postulated following the finding that compressive loading of bovine chondrocytes in chondrons or in agarose pellets leads to ATP release (Chowdhury & Knight, 2006). ATP is an important mediator involved in autocrine/paracrine signalling and it can be released following cell damage and as well as being directly involved in signalling via release.

Chondrocytes have been shown to express P2Y2 receptors (Millward-Sadler et al., 2004) and normal chondrocytes release ATP after mechanical stimulation involving calcium signaling. Recently, Varani et al., (2008) characterised the expression of $P2X_1$ and $P2X_3$ receptors in bovine chondrocytes. Unlike P2Y receptors that are G-protein coupled, P2X receptors are membrane ligand-gated ion channels that open in response to binding of extracellular ATP. Stimulation of purinergic pathways (via P2X receptors) may be important in the response to joint inflammation since ATP further stimulates NO and PGE_2 production in chondrocytes following IL-1β stimulation.

The link between P2 receptors and cell signalling may involve connexin hemichannel expression (Knight et al., 2009). Connexins are membrane proteins that form hemichannels and hemichannels are one of the potential ways of releasing ATP (as well as through anion channels and via exocytosis of ATP-filled vesicles). Cyclic loading leads to hemichannel opening and ATP release in chondrocyte constructs (Garcia & Knight, 2010). In human cartilage, connexion 43 has been found in cells in the superficial region. The presence of these potential mechanosensitive cells primarily in the superficial/middle zones may indicate different mechanotransduction pathways than deeper zone cells. Since hypoxia is known to regulate connexins 43 dephophosphorylation, translocation and proteosomal degradation in other cells the response to mechanical stimulation may be related to the oxygen environment of cartilage.

The primary cilium, a membrane-coated axoneme that projects from the cell surface into the extracellular microenvironment could also be involved in chondrocyte mechanotransduction. The function of primary cilium in chondrocytes has not established but in the study by Knight et al., (2009) approximately 50% of primary cilia had co-expression of connexin 43. It is postulated that deflection of the cilium may activate ATP release via hemichannels and once released, ATP may activate P2 receptors, triggering intracellular Ca^{2+} signalling cascades and mediate effects on proteoglycan and collagen synthesis and MMP expression and NO release.

In osteoarthritic chondrocytes, a reduction in purinergic signalling following mechanical stimulation has been reported. This could be due to desensitisation by ATP released into synovial fluid (increased ATP levels in synovial fluid are reported in OA patients) or by receptor down regulation (since reduction in receptor numbers has been described at the cell surface in OA chondrocytes). The changes in ATP-mediated signalling in OA cartilage is of importance since ATP is normally chondroprotective against proteoglycan loss.

4.1.7 Transient receptor potential (TRP) channels

Transient receptor potential (TRP) channels comprise a superfamily of more than 50 different ion channels with a preference of Ca^{2+}, playing a role in the transduction of several physical stimuli such as temperature, osmotic and mechanical stimuli. TRP channel opening induces membrane depolarisation while increasing cytosolic Ca^{2+} and/or Na^+ concentrations. Most, but not all TRPC members act as store-operated Ca^{2+} channels whereas TRPV channels may be involved in a nonselective conductance of cations with a preference for Ca^{2+}. Since calcium entry through plasma membrane channels is recognised as a cellular signalling event per se, TPR channels provide an ideal candidate to link between mechanical stimuli and cellular response.

In human osteoarthritic chondrocytes, the majority of the investigated TRP genes are expressed (Gavenis et al., 2009) and a correlation appears between the degree of differentiation of chondrocytes and the expression of various members of the TRP family. Their role in cartilage health and disease is, as yet, unknown (Mobasheri &Barrett-Jolley, 2011).

5. Oxygen, mitochondria and reactive oxygen species in articular cartilage

Adult articular cartilage is avascular and hence long diffusion pathways exist for nutrients solutes and oxygen to cross. Synovial fluid has low oxygen tension (6-10%) and articular chondrocytes experience relatively low levels of oxygen, compared to other cell-types, with chondrocytes operating at oxygen tensions ranging from 6-10% at the articular surface to around 2% in the deep zones (Zhou et al., 2004). Despite this, articular chondrocytes not only survive but regulate extracellular matrix synthesis. Although energy production appears to be primarily via a glycolysis in this low oxygen environment, it is being recgonised that mitochondria might play an important role in the health and disease of the joint through their involvement in reactive oxygen species generation, calcium regulation and the intimate role in cell death/survival pathways in cartilage.

5.1 Cartilage oxygen tension and cell metabolism

The oxygen tension gradient in cartilage is determined by cell density and distribution, cartilage thickness, oxygen tension in synovial fluid, oxygen supply from subchondral surface and oxygen consumption rate per cell (Zhou et al., 2004). Articular chondrocytes have a characteristic morphology and metabolism depending on their position in cartilage and part of this may be due to the oxygen gradients that exist. Although the majority of diffusion of oxygen appears to come from the articular surface facing the synovial fluid, there is thought to be a component of diffusion from vessels in the subchondral bone plate and therefore extreme levels of hypoxia (i.e. 1% or less) may not exist *in situ* in cartilage (but could do in disease where subchondral bone plate thickening is a feature of osteoarthritis).

Despite these low oxygen conditions, articular chondrocytes do survive and are able to maintain their cartilage phenotype (Grimshaw & Mason, 2000; Pfander & Gelse, 2007). To survive low oxygen conditions cells possess highly conserved adaptive mechanisms. The most important component is mediated by transcriptional activation involving binding of the transcription factor hypoxia-inducible factor-1 (HIF-1). In cartilage, during physiological hypoxia, HIF-1α is expressed (Lin et al., 2004) and it appears to act as a survival factor since necrotic cartilage occurs in HIF-1 knock-out mice (Gelse et al., 2008).

Although articular chondrocytes reside in low oxygen levels, they are not unresponsive to hypoxia since changes in oxygen tension can have significant effects on matrix synthesis and cell growth. Indeed, matrix synthesis by articular chondrocytes may be optimal at lower tissue oxygen tensions, for example at 5% O_2, Sox9, type II collagen and aggrecan expression is higher than at 21% O_2 (Marty-Hartert et al., 2005). Oxygen diffusion and movement through cartilage may occur at differential rates in response to biochemical and loading differences in different regions and this could lead to local oxygen gradients within pockets of cartilage which could influence cell metabolism as well as differential gene expression.

5.1.1 Articular cartilage metabolism

Within the hypoxic environment of cartilage, articular chondrocytes predominately undergo glycolytic metabolism. Lactate is the major end-product of this process and this adds to the already acidic load experienced by these cells. ATP is generated by substrate level phosphorylation, whereas, apart from superficial layers where relatively higher oxygen levels can exist, oxidative phosphorylation appears to be a lesser component of ATP production.

Reduction of oxygen levels in other cells results in an increase in glucose usage and lactate production, thereby increasing ATP production - this is commonly known as the Pasteur effect. Articular chondrocytes, however, appear to display a negative Pasteur effect where reductions in oxygen levels result in suppression of carbohydrate breakdown (Lee & Urban, 1997). This effect appears to be peculiar to articular cartilage since in fibrocartilaginous intervertebral disc, glucose uptake and lactate production increases under lowered oxygen levels.

5.1.2 Changes in oxygen tension in joint disease

Despite increased blood vessel formation in the synovial membrane and neoangiogenesis from the underlying bone into the deep zone of osteoarthritic cartilage, the hypoxic environment of cartilage appears more pronounced in osteoarthritis. Synovial fluid from osteoarthritic joints contains less oxygen than synovial fluids from healthy joints (Pflander & Gelse, 2007). Reductions in oxygen tension in joint disease could be due to increased oxygen usage by the synovial membrane, alterations in blood flow and gas exchange by fibrosis in the joint capsule and subchondral bone sclerosis (Svalastoga & Kiaet, 1989). Additionally, alterations in diffusion gradients caused by changes in matrix structure, altered biomechanical forces through the cartilage and alterations in oxygen consumption in inflammation (e.g. reactive oxygen species generation) contribute to the reduction in cartilage oxygen levels.

5.1.3 Hypoxia and HIF-1 in osteoarthritis

Chronic hypoxia in the osteoarthritic joint is associated with increased levels of HIF-1 in both synoviocytes and chondrocytes and related HIF-1 targeted genes, such as VEGF and iNOS. Additionally, HIF-1α accumulation can also be increased by other factors such as pro-inflammatory cytokines and changes in mechanical loading, as well as hypoxia (Pfander & Gelse, 2007). HIF-1α is important for anaerobic energy production and matrix synthesis by chondrocytes and appears to have a pivotal role for maintaining chondrocytic phenotype.

As well as the increased synthesis of matrix destructive enzymes, osteoarthritic chondrocytes show enhanced gene expression of type II collagen. This latter feature may be related to oxygen levels since increased accumulation of type II collagen induced by 1% oxygen is accompanied by stabilisation, nuclear translocation and increased activity of HIF-1α. The increase in posttranslational modification of type II collagen may contribute to the increased synthesis of collagen type II seen during osteoarthritis as an effort to restore extracellular matrix.

5.2 The role of mitochondria in articular chondrocytes

Mitochondria are extremely important cellular organelles traditionally seen as the source of cellular energy production (Duchen, 2004). Articular chondrocytes contain fewer mitochondria compared to other, more metabolically active cell types, and this difference may reflect the cellular environment (i.e. hypoxia) and reliance on glycolytic metabolism rather than oxidative phosphorylation for energy production. Despite this, mitochondrial physiology and function in the chondrocyte is still critical to cellular function and they are involved in many important aspects of cell physiology in both health and disease such as ROS generation, Ca^{2+} homeostasis and cell death and survival pathways. Indeed, mitochondrial dysfunction is a key component of a number of diseases, such as diabetes and cancer, and the role of the mitochondrion in osteoarthritis is now beginning to be more fully appreciated (Terkeltaub et al., 2002).

5.2.1 Mitochondria and the chemiosmotic principle of energy production

Mitochondria contain two membrane systems, an outer and inner mitochondrial membrane (Duchen, 2004). The inner mitochondrial membrane is folded into cristae and it is here that the membrane bound enzymes (a series of complexes) of the respiratory chain are located. The chemiosmotic principle of energy production involves the oxidation of cellular substrates to produce ATP. The reductants NADH and $FADH_2$, generated from the tricarboxylic acid (TCA) cycle, enter the mitochondrial electron transport chain. NADH is oxidised to NAD^+ at complex I and $FADH_2$ is oxidised to FAD^{2+} at complex II to provide electrons for ubisemiquinone at complex III. The electron chain complexes catalyse a series of redox reactions creating an electrochemical drive to transfer H^+ from the mitochondrial matrix into the intermembrane space across the inner mitochondrial membrane. This results in a large mitochondrial transmembrane potential of around-150 to -200mV and it is this membrane potential that provides the "protonmotive force" to cause H^+ influx through F_1-F_0 ATP synthase and drive the ATPase "backwards" thus phosphorylating ADP to release ATP. The respiratory rate is regulated by this proton gradient which in turn is dependent on substrate availability, inhibitors of respiration (for example anoxia) and any mechanism that results in the uncoupling of the enzyme complexes.

In articular chondrocytes, both mitochondrial density and activity appears to be lower than other cell types with mitochondrial density significantly reduced in the deep zones compared with the upper zones of articular cartilage, likely to reflect oxygen levels in these zones. There is also evidence that the cytochrome component of the electron transport chain in articular chondrocytes may be incomplete *in situ* and provides further evidence that ATP derived from mitochondrial oxidative phosphorylation is not a major component of energy production in cartilage. Interestingly though, following transfer of cells to a relatively "oxygen-rich" environment (for example during culturing of cartilage explants or isolated cells in ambient conditions), mitochondrial biogenesis occurs (Mignotte et al., 1991). This change within the chondrocyte appears to result in a switch to oxidative phosphorylation. It has to be noted, therefore, that these conditions may not represent *in vivo* conditions of the chondrocyte and interpretation of data on cartilage metabolism requires an appreciation of these potential changes.

5.2.2 Mitochondria and reactive oxygen/nitrogen species

The process of electron transfer along the electron transport chain in mitochondria is not completely efficient and electrons may be "lost" during the redox reactions, resulting in the transfer of electrons to oxygen and the generation of oxygen radicals (reactive oxygen species, ROS). These highly reactive species can result in cellular damage due to lipid peroxidation and DNA damage so efficient mechanisms in the mitochondrium (for example superoxide dismutase) and cytoplasm (for example catalase) exist to reduce the risk of this occurring. In mitochondria of articular chondrocytes, it seems that the main site of ROS generation is complex III (Milner et al., 2007).

As well as being a potential source of cellular damage if left unchecked, reactive oxygen species are now thought to be important mediators of cell signalling. A large number of intracellular signalling pathways are regulated by ROS including cytokine receptors, receptor tyrosine kinases, receptor serine/threonine kinases and p38 MAPK cascades. This can be through the redox status of component proteins. Oxidation and reduction of –SH groups on amino acids can result in conformational change and alteration in enzyme activity.   ROS may also directly regulate activity of transcription factors through oxidative modifications of conserved cysteines. Redox-sensitive transcription factors include NF-kB, AP-1, sp-1, c-myb, p53 , egr-1, HIF-1α and c-fos (Lo & Cruz, 1995).   DNA-binding by AP-1 is also regulated by post-translational modifications which are redox-sensitive and this is also seen with GTP-binding protein Ras.

Nitric oxide appears to have an important role in mitochondrial function (Duchen, 2004). Complex IV has a high affinity for NO and at low O_2 competes with oxygen to inhibit mitochondrial respiration and this may be of relevance in a low oxygen system. Mitochondria may also generate NO themselves and a specific NOS has been shown to be expressed by the mitochondrium.   It appears that an intricate feedback mechanism involving NO, calcium, mitochondrial electron chain activity and ROS levels may exist in the mitochondrium that may be of particular importance in low-oxygen environments such as cartilage.

Cellular antioxidant mechanisms exist though, and it is seen as a balance between ROS production and removal that determine the difference between physiological and pathological ROS levels within the cell.   As with ROS, the balance between physiological and pathological NO levels are also likely to be an important factor since high NO levels react with ROS resulting in peroxynitrite production and damage to the electron chain - a feature present in disease such as osteoarthritis.

5.2.3 Mitochondria and calcium uptake

Mitochondrial calcium handling is an important component of cellular calcium homeostasis since calcium "overload" is thought to be implicated in a number of pathological states including osteoarthritis.   Mitochondrial calcium uptake is driven primarily by the electrochemical gradient established by the mitochondrial potential and the relatively low Ca^{2+} concentration (Duchen, 2004).   When cytosolic calcium increases, calcium moves into the mitochondrial matrix. Intramitochondrial calcium concentration is kept low under "resting" conditions by the Na^+/Ca^{2+} exchanger that results in calcium efflux. Ca^{2+} appears to be taken up into the matrix through the IMM by a uniporter.   Additionally, voltage-dependent anion channels (VDAC) permeant to calcium exist in the outer mitochondrial membrane and may affect inner mitochondrial membrane calcium uptake by acting as a fast filter.   The VDAC also appears to form part of the mitochondrial membrane permeability pore in initiating apoptosis. Calcium microdomains can exist within cells and the proximity of mitochondria to endoplasmic reticulum calcium release sites may result in mitochondria experiencing relatively high local concentrations, promoting rapid calcium uptake to allow direct transfer of calcium between mitochondria and ER (Contreras et al., 2010). In addition, the proximity to the plasma membrane by mitochondria also could allow regulation of calcium influx and therefore mitochondrial positioning could be important regulators of signalling pathways involving calcium.

5.2.4 Mitochondria and cell death

Mitochondria are intimately involved in cell death pathways.   In many cells a reduction in mitochondrially derived ATP leads to loss of maintenance of ion gradients and regulation of calcium and intracellular osmolarity causing cell swelling and death. Cell swelling is an early feature of osteoarthritis and mitochondrial dysfunction is likely to be a significant component of cell death in cartilage disease.

The opening of a large conductance pore (mPTP) occurs through a conformational change of several proteins of the mitochondrial membrane due to a number of conditions such as high $[Ca^{2+}]_m$, oxidative stress, ATP depletion, high inorganic phosphate (P_i) and mitochondrial depolarisation (Duchen 2004). This irreversible high conductance opening causes mitochondrial swelling, cytochrome c release, caspase activation and apoptotic cell death. Apoptotic cell death may be a normal feature of cartilage growth and development, particularly in the hypertrophic zone of the growth plate but factors resulting in abnormal activation are important causes of cellular death and subsequent loss of cartilage integrity in joint disease.

5.2.5 Mitochondria and osteoarthritis

Mitochondria are implicated in the pathogenesis of many diseases, including osteoarthritis and mitochondrial mediated diseases are often due to hypoxic cell stress or aging – relevant factors in joint disease. In diabetes mellitus, defects in the electron chain are described (especially Complexes I and IV) and in neuronal injury (ischaemia/reperfusion injury), mitochondrial injury leads to impaired intracellular Ca^{2+} buffering, increased ROS generation and promotion of apoptosis via release of cytochrome c. Additionally, ETC complex defects are present in Alzheimer's, Parkinson's and Huntingdon's disease and peroxynitrite-mediated nitration of tyrosines in Alzheimer's disease neurons are due to increased NO.

In osteoarthritis, mitochondrial content increases in number and size and mitochondrial swelling has been noted (Terkeltaub et al., 2002). Mitochondrial numbers increase at sites of crystal formation and matrix calcification is a feature of osteoarthritis. It appears that calcification is stimulated by NO/peroxynitrite and chondrocyte apoptosis and this is in turn is modulated by ATP metabolism. Mitochondrial energy reserve is required for matrix synthesis and crystal suppression and therefore altered mitochondrial energy metabolism may lead to crystal formation.

Mitochondrial dysfunction of the electron chain (particularly complexes II and III) has been described in osteoarthritic chondrocytes and this will alter the respiratory state and mitochondrial membrane potential of the mitochondrium (Maniero et al., 2003). A collapse of the mitochondrial membrane potential results in mitochondrial swelling, disruption of the outer mitochondrial membrane and release of pro-apoptotic factors such as cytochrome c, AIF and procaspases from the intermembrane space and hence cell death.

5.3 Oxidative stress and reactive oxygen/nitrogen species in joint disease

When ROS levels exceed the cellular defence mechanisms, cellular damage can occur. This is known as oxidative stress. Increased oxygen consumption by the synovium during inflammation and the exposure to inflammatory mediators can lead to increase in ROS and RNS generation to levels that can induce cellular damage. In the inflamed joint synoviocytes appear to be the key cell driving this response, as opposed to chondrocytes, although it is the effect on the chondrocyte that will lead to compromise in cartilage integrity and hence disease (Schneider et al., 2005). In synoviocytes there are a number of sources of ROS generation, as well as mitochondrial derived ROS including xanthine oxidoreductase and membrane-bound NADPH oxidase (Henroitin et al., 2003).

Oxidative stress results in protein, lipid membrane, DNA damage and therefore cell injury and death (Finkl 2003). Lipid peroxyl radical formation can result in lipid bond cross-linking and alteration in membrane properties as well as forming products, such as aldehydes and saturated hydrocarbons that are toxic to cells. Fragmentation of hyaluronic acid is reported following oxidative damage to the glycosidic bonds. Since hyaluronic acid is a key cartilage biomolecule both in structure and cell signalling, alterations to HA structure will lead to alterations in cytoskeletal polymerisation, for example and affect cell adhesive properties. Oxidative damage to other extracellular components and ROS-induced activation of matrix metalloproteinases can add to the degradative element of these molecules and additionally, the action of IL-1 on proteoglycan loss appears to be mediated by ROS and NO (Henroitin et al., 2003). The direct degradation of proteoglycans and collagen by ROS is due to upregulation of collagenases and other MMPs as well as decreased production of TIMPs. Additionally, NO is implicated in cartilage insensitivity to IGF-1 by inhibiting IGF-1 receptor autophosphorylation. Therefore the use of antioxidant therapy has justifiable support in joint disease.

6. Conclusion

Our knowledge of the cellular processes occurring in articular chondrocytes has grown immensely over recent years but it is the appreciation of the interaction and response of these cells to their unusual and challenging environment and how these change in diseases such as osteoarthritis that will open up new exciting opportunities for potential therapeutic modulation in joint disease. How the chondrocyte senses and adapts to the dynamic nature of the extracellular matrix in health and disease makes us realise the complexity of signals involved and the multiplicity of the component parts, such as, for example, the roles of cell volume regulation, intracellular pH homeostasis and mitochondrial function on cell function in cartilage. The challenge for the future then will be to tie all these elements together and be able to paint the big picture that reveals the many complex interactions occurring within the joint.

7. List of abbreviations

AQP	Aquaporin
ATP	Adenosine triphosphate
ECM	Extracellular matrix
ENaC	Epithelial sodium channel
ERK1/2	Extracellular signal-regulated kinase 1/2
ETC	Electron chain transport
$FADH_2$	Flavin adenine dinucleotide H_2
GAG	Glycosaminoglycan
GLUT	Glucose transporter
HA	Hyaluronic acid
HIF-1	Hypoxia-inducible factor-1
Hz	Hertz
kDa	kiloDaltons
IGF-1	Insulin-like growth factor-1
IL-1	Interleukin-1
IMM	Inner mitochondrial membrane

MAPK	*Mitogen-activated protein kinase*
MCT	*Monocarboxylate transporter*
MEK	*Mitogen-activated protein kinase kinase*
MMP	*Matrix metalloproteinase*
MPa	*Megapascals*
mPTP	*mitochondrial permeability transition pore*
NADH	*Nicotinamide adenine dinucleotide H*
NHE	*Na+/H+ exchange*
NO	*Nitric oxide*
OA	*Osteoarthritis*
OMM	*Outer mitochondrial membrane*
PGE$_2$	*Prostaglandin E$_2$*
PKA	*Protein kinase A*
TCA	*Tricarboxylic acid cycle*
TGF-β	*Transforming growth factor-β*
TRP	*Transient receptor potential*
VAHC	*Voltage-activated H+ channel*
VDAC	*Voltage-dependent anion channel*
VGCC	*Voltage-gated calcium channel*
VGSC	*Voltage-gated sodium channel*

8. References

Becerra, J., Adrades, J.A., Guerado, E., Zamora-Navas, P., Lopez-Puertas, J.M. & Reddi, A.H. (2010). Articular cartilage: structure and regeneration. *Tissue Engineering Part B Review,* Vol.16, No.6, (December 2010), pp. 617-627

Berridge, M.J., Bootman, M.D. & Lipp, P. (1998). Calcium - a life and death signal. *Nature,* Vol.395, No. 6703 (October 1998), pp.645-648

Browning, J.A, Walker, R.E., Hall, A.C. & Wilkins, R.J. (1999). Modulation of Na+ x H+ exchange by hydrostatic pressure in isolated bovine articular chondrocytes. *Acta Physiologica Scandinavica,* Vol.166, No.1, (May 1999), pp. 39-45

Bush, P.G. & Hall, A.C. (2001). The osmotic sensitivity of isolated and in situ bovine articular chondrocytes. *Journal of Orthopaedic Research,* Vol.19, No.5, (September 2001), pp. 768-778

Bush, P.G. & Hall, A.C. (2005) Passive osmotic properties of in situ human articular chondrocytes within non-degenerate and degenerate cartilage. *Journal of Cellular Physiology,* Vol.204, No.1, (July 2005), pp.309-319

Chowdhury, T.T & Knight, M.M. (2006). Purinergic pathway suppresses the release of NO and stimulates proteoglycan synthesis in chondrocyte/agarose constructs to dynamic compression. *Journal of Cell Physiology,*Vol. 290, No.3, (December 2009), pp.845-853

Clarke, R.B., Hatano, N., Kondo, C., Belke, D.D., Brown, B.S., Kumar, S., Votta, B.J. & Giles W.R. (2010). Voltage-gated K+ currents in mouse articular chondrocytes regulate membrane potential. *Channels,* Vol.4, No.3, (May-June 2010), pp. 179-191

Comper, W.D. (1996). Water:Dynamic aspects, *In* Extracellular Matrix Volume 2 Molecular Components and Interactions, Comper W.D., pp.1-21. Harwood Academic Publishers, Amsterdam

Contreras, L., Drago, I., Zampese, E. and Pozzan, T. (2010). Mitochondria: the calcium connection. *Biochimica et Biophysica acta,* Vol.1797, No.6-7, (June-July 2010), pp.607-618

Das, R.H.J., van Osch, G.J., Kreukniet, M., Oostra, J., Weinans, H. & Jahr, H. (2010). Effects of individual control of pH and hypoxia in chondrocyte culture. *Journal of Orthopaedic Research,* Vol.28, No. 4, (April 2010), pp. 537-545

Duchen, M.R.(2004). Role of mitochondria in health and disease. *Diabetes,*Vol.53, Suppl.1, (February 2004), pp. S96-S102

Erickson, G.R., Alexopoulos, L.G. & Guilak, F. (2001). Hyper-osmotic stress induces volume change and calcium transients in chondrocytes. *Journal of Biomechanics,* Vol.34, No.12, (December 2001), pp. 1527-1535

Finkl, T. (2003). Oxidant signals and oxidative stress. *Current Opinion in Cell Biology,* Vol.15, No.2, (February 2003), pp.247-254

Funabashi, K., Fujii, M., Yamamura, H., Ohya, S. & Imaizumi, Y. (2010). Contribution of chloride channel conductance to the regulation of resting membrane potential in chondrocytes. *Journal of Pharmacological Science,* Vol.113, No.1, (April 2010), pp. 94-99

Garcia, M. & Knight, M. (2010). Cyclic Loading Opens Hemichannels to release ATP as part of a chondrocyte mechanotransduction pathway. *Journal of Orthopaedic Research,* Vol.28, No.4, (April 2010), pp. 510-515

Gavenis, K., Schumacher, C., Schneider, U., Eisfeld, J., Mollenhauer, J. and Schmidt-Rohlfing, B. (2009). Expression of ion channels of the TRP family in articular chondrocytes from osteoarthritic patients: changes between native and in vitro propagated chondrocytes. *Molecular Cellular Biochemistry,* Vol.321., No.1-2, (January 2009), pp.135-143

Gelse, K., Pfander, D., Obier, S., Knaup, K.X., Wiesener, M., Hennig, F.F. & Swoboda, B. (2008). Role of hypoxia-inducible factor 1 alpha in the integrity of articular cartilage in murine knee joints. *Arthritis Research Therapy,* Vol.10. No.5, (September 2008), pp. R111

Goldring, M.B. (2006). Update on the biology of the chondrocyte and new approaches to treating cartilage diseases. *Best Practice and Research Clinical Rheumatology,* Vol.20, No.5, (October 2006), pp. 1003-1010

Grimshaw, M.J. & Mason, R.M. (2000). Bovine articular chondrocyte function in vitro depends on oxygen tension. *Osteoarthritis Cartilage,* Vol.8, No.5. (September 2000), pp.386-392

Guilak, F., Zell, R.A., Erickson, G.R., Grande, D.A., Rubin, C.T., McLeod, K.J. and Donahue, H.J. (1999). Mechanically induced calcium waves in articular chondrocytes are inhibited by gadolinium and amiloride. *Journal of Orthopaedic Research,* Vol. 17, No.3, (May 1999), pp.421-429

Guilak, F., Alexopoulos, L.G., Upton, M.L., Youn, I. Choi, J.B., Cao, L., Setton, L.A. & Haider, M.A. (2006). The pericellular matrix as a transducer of biomechanical and biochemical signals in articular cartilage. *Annuals New York Academy of Science,* Vol. 1068, (April 2006), pp. 498-512

Hall, A.C., Horowitz, E.R. & Wilkins, R.J. (1996a). The cellular physiology of articular cartilage. *Experimental Physiology,* Vol.81, No.3, (May 1996), pp.535-545

Hall, A.C., Starks, I, Shoults, C.L. & Rashidbigi, S. (1996b). Pathways for K+ transport across the bovine articular chondrocyte membrane and their sensitivity to cell volume. *American Journal of Physiology*, Vol.270, No.5(Pt 1), (May 1996), pp. C1300-1310

Hall A.C. (1999). Differential effects of hydrostatic pressure on cation transport pathways of isolated articular chondrocytes. *Journal of Cellular Physiology*, Vol.178, No.2, (February 1999), pp. 197-204

Hall, A.C. & Bush, P.G. (2001). The role of a swelling-activated taurine transport pathway in the regulation of articular chondrocyte volume. *Pflugers Archive: European Journal of Physiology*, Vol.442, No.5, (August 2001), pp.771-781

Hardingham, T. & Fosang A.J. (1992) Proteoglycans: many forms and functions. *FASEB Journal*. 6, 861-870.

Hasler, E.M., Herzog, W., Wu, J.Z., Muller, W. & Wyss, U. (1999). Articular cartilage biomechanics: theorectical models, material properties, and biosynthetic response. *Critical Reveiw of Biomedical Engineering*, Vol.27, No.6, pp.415-488

Henroitin, Y.E., Bruckner, P. And Pujol, J.P. (2003). The role of reactive oxygen species in homeostasis and degradation of cartilage. *Osteoarthritis Cartilage*, Vol.11, No.10, (October 2003), pp.747-755

Hoffmann, E.K., Lambert, I.H. & Pedersen SF. (2009). Physiology of cell volume regulation invertebrates. *Physiological Reviews*, Vol.89, No.1, (January 1999), pp. 193-277

Huber, M., Trattnig, S. & Linter, F. (2000). Anatomy, biochemistry and physiology of articular cartilage. *Investigations in Radiology*, Vol.35, No.10, (October 2000), pp. 573-580

Jeffery, A.K., Blunn, G.W., Archer, C.W. & Bentley, G. (1991). Three-dimensional collagen architecture in bovine articular cartilage. *Journal of Bone and Joint Surgery*, Vol.73-B, No.5, (September 1991), pp. 795-801

Kaab, M.J., Ito, K., Clark, J.M., Notzi, H.P. (1998). Deformation of articular cartilage collagen structure under static and cyclic loading. *Journal of Orthopaedic Research*, Vol.16, No.6, (November 1998), pp.743-751

Kerrigan, M.J. & Hall, A.C. (2008). Control of chondrocyte regulatory volume decrease (RVD) by [Ca2+]i and cell shape. *Osteoarthritis and Cartilage*, Vol.16, No.3, (March 2008), pp.312-322

Kim, Y-J., Bonassar, L.J. and Grodzinsky, A.J. (1995). The role of cartilage streaming potential, fluid flow and pressure in the stimulation of chondrocyte biosynthesis during dynamic compression. *Journal of Biomechanics*, Vol.28, No.9, (September 1995), pp.1055-1066

Knight, M.M., McGlashan, S.R., Garcia, M., Jensen, C.G. & Poole, C.A. (2009) Articular chondrocytes express connexin 43 hemichannels and P2 receptors – a putative mechanoreceptor complex involving the primary cilium? *Journal of Anatomy*, Vol.214, No.2, (February 2009), pp.275-283

Kuettner, K.E., Aydelotte, M.B.& Thonar, E.J. (1991). Articular cartilage matrix and structure: a review. *Journal of Rheumatology Supplement*, Vol.27 (February 1991), pp. 46-48

Lai, W.M., Sun, D.D., Ateshian, G.A., Guo, X.E. & Mow, V.C. (2002). Electrical signals in cartilage. *Biorheology*, Vol.39, No.1-2, pp.39-45

Lee, R.B. and Urban J.P. (1997). Evidence for a negative Pasteur effect in articular cartilage. *Biochemical Journal*, Vol. 321, No.1, (January 1997), pp.95-102

Lo, Y.Y. and Cruz, T.F. (1995). Involvement of reactive oxygen species in cytokine and growth factor induction of c-fos expression in chondrocytes. *Journal of Biological Chemistry*, Vol.270., No.20., (May 1995), pp.11727-11730

Loeser, R.F. (1993). Integrin-mediated attachment of articular chondrocytes to extracellular matrix proteins. *Arthritis Rheumatism,* Vol. 36, No.8, (August 1993), pp. 1103-1110

Loeser, R.F. (1994). Modulation of integrin-mediated attachment of chondrocytes to ECM proteins by cations, retinoic acid and TGF-β. *Experimental Cellular Research,* Vol.211, No.1, (March 1994), pp. 17-23

Loeser, R.F. (1997). Growth factor Regulation of chondrocyte integrins. Differential effects of insulin-like growth factor 1 and transforming growth factor beta on alpha 1 beta 1 integrin expression and chondrocyte adhesion to type IV collagen. *Arthritis Rheumatism,* Vol.40, No.2, (February 1997), pp. 270-276

Loeser, R.F. (2000). Chondrocyte integrin expression and function. *Biorheology* Vol.37, No.1-2, pp.109-116

Loeser, R.F. (2002). Integrins and cell signalling in chondrocytes. *Biorheology,* Vol.39, No.1-2, pp. 119-124

Lin, C., McGough, R, Aswad, B, Block, J,A. & Terek, R. (2004) Hypoxia induces HIF-1alpha and VEGF expression in chondrocsarcoma cells and chondrocytes. *Journal of Orthopaedic Research,* Vol.22, No.6, (November 2004), pp. 1175-1181

Lui, K.E., Panchal, A.S, Santhanagopal, A, Dixon, S.J. & Bernier, S.M. (2002) Epidermal growth factor stimulates proton efflux from chondrocytic cells. *Journal of Cellular Physiology,* Vol.192, No.1, pp.102-112

Maneiro, E., Martin, M.A., de Andres, M.C., Lopez-Armada, M.J., Fernandez-Sueiro, J.L., del Hoyo, P., Galdo, F., Arenas, J. and Blanco, F.J. (2003). Mitochondrial respiratory activity is altered in osteoarthritic human articular chondrocytes. *Arthritis Rheumatism,* Vol.48, No.3, (March 2003), pp.700-708

Mathy-Hartert, M. Burton, S., Deby-Dupont, G. Devel, P., Reginster, J.Y. & Henroitin, Y. (2005). Influence of oxygen tension on nitric oxide and PGE2 synthesis by bovine chondrocytes. *Osteoarthritis Cartilage,* Vol.13, No. 1, (January 2005), pp.74-79

Meredith, D., Bell, P., McClure, B. & Wilkins, R.J. (2002). Functional and molecular characterisation of lactic acid transport in bovine articular chondrocytes. *Cellular Physiology and Biochemistry,* Vol.12, No.4, pp.227-234

Meredith, D., Gehl, K.A., Seymour, J., Ellory, J.C. & Wilkins, R.J. (2007). Characterisation of sulphate transporters in isolated bovine articular chondrocytes. *Journal of Orthopaedic Research,* Vol.25, No.9, (September 2007), pp. 1145-1153

Mignotte, F., Champagne, A.M., Froger-Gaillard, B., Benel, L., Gueride, M., Adolphe, M. and Mounolou, J.C. (1991). Mitochondrial biogenesis in rabbit chondrocytes transferred to culture. *Biology of the Cell,* Vol.71., No.1-2., pp.67-72

Miki, T. & Seino, S. (2005). Role of KATP channels as metabolic sensors in acute metabolic changes. *Journal of Molecular and Cellular Cardiology,* Vol.38, No.6., (June 2005), pp. 917-925

Milner, P.I., Fairfax, T.P., Browning, J.A., Wilkins, R.J. & Gibson, J.S. (2006). The effect of O2 on pH homeostasis in equine articular chondrocytes. *Arthritis Rheumatism,* Vol.54, No.11, (November 2006), pp.3523-3532

Milner, P.I., Wilkins, R.J. & Gibson, J.S. (2007). The role of mitochondrial reactive oxygen sepcies in pH regulation in articular chondrocytes. *Osteoarthritis Cartilage,* Vol.15, No.7, (July 2007), pp.735-742

Millward-Sadler S.J., Wright, M.O. Flatman, P.W. & Salter, D.M. (2004). ATP in the mechanotransduction pathway of normal human articular chondrocytes. *Biorheology,* Vol. 41, No.3-4, pp. 567-575

Mobasheri, A., Carter, S.D., Martin-Vasallo, P. & Shakibaei, M. (2002) Integrins and stretch activated ion channels; putative components of functional cell surface mechanoreceptors in articular chondrocytes . *Cell Biology International*. Vol.26, No. 1, pp. 1-18

Mobasheri, A., Trujillo, E., Bell, S., Carter, S.D., Clegg, P.D., Martin-Vasallo, P. & Marples, D. (2004) Aquaporin water channels AQP1 and AQP3 are expressed in equine articular chondrocytes. *The Veterinary Journal*, Vol.168, No. 2, (September 2004), pp.143-150

Mobasheri, A., Gent, T.C., Nash, A.I., Womack, M.D., Moskaluk, C.A. and Barrett-Jolley, R.B. (2007) Evidence for functional ATP-sensitive (K(ATP)) potassium channels in human and equine articular chondrocytes. *Osteoarthritis Cartilage*, Vol.15, No.1, (January 2007), pp.1-8

Mobasheri, A. & Barrett-Jolley, R.B. (2011) Transient receptor potential channels: emerging roles in health and disease. *The Veterinary Journal*, Vol. 187, No.2, (February 2011), pp. 145-146

Morris, N.P., Keene, D.R. & Horton, W.A. (2002) Morphology of Connective tissue: Cartilage, *In* Connective Tissue and Its Heritable Disorders, Royce, P.M. and Steinmann, B. pp. 41-66. Wiley-Liss Inc., New York

Mow, V.C., Holmes, M.H. & Lai,W.M. (1984). Fluid transport and mechanical properties of articular cartilage: a review. *Journal of Biomechanics*, Vol.17, No.5, pp.377-394

Palmer, J.L. & Bertone, A.L. (1994). Joint structure, biochemistry and biochemical disequilibrium in synovitis and equine joint disease. *Equine Veterinary Journal*, Vol.26, No.4, pp. 263-277

Pedersen, S.F. & Cala, P.M. (2004). Comparative biology of the ubiquitous Na+/H+ exchanger, NHE1: lessons from erthrocytes. *Journal of Experimental Zoology A Experimental Biology*, Vol.301, No.7, (July 2004), pp. 569-578

Pfander, D. and Glese, K. (2007). Hypoxia and osteoarthritis: how chondrocytes survive hypoxic environments. *Current Opinion in Rhuematology*, Vol.19., No.5., (September 2007), pp.457-462

Sanchez, J.C. and Wilkins, R.J. (2003). Effects of hypotonic shock on intracellular pH in bovine articular chondrocytes. *Comparative Biochemistry Physiology A Molecular Intregrated Physiology*, Vol.135, No.4, (August 2003), pp575-583.

Sanchez, J.C., Danks, T.A. & Wilkins, R.J. (2003). Mechanisms involved in the increase in intracellular calcium following hypotonic shock in bovine articular chondrocytes. *General Physiology Biophysics*, Vol.22, No.4, (December 2003), pp. 487-500

Sanchez, J.C. & Lopez-Zapata, D.F. (2010). Effects of osmostic challenges on membrane potential in human articular chondrocytes from healthy and osteoarthritic cartilage. *Biorheology*, Vol.47, No.5-6, pp. 321-331.

Shikhman, A.R., Brinson, D.C. & Lotz, M.K. (2004). Distinct pathways regulate facilitated glucose transport in human articular chondrocytes during anabolic and catabolic responses. *American Journal of Physiology Endocrinology and Metabolism*, Vol.286, No.6, (June 2004), pp.E980-E985

Solomon, D.H., Wilkins, R.J., Meredith, D. And Browning, J.A. (2007) Characterisation of inorganic phosphate transport in bovine articular chondrocytes. *Cellular Physiology and Biochemistry*, Vol.20, No.1-4, pp.99-108

Svalastoga, E. & Kiaet, T. (1989). Oxygen consumption, diffusing capacity and blood flow of the synovial membrane in osteoarthritic rabbit knee joints. *Acta Veterinaria Scandinavica*, Vol.30, No.2, pp. 121-125

Tattersall, A., Meredith, D., Furla, P., Shen, M. R., Ellory, C. & Wilkins, R.J. (2003). Molecular and functional identification of the NHE isoforms NHE1 and NHE3 in isolated bovine articular chondrocytes. *Cellular Physiology and Biochemistry* Vol. 13, No.4. pp. 215-222

Tattersall A.L. & Wilkins, R.J. (2008) Modulation of Na$^+$-H$^+$ exchange isoforms NHE1 and NHE3 by insulin-like growth factor-1 in isolated bovine chondrocytes. *Journal of Orthopaedic Research.*, Vol.26, No.11, pp. 1428-1433

Terkeltaub, R., Johnson, K., Murphy, A. and Ghosh, S. (2002). Invited review: the mitochondrion in osteoarthritis. *Mitochondrion,* Vol.1, No.4, (February 2002), pp.301-319

Urban, J.P. (1994) The chondrocyte: a cell under pressure. *British Journal of Rhuematology,* Vol.33, pp. 901-908

Urban, J.P. (2000) Present perspectives on cartilage and chondrocyte mechanobiology/ *Biorheology*, Vol.37, No.1-2, pp.185-190

Van der Kraan, P.M. & van den Berg, W.B. (2000) Anabolic and destructive mediators in osteoarthritis *Current opinion in clinical nutrition and metabolic care*, Vol. 3, pp. 205-211

Varani, K., De Mattei, M., Vincenzi, F, Tosi, A., Gessi, S, Merghi, S, Pellati, A, Masieri, F., Ongaro, A.& Borea, P.A. (2008). Pharmacological characterisation of P2X1 and P2X3 purinergic receptors in bovine chondrocytes . *Osteoarthritis and Cartilage,* Vol.16, No. 11, (November 2008), pp 1421-1429

Wang, Q.G., El Haj, A.J. & Kuiper, N.J. (2008). Glycosaminoglycan in the pericellular matrix of chondrons and chondrocytes. *Journal of Anatomy,* Vol.213, No.3., (September 2008), pp.266-273

Wilkins, R.J. and Hall, A.C. (1992). Measurement of intracellular pH in isolated bovine articular chondrocytes. *Experimental Physiology* Vol.77, pp. 521-524

Wilkins, R.J. and Hall, A.C. (1995) Control of matrix synthesis in isolated bovine chondrocytesby extracellular and intracellular pH. *Journal of Cell Physiology,* Vol.164, No.3, (September 1995), pp.474-481

Wilkins, R.J., Browning, J.A. & Ellory, J.C. (2000). Surviving in a matrix: membrane transport in articular chondrocytes. *Journal Membrane Biology.* Vol.177, No.2 (September 2000), pp. 95-108

Wilkins, R.J., Fairfax, T.P. Davies, M.E., Muzamba, M.C. & Gibson, J.S. (2003). Homeostasis of intracellular Ca^{2+} in equine chondrocytes: response to hypotonic shock. *Equine Veterinary Journal,* Vol.35, No.5, (July 2003), pp. 439-443

Wilson. J.R., Duncan, N.A., Giles, W.R. and Clark, R.B. (2004) A voltage-dependent K+ current cotributes to membrane potential of acutely isolated canine articular chondrocytes. *Journal of Physiology,* Vol.557, No.1, pp93-104

Windhaber, R.A., Wilkins, R.J. & Meredith, D. (2003). Functional characterisation of gluocse transport in bovine articular chondrocytes. *Pflugers Archive: European Journal of Physiology,* Vol.446, No.5, (August 2003), pp. 572-577

Yamazaki, N., Browning, J.A. & Wilkins, R.J. (2000) Modulation of NHE by osmotic shock in isolated articular chondrocytes. *Acta Physiologica Scandinavica* Vol.169. No. 3, (July 2000), pp. 221-228

Yellowley, C.E., Hancox, J.C. & Donahue, H.J. (2002). Effects of cell swelling on intracellular calcium and membrane currents in bovine articular chondrocytes. *Journal of Cellular Biochemistry,* Vol.86, No.2, pp. 290-301

Zhou, S., Cui, Z. & Urban, J.P. (2004). Factors affecting the oxygen concentration gradient from the synovial surface of articular cartilage to the cartilge-bone interface: a modelling study. *Arthritis Rhuematism,* Vol.50, No.12, (December 2004), pp. 3915-3924

12

The Role of Synovial Macrophages and Macrophage-Produced Mediators in Driving Inflammatory and Destructive Responses in Osteoarthritis

Jan Bondeson[1], Shane Wainwright[2],
Clare Hughes[2] and Bruce Caterson[2]
[1]Department of Rheumatology, Cardiff University,
Heath Park, Cardiff,
[2]Connective Tissue Biology Laboratories, Cardiff School of Biosciences,
Cardiff University, Museum Avenue, Cardiff,
UK

1. Introduction

Osteoarthritis (OA), one of the most common diseases among humans, is characterised pathologically by focal areas of damage on articular cartilage centred on load-bearing areas, associated with formation of new bone at the joint margins and changes in subchondral bone. Given the huge economic and personal burden of OA, and the fact that this disease is the major cause for the increasing demand for joint replacements, there is urgent need for disease modifying treatments to stop or at least slow the development and progression of OA.

But for this to be possible, we need further knowledge about the pathogenesis of disease initiation and progression in OA. The great success of targeted biologic therapy against rheumatoid arthritis (RA) in recent years has meant that much research has been devoted to investigating the pathophysiology of osteoarthritis (OA), in the hope of defining novel therapeutic targets. In contrast to RA, with its pannus and erosions, OA has long been thought of as a degenerative disease of cartilage, with secondary bony damage and osteophytes. In recent years, the importance of the synovium, and in particular the synovial macrophages, in OA, has been highlighted in both in vitro and in vivo studies. This article will give an overview of some important recent findings concerning the ability of macrophages to drive inflammatory and destructive disease mechanisms in OA, the role of their proinflammatory cytokines in doing so, and the potential for macrophages and macrophage-produced cytokines to be used as therapeutic targets for the development of disease-modifying anti-ostroarthritic drugs (DMOADs). There is also an abundance of potential downstream therapeutic targets in OA, including the matrix metalloproteinases, the aggrecanases, the inducible nitric oxide synthetase, and elements of the Wnt pathway.

2. Synovial macrophages and macrophage-produced mediators in driving inflammatory and destructive responses in osteoarthritis

2.1 Macrophage biology in RA and OA

In rheumatoid arthritis (RA), it is today accepted that both inflammatory and destructive features of the disease are driven through synovitis. The RA synovium has a plentiful infiltrate of activated macrophages, particularly at the cartilage-pannus junction (Kinne et al., 2007). These macrophages produce tumour necrosis factor α (TNFα), interleukin (IL)-1β and other proinflammatory cytokines. Since there is a 'cytokine cascade' with TNFα driving the other inflammatory mediators, this cytokine has become a key therapeutic target in RA, with several anti-TNFα biologic agents being used with considerable success (Feldmann & Maini, 2008). Although biologics with anti-B cell and anti-T cell co-stimulation properties have since been introduced, the anti-TNFα agents remain a mainstay of RA therapy. They have shown long-term sustained efficacy and safety, and are used all over the world with excellent results.

Clinically, RA and OA are usually easy to differentiate. X-rays of affected joints show erosions and periarticular osteoporosis in RA; in OA, they show reduction of joint space as a sign of cartilage degradation, and in later stages of the disease bony sclerosis and osteophytes. The joint pattern differs, with early RA affecting the proximal interphalangeal, metacarpophalangeal and metatarsophalangeal joints, and OA usually affecting the large joints, like the hips and knees, and also the distal (and sometimes proximal) interphalangeal joints. The typical RA patient has an elevated erythrocyte sedimentation rate, C-reactive protein and IL-6, the vast majority of OA patients do not. In RA patients, synovitis is a major feature of the disease, causing joint swelling and exudation, and driving cartilage degradation and the formation of pannus and erosive changes. In OA, there is much less joint swelling and exudation, and no pannus or erosions.

Many OA patients also have a variable degree of synovitis. Synovial inflammation is likely to contribute to disease progression in OA, as judged by the correlation between biological markers of inflammation and the progression of structural changes in OA (Clark et al., 1999; Sowers et al., 2002). Histologically, the OA synovium shows hyperplasia with an increased number of lining cells and a mixed inflammatory infiltrate mainly consisting of macrophages [Benito et al., 2005; Farahat et al., 1993]. Synovial biopsies from patients with early inflammatory OA may even resemble RA biopsies morphologically, although the percentage of macrophages is lower (1-3% as compared with 5-20%) and the percentages of T and B cells much lower [Bondeson et al., 1999a; Amos et al., 2006; Blom & van den Berg, 2007]. The synovial fluid of patients with active RA synovitis contains numerous polymorphonuclear leucocytes, something that is not the case in OA; another indicator that there is difference in pathophysiology between RA and OA synovitis.

In RA, it is today accepted that the synovitis is cytokine driven, through an disequilibrium between proinflammatory (TNFα, IL-1) and anti-inflammatory (IL-10, the IL-1 receptor antagonist, soluble TNF receptors). These proinflammatory cytokines are largely produced from a considerable infiltrate of synovial macrophages, which are particularly numerous and highly activated at the cartilage-pannus junction. Since macrophage-produced TNFα is the main mediator of disease, driving the other proinflammatory cytokines through a cytokine cascade, neutralisation of this one cytokine can reverse both synovitis and progression of joint damage (Brennan & McInnes, 2008).

Until recently, very little was known about the pathophysiology of synovitis in OA, or its role in promoting cartilage degradation, osteophytes and other features of the disease. The marked

differences in cell percentages in the inflammatory infiltrate between RA and OA would speak
in favour of differences also in the cytokine interdependence in these two diseases. For example,
the great scarcity of T cells in the OA synovium would tend to rule them (and their cytokines)
out as potential drivers of synovitis in this disease. Instead, it has been proposed that this OA
synovitis is cytokine driven, possibly through macrophage-produced TNFα and/or IL-1β,
although the levels of proinflammatory cytokines are lower than in RA. These cytokines can
stimulate their own production and induce synovial cells and chondrocytes to produce IL-6, IL-
8 and leukocyte inhibitory factor, as well as stimulate protease and prostaglandin production
(Fernandes et al., 2002). The hypothesis that TNFα and IL-1 are key mediators of inflammation
and articular cartilage destruction has raised the possibility of anti-cytokine therapy in OA, or
the design of specific disease-modifying osteoarthritic drugs (Abramson & Yazici, 2006; Pelletier
& Martel-Pelletier, 2005; Berenbaum, 2007; Qvist et al., 2008).

If it is accepted that synovial inflammation, and the production of proinflammatory and
destructive mediators from the OA synovium, are of importance for the symptoms and
progression of osteoarthritis, it is a key question which cell type in the OA synovium is
responsible for maintaining synovial inflammation. In RA, where the macrophage is the
main promoter of disease activity, macrophage-produced TNFα is a major therapeutic
target. Much less is known about macrophage biology in OA, however, although
histological studies have demonstrated that OA synovial macrophages exhibit an activated
phenotype, and that they produce both proinflammatory cytokines and vascular endothelial
growth factor (Benito et al., 2005; Haywood et al., 2003).

The spontaneous production of a variety of pro- and anti-inflammatory cytokines,
including TNFα, IL-1β and IL-10, is one of the characteristics of synovial cell cultures
derived from digested RA or OA synovium. In addition, the major MMPs and TIMPs are
spontaneously produced by these cell cultures (Foxwell et al., 1998; Bondeson et al., 1999a;
Amos et al., 2006). Less TNFα and IL-10 is produced from OA samples but the levels are
still easily detectable by ELISA (Amos et al., 2006). It is possible to use effective
adenoviral gene transfer in this model without causing apoptosis or disrupting
intracellular signalling pathways. Using an adenovirus effectively transferring the
inhibitory subunit IκBα, it was possible to selectively inhibit the transcription factor NFκB
in synovial cocultures from RA or OA patients. Macrophage-produced TNFα and IL-1β
was very strongly NFκB dependent in the RA synovium, but in OA synovium, adenoviral
transfer of IκBα did not affect IL-1β production and had only a partial effect on TNFα.
Effects on other cytokines were similar in RA and OA synovium, with IL-6 and IL-8 both
being NFκB dependent, as well as the p75 soluble TNF receptor, whereas IL-10 and the IL-
1 receptor antagonist were both NFκB independent. In addition, the matrix
metalloproteinases (MMP) 1,3, and 13 were strongly NFκB dependent in both RA and OA,
whereas their main inhibitor, tissue inhibitor of metalloproteinases (TIMP)-1 was not
(Bondeson et al., 1999a; Amos et al., 2006).

The differential effect of NFκB downregulation on the spontaneous production of TNFα and
IL-1β on RA and in OA would indicate that the regulation of at least one key intracellular
pathway differs fundamentally between these diseases. It is known that both TNFα and IL-
1β have functional NFκB elements on their promoters and that in various macrophage
models, there are both NFκB dependent and NFκB independent ways of inducing TNFα
and IL-1β (Bondeson et al., 1999b; Hayes et al., 1999). It would seem as if there are
fundamental differences in the regulation of macrophage-produced TNFα and IL-1β

between RA and OA, with cytokine levels being higher and NFκB playing a more important role in RA (Bondeson et al., 1999a; Amos et al., 2006; Brennan et al., 2002; Andreakos et al., 2003). The differential effect of NFκB downregulation on the spontaneous production of TNFα and IL-1β on RA and in OA would indicate that the regulation of at least one key intracellular pathway differs fundamentally between these diseases. There are not many other studies comparing RA and OA intracellular signalling, although a recent study demonstrated differences in the phosphorylation of the Pyk2 and Src kinases, belonging to the focal adhesion kinase family, between RA and OA (Shahrara et al., 2007).

2.2 Macrophages drive both inflammatory and destructive responses in the OA synovium

In cultures of osteoarthritis synovial cells, specific depletion of synovial macrophages could be achieved using incubation of the cells with anti-CD14-conjugated magnetic beads (Bondeson et al., 2006). These CD14+-depleted cultures of synovial cells no longer produced significant amounts of macrophage-derived cytokines like TNFα and IL-1β. Interestingly, there was also significant inhibition (40-70%) of several cytokines produced mainly by synovial fibroblasts, like IL-6 and IL-8, and also significant downregulation of MMP-1 and MMP-3 (Figure 1). This would indicate that OA synovial macrophages play an important role in activating fibroblasts in these densely plated cultures of synovial cells, and in perpetuating the production of proinflammatory cytokines and destructive enzymes (Bondeson et al., 2006). That the regulation is not tighter than observed is probably because the fibroblasts have an activated phenotype when put into culture, with considerable spontaneous production of cytokines and other mediators. It can be speculated that once the macrophages are removed, the synovial fibroblasts change their phenotype and downregulate their production of both proinflammatory cytokines and destructive MMPs.

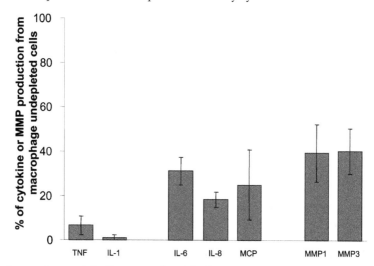

Fig. 1. OA cultures of synovial cells were either left intact or macrophage depleted. Cells were left to adhere for 24 h before the supernatants were removed for ELISA analysis of cytokines and MMPs, with data expressed as the percentage of cytokine/MMP production in the depleted culture as compared with the undepleted one, with the SEM given. Adapted from [23].

An important series of papers, using injections of liposome-encapsulated clodronate to induce depletion of synovial lining macrophages, has provided some intriguing new information about the role of macrophages in driving degenerative changes in a mouse model of experimental OA induced by injection of collagenase (Blom et al., 2004, 2007a). The collagenase injection causes weakening of ligaments leading to gradual onset of OA pathology within six weeks of induction, without any direct collagenase-induced cartilage damage being observed. If macrophage depletion had been achieved prior to the elicitation of experimental OA, there was potent reduction of both fibrosis and osteophyte formation (Blom et al., 2004, 2007a; van Lent et al, 2004). This would indicate that in this murine model of OA, synovial macrophages control the production of the growth factors that promote fibrosis and osteophyte formation, both key pathophysiological events in OA.

In this model of murine experimental OA, it was also possible to monitor the effect of macrophage depletion on the formation of the VDIPEN neoepitope that indicates MMP-induced cleavage of aggrecan (Blom et al., 2007). Between day 7 and day 14, however, VDIPEN expression more than doubled in non-depleted joints, whereas it remained unchanged in depleted ones. This would indicate that, in agreement with the data from human OA synovium discussed above, the production of MMPs in this murine model of OA is macrophage dependent. Analysis of samples of synovium and cartilage from the murine OA joints in this model demonstrated that MMP-2,3 and 9 were induced in both these tissues when murine OA was induced by collagenase. But whereas the MMP levels in the cartilage were unaffected by macrophage depletion, those in the synovium were inhibited, suggesting that removal of the macrophages would downregulate the production of MMPs from the synovial fibroblasts, and that the gradual decrease in the diffusion of these MMPs to the cartilage would prevent aggrecanolysis, as evidenced by the reduction in VDIPEN expression.

2.3 Macrophage-produced cytokines as therapeutic targets in OA

To investigate the mechanisms involved in this macrophage driven stimulation of inflammatory and degradative pathways in the OA synovium, specific neutralisation of the endogenous production of TNFα and/or IL-1β could be used in the cultures of OA synovial cell (Bondeson et al., 2006). OA synovial cell cultures were either left untreated, incubated with the p75 TNF soluble receptor Ig fusion protein etanercept (Enbrel), incubated with a neutralizing anti-IL-1β antibody, or incubated with a combination of Enbrel and anti-IL-1β. As could be expected, TNFα production was effectively neutralised by Enbrel treatment, and IL-1β by treatment with the neutralizing anti-IL-1β antibody (Figure 2). There was no effect of Enbrel on IL-1β production, nor did the neutralizing anti-IL-1β antibody affect the production of TNFα. This is in marked contrast to the situation in RA, where IL-1β is strongly TNFα dependent in these cultures of synovial cells (Brennan et al., 1989). This finding would seem to indicate yet another difference in macrophage cytokine biology between RA and OA: whereas TNFα is the 'boss cytokine' in the RA synovium, regulating the production of IL-1β, there is a redundancy between these two cytokines in the OA synovium, with neither TNFα nor IL-1β regulating the production of the other (Figure 2).

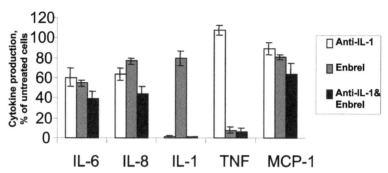

Fig. 2. Effect of neutralisation of TNFα and/or IL-1β on cytokine production in OA synovial cells. In these experiments, 2×10^6 cells per well were plated into 4 wells on a 24 well plate in 1 ml RPMI 1640 supplemented with 10% FCS. The cells in these 4 wells were either left untreated, incubated with the p75 TNF soluble receptor Ig fusion protein etanercept (Enbrel), incubated with a neutralizing anti-IL-1β antibody, or incubated with a combination of etanercept and anti-IL-1β. After incubation for 48 h the supernatants were removed for ELISA analysis of various cytokines. The data is expressed as percentage of the production of untreated cells, with the SEM given.

Both Enbrel and the neutralizing anti-IL-1β antibody inhibited IL-6 and IL-8, with 60% inhibition achieved when both IL-1β and TNFα were neutralized (Figure 2). The production of MCP-1 was not affected by the neutralizing anti-IL-1β antibody, but it was significantly decreased by Enbrel and by the combination of the two. It was also possible to study the effect of neutralizing IL-1β and/or TNFα on the mRNA expression and protein production of the major MMPs and aggrecanases, using RT-PCR and ELISA analysis in parallel (Bondeson et al., 2006, 2008). The results indicate that although neither Enbrel nor the neutralizing anti-IL-1β antibody had an impressive effect on the important collagenases MMP-1 and MMP-13, combination of the two led to significant inhibition both on the mRNA and protein levels (Figure 3). These findings indicate that in the OA synovium, the macrophages potently regulate the production of several important fibroblast-produced cytokines and MMPs, via a combined effect of IL-1β and TNFα.

There was no effect of either Enbrel or the neutralizing anti-IL-1β antibody on ADAMTS5 expression, nor was it at all affected by a combination of these treatments (Figure 3). Thus ADAMTS5 appears to be constitutive in OA synovial cells. In contrast, ADAMTS4 was significantly ($p<0.05$) inhibited by Enbrel, and more potently ($p<0.01$) inhibited by a combination of Enbrel and the neutralizing anti-IL-1β antibody (Figure 3). This would indicate that in the human OA synovium, the upregulation of ADAMTS4 is dependent on TNFα and IL-1 produced by the synovial macrophages, whereas ADAMTS5 is constitutive, and not changed by these cytokines (Bondeson et al., 2006, 2008).

After the success of targeted biological therapy in RA, there has been a good deal of interest in investigating anti-cytokine strategies also in OA (Malemud, 2004; Blom et al., 2007b). In RA, TNFα has become the major therapeutic target, whereas strategies targeting IL-1 have met with only moderate success. From the clinical data available, the same appears to be true for psoriasis, psoriatic arthritis, ankylosing spondylitis and juvenile chronic arthritis. In juvenile chronic arthritis, strategies directed against either TNFα or the IL-1 receptor antagonist have been successful (Burger et al., 2006; Kalliolas & Liossis, 2008). This may

The Role of Synovial Macrophages and Macrophage-Produced Mediators in Driving Inflammatory and Destructive
Responses in Osteoarthritis

241

indicate that there are subtle differences in cytokine biology between these inflammatory arthritides, with IL-1 having a relatively more prominent role in juvenile chronic arthritis, and in adult Still's disease. Some of the potential small molecule disease-modifying anti-osteoarthritic drugs, like pralnacasan and diacerein, would appear to act at least in part as inhibitors of interleukin-1 (Rudolphi et al., 2003; Pavelka et al., 2007; Qvist et al., 2008).

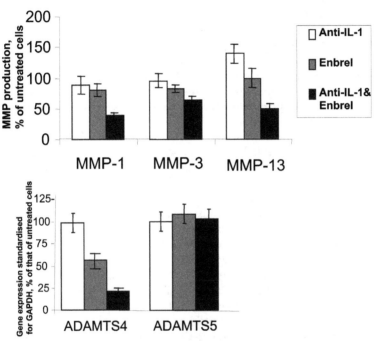

Fig. 3. Effect of neutralisation of TNFα and/or IL-1β on MMP production and ADAMTS gene expression in OA synovial cells. Experimental conditions were as in the Legend to Figure 2. After incubation for 48 h the supernatants were removed for ELISA analysis of MMPs. The cells were washed with PBS and the RNA extracted using Tri-reagent for RT-PCR analysis using oligonucleotide primers specific for ADAMTS4 and ADAMTS5. Analyis of GAPDH was used for comparison of gene expression, and in the right panel. ADAMTS4 and ADAMTS5 mRNA levels, expressed as percentage of the gene expression in untreated cells, as standardised for GAPDH, are given (n=4).

The experimental data described above would hint that unlike the situation in RA, there is redundancy between TNFα and IL-1 in the OA synovium. Both these cytokines appear to play important roles in driving the production of other proinflammatory cytokines, as well as MMPs and aggrecanases, however (Bondeson et al., 2006, 2010). In a patient with inflammatory knee OA, with synovitis visible on an MRI scan, an anti-TNF drug had marked benefit on pain and walking distance, as well as synovitis, synovial effusion and bone marrow oedema (Grunke & Schulze-Koops, 2006). In a pilot study involving 12 patients with inflammatory hand OA, the anti-TNFα antibody adalimumab had no significant effect (Magnano et al., 2007). Another pilot study involving 10 patients indicated that intra-articular injection of the anti-TNFα antibody infliximab caused significant symptomatic relief compared with placebo, although there was no significant difference in the radiological progression score after 12 months (Fioravanti et al., 2009). Interestingly, another study looked at the radiological progression of interphalangeal OA in a large cohort of RA patients treated with various disease-modifying drugs or with the anti-TNF antibody infliximab found that OA progression was significantly reduced in the patients receiving infliximab (Güler-Yüksel et al., 2008, 2010). An early study in 13 patients with knee OA indicated that intra-articular administration of the interleukin-1 receptor antagonist anakinra had some degree of analgesic effect (Chevalier et al., 2005; Goupille et al., 2007). Disappointingly, a later double-blind, placebo-controlled study could demonstrate no improvement in knee OA symptoms after intra-articular injection of anakinra, however (Chevalier et al., 2009). This may well be related to the short half-life of the drug, and the invention of an effective sustained-release system, or another alternative anti-IL-1 strategy that works intra-articularly, might still be worth trying (Martel-Pelletier & Pelletier, 2009).

There is a need for further clinical trials, with larger numbers of patients, to compare the effect of anti-cytokine strategies in large joint (knee/hip) with small joint (hand) OA, as well as correlating the results of targeted cytokine inhibition with the clinical amount of synovitis and macrophage infiltration. It would seem likely that inhibition of either TNFα or IL-1 would be much more efficacious in patients with significant inflammatory OA, as evidenced by joint exudation and active synovitis. In patients who already have significant irreversible bone and cartilage damage, the effect of these biologics would be less impressive. Since a combination of the anti-TNF biologic etanercept and the recombinant IL-1 receptor antagonist anakinra provided no added benefit and increased risk of infection and other side effects, such combination therapy is not recommended in RA (Genovese et al., 2004). In OA, however, such a combination could potentially be more attractive, due to the evidence that there is redundancy between TNFα and IL-1 in the OA synovium, if there is a way to solve the obvious safety concerns. As with all potential disease-modifying strategies in OA, a major obstacle for anti-cytokine therapy in OA will be the difficulty of recruiting patients with early inflammatory OA, before gross bone and cartilage loss is obvious on X-rays and clinical examination. In recent years, some exciting molecular imaging techniques, involving a tracer binding to the macrophage peripheral benzodiazepine receptor, or alternatively folate receptor β, have been invented (van der Laken et al., 2008; van der Heijden et al., 2009). Although hitherto published only for RA, there is no reason these methods could not be used also in OA, with the potential to identify a sub-group of patients with a higher degree of macrophage infiltration, or alternatively to correlate success with anti-cytokine approaches with the amount of macrophages detected.

2.4 Some potential downstream therapeutic targets in OA

Nitric oxide (NO) has been demonstrated to be a pathogenic mediator in OA. NO and its metabolites plays a role in the cyclooxygenase-2 activation leading to prostaglandin production, in activation of MMPs, in DNA damage, lipid peroxidation, chondrocyte apoptosis, and reduction of proteoglycan synthesis. NO production is regulated by the enzyme inducible NO synthetase (iNOS), which is in turn driven by proinflammatory cytokines and other pathologic stresses. In animal models of OA, the presence of iNOS and NO production was correlated with a higher rate of chondrocyte apoptosis and meniscal degeneration (Hashimoto et al., 1998; Hellio le Graverand et al., 2000). iNOS is overexpressed in human OA synovium and cartilage, and the levels of 3-nitrotyrosine and other NO metabolites is elevated in OA patients. Sustained high levels of NO leads to the formation of various harmful NO-derived metabolites, of which the radical peroxynitrite is an inducer of cytotoxicity and tissue damage.

Due to its many harmful effects on joint integrity, iNOS has long been of interest in both inflammatory and degenerative arthritis. It was defined as a potential therapeutic target in OA after a study in a murine model of joint instability-induced experimental OA showed that iNOS-deficient mice developed significantly less OA than wild-type animals, with about 50% reduction of both osteophytes and cartilage lesions (van den Berg et al., 1999). In a canine model of joint instability-induced experimental OA, treatment with a small-molecule iNOS inhibitor led to impressive inhibition of 3-nitrotyrosine formation, and significant (nearly 50%) reduction of OA lesions. A two-year Phase IIb/III clinical trial (Pfizer) is ongoing to evaluate the safety and efficacy of a selective iNOS inhibitor in the treatment of obese or overweight patients with knee OA (Hellio le Graverand-Gastineau, 2010).

An interesting and novel therapeutic target in OA is osteogenic protein-1 (OP-1), which exhibits potent anabolic activity in models of cartilage homeostasis and repair. This growth factor also has anti-catabolic actions, including MMP and aggrecanase inhibition (Badlani et al., 2008). It has been investigated in various animal models of OA with positive results: injected intra-articularly, it inhibited cartilage degeneration and the progression of OA (Sekiya et al., 2009). A Phase I clinical trial of intra-articular recombinant OP-1 (Stryker), assessing safety and effect on signs and symptoms, with dose escalation over 24 weeks, has been completed (Hellio le Graverand-Gastineau, 2010).

Another potential therapeutic target in OA is fibroblast growth factor (FGF)-18, which plays a role in chondrogenesis and osteogenesis during skeletal development and growth. In a rat model of meniscal tear-induced OA, bi-weekly intra-articular injections of recombinant FGF-18 induced a significant, dose-dependent reduction in cartilage degeneration, as well as an increased in chondrocyte size and subchondral bone remodelling (Moore et al., 2005). Intra-articular, recombinant FGF-18 (Merck Serono) has undergone a 12-month Phase II clinical trial in knee OA, and another Phase II study in acute cartilage injury is under way (Hellio le Graverand-Gastineau, 2010).

In recent years, the Wnt signalling pathways has been implicated in the pathophysiology of OA. The Wnts are a complex family of lipid modified, secreted glycoproteins that play a role in synovial joint formation, and are involved in the transcription of many proteins. Wnt signalling occurs through at least three pathways. Best known is the canonical Wnt pathway that induces β-catenin, but there is also a Wnt-Ca^{2+} pathway and a planar cell polarity pathway. It is canonical Wnt that is thought to play a role in OA, however. In this pathway, Wnt binds to the Frizzled receptor, and through several signalling steps this leads to accumulation of cytoplasmic β-catenin, which translocates to the nucleus and binds to TCF/LEF transcription factors, converting them from repressors to activators of the transcription of a great variety of genes, important MMPs, growth factors and chondrocyte hypertrophy markers among them (Blom et al., 2010). Whereas low levels of β-catenin are of importance to prevent chondrocyte apoptosis, intracellular accumulation of β-catenin appears to induce OA-like changes. In particular, increased levels of β-catenin are observed in areas of cartilage degeneration.

Recent data suggest a role for wnt-1 induced signalling protein 1 (WISP-1), a wnt-induced secreted protein, in the synovium during OA (Blom et al., 2009). During experimental OA wnt-signalling is not only occurring in the cartilage but also in the synovium, as was found by β-catenin staining. WISP-1, a gene in which a polymorphism was shown to be associated with spinal OA (Urano et al., 2007) was strongly upregulated in the synovium of two models for OA. Further investigation indicated that WISP-1 is a potent inducer of MMPs in macrophages, whereas the short term effect on chondrocytes is less pronounced. In addition, overexpression of WISP-1 specifically in the synovium induced MMP and aggrecanase mediated neoepitopes VDIPEN and NITEGE in the cartilage, indicating that WISP-1 expression in synovial cells leads to cartilage degradation. Interestingly, these effects were independent of IL-1, since WISP1 did not induce IL-1 production in macrophages, nor was cartilage damage decreased in IL-1 deficient mice after synovial WISP-1 overexpression. Blocking studies are needed in order to substantiate this role for WISP-1 in (experimental) OA.

The targeting of Wnt signalling in OA drug discovery is likely to be impaired by the lack of knowledge concerning the normal function of these signalling pathways. For example, the direct targeting of β-catenin is likely to be hazardous, considering its importance for normal chondrocyte physiology, and its role in carcinogenesis. Whereas intracellular accumulation of β-catenin is linked to the induction of OA-like pathology, conditional knockdown of β-catenin signalling is equally harmful, since it induces chondrocyte apoptosis (Blom et al., 2010). Importantly, there is an increasing amount of data concerning the change of expression of certain Wnt protein and their inhibitors in the OA synovium. For example, Wnt16 is strongly upregulated in the synovium in a model of experimental OA, and also as a result of cartilage injury. Although both WISP-1 and Wnt16 have promise, more knowledge of Wnt signalling in health and disease is needed before any member of this family of protein can be defined as a therapeutic target in OA.

2.5 Matrix metalloproteinases as potential therapeutic targets in OA

Matrix metalloproteinases (MMPs) are a family of zinc-dependent endopeptidases that are synthesized as inactive proenzymes and activated extracellularly through cleavage of their prodomains by other proteases. Since MMPs cleave many of the structural components of the extracellular matrix, they have long been known to play a part in both inflammatory and degenerative arthritis. Inhibition of their activity through various broad-spectrum MMP inhibitors was effective in both mouse and guinea-pig models of osteoarthritis, but in humans these nonspecific MMP inhibitors caused musculoskeletal side effects, with painful joint stiffening and adhesive capsulitis (Hutchinson et al., 1998). Since no specific MMP has been pointed out as being involved in this musculoskeletal syndrome, the lack of selectivity of these broad-spectrum MMP inhibitors has been blamed for this side effect.

Since there is evidence that MMP-13 may well be the dominant collagenase in OA cartilage, with higher activity against type II collagen than any of the others, this MMP has been a main target for drug discovery. In a mouse model, overexpression of MMP-13 via an inducible transgene caused an OA-like phenotype (Neuhold et al., 2001). Recently, a group of compounds with a high degree of potency against MMP-13, as well as selectivity against other MMPs, were presented as a novel class of MMP-13 inhibitors. In the rat medial meniscal tear model of OA, one of these compounds protected articular cartilage as effectively as a broad-spectrum MMP inhibitor (Baragi et al., 2009). Numerous MMP-13 inhibitors are in early phase clinical development as DMOADs.

In osteoarthritis, aggrecan degradation, caused by increased activity of proteolytic enzymes that degrade macromolecules in the cartilage extracellular matrix, is followed by irreversible collagen degradation. The degradation of aggrecan is mediated by various matrix proteinases, mainly the aggrecanases, multidomain metalloproteinases belonging to the ADAMTS family. There has been much interest in the possible role of these aggrecanases, mainly ADAMTS4 and ADAMTS5, as therapeutic targets in osteoarthritis. It has long been debated which of the ADAMTSs is the main aggrecanase in human OA. Due to observations of ADAMTS4 mRNA being inducible through interleukin (IL)-1 and other stimuli in human OA chondrocytes and synovial fibroblasts, this enzyme attracted a good deal of attention (Bondeson et al., 2008).

But in models of murine OA induced by antigen or surgical joint destabilisation, ADAMTS5 is the pathologically induced aggrecanase. ADAMTS4 deficient mice develop normally and develop surgically induced degenerative arthritis in a similar manner to wild-type mice, but deletion of ADAMTS5 protects mice from developing arthritis (Glasson et al., 2004, 2005; Stanton et al., 2005). These results suggest that at least in murine models of OA, ADAMTS5 is the major aggrecanase. The only caveat to this conclusion is that there is a discrepancy between human and murine cells with regard to the regulation of ADAMTS5: the murine, but not the human, ADAMTS5 gene responds to IL-1 stimulation. Furthermore, a study using a small interfering RNA approach could demonstrate that both ADAMTS4 and ADAMTS5 contribute to the aggrecanase activity in human cartilage explants (Song et al., 2007). The search for the primary aggrecanase in human OA is still ongoing (Bondeson et al., 2008; Tortorella & Malfait, 2008).

The available data on ADAMTS5 gene promoters would suggest that this enzyme is the antithesis of ADAMTS4, with regard to its regulation. ADAMTS5 activity is reduced by C-terminal processing, whereas ADAMTS4 activity is enhanced (Gendron et al., 2007; Fosang et al., 2008). Then, in human cartilage and synovium, ADAMTS5 is constitutive whereas ADAMTS4 is the inducible aggrecanase, responding to IL-1 and TNFα in an NFκB dependent manner (Bondeson et al., 2008). The contrast between murine and human chondrocyte studies indicates that the situation may well be profoundly different in mice, something that of course would affect the validity of OA animal studies using these animals.

Several pharmaceutical companies (Wyeth/Pfizer, Schering-Plough, Rottapharm SpA, Alantos Pharm, Japan Tobacco) have patented small-molecule inhibitors of ADAMTS4 and ADAMTS5, developed mainly as potential DMOADs. Some of these compounds are claimed to be specific, whereas others have effect against both enzymes, against other ADAMTS members, or even against MMPs (Wittwer et al., 2007; Tortorella et al., 2009). The Wyeth/Pfizer compound was recently used in a phase I clinical trial in osteoarthritis (Hellio le Graverand-Gastineau, 2010; Gilbert et al., 2011).

The main endogenous inhibitor of ADAMTS4 and ADAMTS5 is tissue inhibitor of metalloproteinases (TIMP)-3, with K_i values in the subnanomolar range (Kashiwagi et al., 2001). This inhibition may well be modulated by interactions between aggrecan and the C-terminal domain of ADAMTS4 (Wayne et al., 2007). Interestingly, reactive-site mutants of the N-terminal inhibitory domain of TIMP-3, also inhibit ADAMTS4 (Lim et al., 2010). TIMP-3 knockout mice spontaneously lose their articular cartilage (Sahebjam et al., 2007). There is a good deal of interest in recombinant full-length or N-terminal TIMP-3 as a potential DMOAD, to be delivered intra-articularly, although it is yet to enter clinical trials.

3. Conclusions

In a recent editorial about the development of biologic therapy in RA, its distinguished authors pointed out that two of the greatest impediment for drug discovery were preconceived ideas about disease mechanisms and vested interests among those responsible for investigating potential therapeutic targets (Maini & Feldmann, 2007). In the early 1990s, it was generally accepted that 'autoimmune' diseases like RA were T cell driven. The synovial T cells were driving both inflammatory and destructive pathways, it was presumed, and although immunosuppression with drugs like cyclosporine or azathioprine could ameliorate symptoms, the disease remained incurable. Although this concept was successively undermined by the demonstration of low levels of lymphokines in RA synovial tissue and exudates, and later by the failure of anti-CD4 therapy in RA, it was adhered to with a rigidity that today seems quite inexplicable. Another both unconstructive and nihilistic notion popular at this time was that there was redundancy between proinflammatory cytokines and other inflammatory mediators, meaning that the targeting of an individual cytokine would be pointless. The notion of TNFα as a therapeutic target was initially greeted with incredulity, leading to a significant delay in the clinical development of these strategies (Feldmann, 2009). An idea originating in Britain was overlooked by the biotech and pharmaceutical industry of that country, and later commercialized in the United States with remarkable success.

The discovery that the neutralization of a single cytokine could lead to lasting remission in RA, with regard to both inflammation and development of erosions, had several beneficial effects for medical research. Firstly, it inspired further research into the disease mechanisms of other forms of chronic inflammation, leading to the establishment of anti-TNFα biologic therapy also in inflammatory bowel disease, psoriatic arthritis, ankylosing spondylitis, juvenile chronic arthritis and psoriasis. Secondly, it blew aside the concept that RA was an incurable 'autoimmune' disease, and inspired intensive research into RA pathophysiology, with the aim to find other targets for directed biologic therapy. This research has been rewarded with considerable success, with effective anti-CD20 and anti-T cell costimulation biologics now being available for use in RA, and many other biologics on their way in clinical development. Thirdly, the successes for biologic therapy of RA opened the door for more energetic work to identify potential therapeutic targets also in other chronic diseases. Even OA, the 'ugly sister' of rheumatology, received considerable attention, since here was a disease with immense unmet need and no disease modifying strategies on the market.

It is of course important that the lessons learnt from the successful drug development for RA and other forms of inflammatory arthritis are implemented in the search for therapeutic targets in OA. First to go should be the counterproductive notion of OA as the incurable result of 'wear and tear'. Although mechanical trauma and strain definitely play a part in the pathogenesis of OA, it remains a multifactorial disease. Many sick and obese people never develop OA; some fit and healthy ones do. It would also be beneficial if the concept of OA an primarily a disease of cartilage was challenged. A more promising approach, conducive to the definition of potential therapeutic targets, would be to consider the pathophysiological contributions of both synovium and cartilage (Figure 4). Activated synovial macrophages stimulate synovial fibroblasts, leading to the production of proinflammatory cytokines and that will have the ability to activate chondrocytes into producing further degradative enzymes. Furthermore, the production of MMPs, and quite possible aggrecanases, from the synovium, would also have a pathophysiological potential.

Since OA is a heterogenous disease, with variable degree of synovitis and macrophage infiltration, this simplified diagram of inter-cell and inter-tissue signalling (Figure 4) is likely to differ between patients: some have a higher degree of macrophage activation, synovitis and joint exudation, whereas others have 'dry' OA.

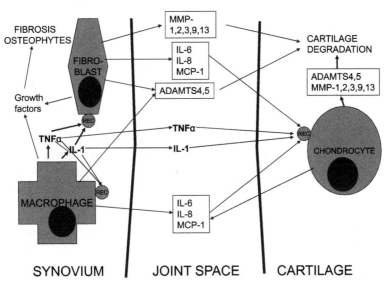

Fig. 4. A simplified view of the role of synovial macrophages in OA, in activating synovial fibroblasts and driving inflammatory and destructive responses. In this figure, 'REC' signifies all kinds of cell surface-related receptors. It remains unproven, although not unlikely, that ADAMTS4 and/or ADAMTS5 produced by synovial cells can be secreted into the synovial fluid, to influence cartilage degradation. Nor is it entirely clear that synovial macrophages produce ADAMTS4, although some preliminary data hints that this is possible.

Both in vitro and in vivo data point out the synovial macrophages and their main proinflammatory cytokines as potential therapeutic targets in OA. Macrophages drive the production of IL-6 and IL-8, the main MMPs (1,3,9,13) and ADAMTS4 from the synovial fibroblasts, and they are also crucial for the development of OA-related pathology, such as osteophyte formation and MMP-mediated cartilage breakdown (Bondeson et al., 2006, 2010; Blom et al., 2004, 2007). It should be remembered that the biology of OA synovitis is quite dissimilar from that in RA, with different cell composition, fewer macrophages, less synovial proliferation and synovial cell transformation, and no pannus or erosions. There are also differences in the regulation of key intracellular pathways between RA and OA macrophages (Amos et al., 2006) and important differences in cytokine biology (Bondeson et al., 2006), indicating that on the molecular as well as the clinical and histopathological levels, RA and OA are quite different diseases. The finding that there is redundancy between TNFα and IL-1 in the OA synovium, whereas TNFα drives IL-1 in RA, may well have some importance for the potential of anti-cytokine biologic treatment of OA. The concept of OA as a heterogenous disease would seem to be crucial for the application of anti-TNFα and/or anti-IL-1 strategies in this disease: in a patient with synovitis, exudation and bone marrow oedema, these strategies are likely to be more successful than in a patient with 'dry' OA secondary to obesity, or non-inflammatory OA of the distal interphalangeal joints. Had the clinical trials concerning anti-IL-1 and anti-TNFα strategies in OA selected patients with inflammatory knee OA verified by MRI, instead of patients with OA of the distal interphalangeal joints, the results may well have been different.

Disappointingly, there are currently no approved disease-modifying therapeutic strategies for OA. The three main impediments of drug development in OA have been the inadequacy of animal models of the disease, the difficulty in defining endpoints, finding validated biomarkers, and conducting worthwhile clinical trials in a disease that is so very slowly progressive, and the selection of patients for these clinical trials. Early OA is often asymptomatic, and the denudation of articular cartilage in advanced OA is likely to be an irreversible process. Many patients are likely to have some degree of denudation of cartilage, and exposure of subchondral bone, already at the time they exhibit radiographically obvious OA. Due to the slow progression of the disease, OA clinical trials need to take between one and three years, and use large numbers of patients. It would have been important to recruit patients with early disease, and a high risk of rapid progression, but the criteria currently used to define inclusion into clinical studies, and the lack of reliable predictors of disease progression, renders this very difficult. Furthermore, the commonly used measurement of OA progression, joint space narrowing on plain radiographs, is something of a blunt instrument, due to the slow progression of the disease.

The first criterium a DMOAD must fulfil is that its safety profile must be impeccable. Various drug companies and research organizations have performed clinical trials with existing drugs of proven safety, like the bisphosphonate drug Risedronate and the antibiotic Doxycycline but with unimpressive results. Nor has Diacerein, a compound with some degree of interleukin-1β inhibitory effect in vitro, or Licofelone, supposed to act as a combined cyclooxygenase and 5-lipoxygenase inhibitor, any obvious disease modifying potential in OA (see review by Hellio le Graverand-Gastineau, 2010). There is also a good deal of data concerning the widely available over-the-counter 'nutraceuticals' glucosamine and chondroitin sulphate. Although some early studies indicated that these substances at least had an analgesic effect, a recent meta-analysis found no evidence of them affecting neither joint pain, nor joint space narrowing, in OA (Wandel et al., 2010). Worryingly, there was also a discrepancy between industry sponsored and industry independent clinical trials, the latter indicating that the substances were close to worthless.

The situation appears to be that the existing drugs can provide little help to OA drug discovery: not only are they ineffective, but they provide no worthwhile clues as to future therapeutic targets in this disease. For some of them, their mechanisms are unknown, whereas others have been introduced from elements of serendipity rather than from understanding of the basic principles of OA pathophysiology. For OA drug discovery to move in the right direction, new ideas are required. Three compounds in phase III or phase IV development, namely calcitonin, vitamin D3 and avocado-soybean unsaponifiable; it would be an agreeable surprise if either of them has success as a DMOAD. Some more promising candidates are currently in phase II clinical trials. The Pfizer iNOS inhibitor benefits from quite solid preclinical data, and there is nothing to suggest it would be unsafe. Even a DMOAD leading to 20-30% slowing of the progression of OA would be in a strong market position, due to the absence of any competitor. Both OP-1 and FGF-18 are also in Phase II clinical trials. Albeit showing enormous future as a potential therapeutic target in OA, the canonical Wnt pathway is currently insufficiently understood, due to its complexity and its role in maintaining physiological function.

Non-selective MMP inhibitors are unlikely to have any future as potential DMOADs, but the selective MMP-13 inhibitors may well feature, although they do not appear to have progressed into clinical trials. Theoretically, the aggrecanase inhibitors have considerable promise as DMOADs. In mice, ADAMTS5 is clearly the dominant aggrecanase with regard to the development of OA in mice, but the dominant aggrecanase in human OA has not yet been identified. It is an important task for OA drug development that this is achieved, due to the need for an aggrecanase inhibitor used as a DMOAD to be as selective as possible. Another problem is that the normal function of ADAMTS4 and ADAMTS5 has not been elucidated. Both ADAMTS4 and ADAMTS5 knockout mice are fertile and phenotypically normal, speaking against these enzymes influencing the natural murine skeletal or joint development (Glasson et al., 2004, 2005). However, a recent study has indicated that ADAMTS5-deficient mice in fact had reduced apoptosis and decreased versican cleavage in the interdigital webs (McCulloch et al., 2010).

The search for a future DMOAD is reaching a critical time. There is a need for one of the abovementioned strategies to show definite promise in clinical trials, for the pharmaceutical industry to become convinced that the enormous effort and very considerable dollar costs to conduct preclinical and clinical OA research can be worth the effort. Some companies have already has OA projects, or even entire OA research departments, axed due to disappointing results in spite of vast financial spending. The window of opportunity for the search for therapeutic targets in OA, opened by the success of the anti-TNFs and other biologics for use in RA and other forms of inflammatory diseases, might be in danger of closing fast if some of the potential DMOADs in clinical development would join the long list of compounds used in 'failed' clinical studies in OA.

4. Acknowledgements

Address correspondence to Dr J. Bondeson at the Department of Rheumatology, Cardiff University, Heath Park, Cardiff CF14 4XN, UK; E-mail: BondesonJ@cf.ac.uk. This work has been supported by the Arthritis Research UK, grants no. W0596, 13172, 14570 and 18893.

5. Abbreviations

ADAMTS, A Disintegrin And Metalloproteinase with Transspondin Motives.
DMOAD, Disease-modifying anti-osteoarthritis drug
IL, Interleukin
MMP, Matrix metalloprotease.
NFκB, Nuclear factor κB.
OA, Osteoarthritis.
RA, Rheumatoid arthritis.
TIMP, Tissue inhibitor of metalloproteases.
TNF, Tumour necrosis factor.

6. References

Abramson, S.B. & Yazici, Y. (2006) Biologics in development for rheumatoid arthritis: relevance to osteoarthritis. *Advanced Drug Delivery Reviews* Vol. 58, No. 2 (May 2006), pp. 212-225. ISSN 0169-409X

Amos, N., Lauder, S., Evans, A., Feldmann, M. & Bondeson, J. (2006) Adenoviral gene transfer into osteoarthritis synovial cells using the endogenous inhibitor IκBα reveals that most, but not all, inhibitory and destructive mediators, are NFκB dependent. *Rheumatology* Vol. 45, No. 3 (March 2006), pp. 1201-1209. ISSN 1462-0324

Andreakos, E., Smith, C., Kiriakidis, S., Monaco, C., de Martin, R., Brennan, F.M., Paleolog, E., Feldmann, M. & Foxwell, B.M. (2003) Heterogenous requirement of IkappaB kinase 2 for inflammatory cytokine and matrix metalloproteinase production in rheumatoid arthritis: implications for therapy. *Arthritis and Rheumatism* Vol. 48, No. 7 (July 2003), pp. 1901-1912. ISSN 1529-0131

Badlani, N., Inoue, A., Healey, R., Coutts, R. & Amiel, D. (2008) The protective effect of OP-1 on articular cartilage in the development of osteoarthritis. *Osteoarthritis and Cartilage* Vol. 16, No. 5 (May 2008), 600-606. ISSN 1063-4584

Baragi, V.M., Becher, G., Bendele, A.M., Biesinger, R., Bluhm, H., Boer, J., Deng, H., Dodd, R., Essers, M., Feuerstein, T., Gallagher, B.M. Jr, Gege, C., Hochgürtel, M., Hofmann, M., Jaworski, A., Jin, L., Kiely, A., Korniski, B., Kroth, H., Nix, D., Nolte, B., Piecha, D., Powers, T.S., Richter, F., Schneider, M., Steeneck, C., Sucholeiki, I., Taveras, A., Timmermann, A., Van Veldhuizen, J., Weik, J., Wu, X. & Xia, B. (2009) A new class of potent matrix metalloproteinase 13 inhibitors for potential treatment of osteoarthritis: Evidence of histologic and clinical efficacy without musculoskeletal toxicity in rat models. *Arthritis and Rheumatism* Vol. 60, No. 7 (July 2009), pp. 2008-2018. ISSN 1529-0131

Benito, M.J., Veale, D.J., FitzGerald, O., van den Berg, W.B. & Bresnihan, B. (2005) Synovial tissue inflammation in early and late osteoarthritis. *Annals of the Rheumatic Diseases* Vol. 64, No. 9 (September 2005), pp. 1263-1267. ISSN 0003-4967

Berenbaum, F. (2007) The quest for the holy grail: a disease-modifying osteoarthritis drug. *Arthritis Research and Therapy* Vol. 9, No. 6 (December 2007), article no. 111. ISSN 1478-6354

Blom, A.B., van Lent, P.L.E.M., Holthuysen, A.E.M., van der Kraan, P.M., Roth, J., van Rooijen, N. & van den Berg WB. (2004) Synovial lining macrophages mediate osteophyte formation during experimental osteoarthritis. *Osteoarthritis and Cartilage* Vol. 12, No. 8 (August 2004), pp. 627-635. ISSN 1063-4584

Blom, A.B. & van den Berg, W.B. (2007) The synovium and its role in osteoarthritis. In: *Bone and Osteoarthritis*, F. Bronner & M.C. Farach-Carson (Eds.), Vol. 4, pp. 65-79, Springer Verlag, ISBN 9781846285134, Berlin, Germany.

Blom, A.B., van Lent, P.L., Libregts, S., Holthuysen, A.E., van der Kraan, P.M., van Rooijen, N. & van den Berg, W.B. (2007a) Crucial role of macrophages in matrix metalloproteinase-mediated cartilage destruction during experimental osteoarthritis. *Arthritis and Rheumatism* Vol. 56, No. 1 (January 2007), pp. 147-157. ISSN 1529-0131

Blom, A.B., van der Kraan, P.M. & van den Berg, W.B. (2007b) Cytokine targeting in osteoarthritis. *Current Drug Targets* Vol. 8, No. 2 (February 2007), pp. 283-292. ISSN 1389-4501

Blom, A.B., Brockbank, S.M., van Lent, P.L., van Beuningen, H.M., Geurts, J., Takahashi, N., van der Kraan, P.M., van de Loo, F.A., Schreurs, B.W., Clements, K., Newham, P. & van den Berg, W.B. (2009) Involvement of the Wnt signaling pathway in experimental and human osteoarthritis: prominent role of Wnt-induced signaling protein 1. *Arthritis and Rheumatism* Vol. 60, No. 2 (February 2009), pp. 501-512. ISSN 1529-0131

Blom, A.B., van Lent, P.L., van der Kraan, P.M. & van den Berg, W.B. (2010) To seek shelter from the WNT in osteoarthritis? WNT-signaling as a target for osteoarthritis therapy. *Current Drug Targets* Vol. 11, No. 5. (May 2010), pp. 620-629. ISSN 1389-4501

Bondeson, J., Foxwell, B.M.J., Brennan, F.M. & Feldmann, M. (1999a) Defining therapeutic targets by using adenovirus: blocking NF-κB inhibits both inflammatory and destructive mechanisms in rheumatoid synovium, but spares anti-inflammatory mediators. *Proceedings of the National Acadademy of Sciences of the USA* Vol. 96, No. 5 (May 1999), pp. 5668-5673. ISSN 0027-8424

Bondeson, J., Browne, K.A., Brennan, F.M., Foxwell, B.M.J. & Feldmann, M. (1999b) Selective regulation of cytokine induction by adenoviral gene transfer of IκBα into human macrophages: lipopolysaccharide-induced, but not zymosan-induced, proinflammatory cytokines are inhibited, but IL-10 is NFκB independent. *Journal of Immunology* Vol. 162, No. 5 (March 1999), pp. 2939-2945. ISSN 0022-1767

Bondeson, J., Wainwright, S.D., Lauder, S., Amos, N. & Hughes, C.E. (2006) The role of synovial macrophages and macrophage-produced cytokines in driving aggrecanases, matrix metalloproteinases and other destructive and inflammatory responses in osteoarthritis. *Arthritis Research and Therapy* Vol. 8, No. 6, (2006), article no. R187. ISSN 1478-6354

Bondeson, J., Wainwright, S., Hughes, C. & Caterson, B. (2008) The regulation of ADAMTS4 and ADAMTS5 aggrecanases in osteoarthritis: a review. *Clinical and Experimental Rheumatology* Vol. 26, No. 1 (February 2008), pp. 139-145. ISSN 1593-098X

Bondeson, J., Blom, A.B., Wainwright, S., Hughes, C., Caterson, B. & van den Berg, W.B. (2010) The role of synovial macrophages and macrophage-produced mediators in driving inflammatory and destructive responses in osteoarthritis. *Arthritis and Rheumatism* Vol. 62, No. 3 (March 2010), pp. 647-57. ISSN 1529-0131

Brennan, F.M., Chantry, D., Jackson, A., Maini, R. & Feldmann, M. (1989) Inhibitory effect of TNFa antibodies on synovial cell interleukin-1 production in rheumatoid arthritis. *Lancet* Vol. ii, No. 8657 (July 1989), pp. 244-247. ISSN 0140-6736

Brennan, F.M., Hayes, A.L., Ciesielski, C.J., Green, P., Foxwell, B.M.J. & Feldmann, M. (2002) Evidence that rheumatoid arthritis synovial T cells are similar to cytokine-activated T cells. *Arthritis and Rheumatism* Vol. 46, No. 1 (January 2002), pp. 31-41. ISSN 1529-0131

Brennan, F.M. & McInnes, I.B. (2008) Evidence that cytokines play a role in rheumatoid athritis. *Journal of Clinical Investigations* Vol. 118, No. 11 (November 2008), pp. 3537-3545. ISSN 0021-9738

Burger, D., Dayer, J.-M., Palmer, G. & Gabay, C. (2006) Is IL-1 a good therapeutic target in the treatment of arthritis? *Best Practice and Research: Clinical Rheumatology* Vol. 20, No. 5 (October 2006), pp. 879-896. ISSN 1521-6942

Chevalier, X., Girardeau, B., Conzorier, T., Marliere, J., Kiefer, P. & Goupille, P. (2005) Safety study of intraarticular injection of interleukin 1 receptor antagonist in patients with painful knee osteoarthritis: a multicenter study. *Journal of Rheumatology* Vol. 32, No. 7 (July 2005), pp. 1317-1323. ISSN 0315-162X

Chevalier, X., Goupille, P., Beaulieu, A.D., Burch, F.X., Bensen, W.G., Conrozier, T., Loeuille, D., Kivitz, A.J., Silver, D. & Appleton, B.E. (2009) Intraarticular injection of anakinra in osteoarthritis of the knee: a multicenter, double-blind, placebo-controlled study. *Arthritis Care and Research* Vol. 61, No. 3 (March 2009), 344-352. ISSN 0893-7524

Clark, A.G., Jordan, J.M., Vilim, V., Renner, J.B., Dragomir, A.D., Luta, G. & Kraus, V.B. (1999) Serum cartilage oligomeric protein reflects osteoarthritis presence and severity. *Arthritis and Rheumatism* Vol. 42, No. 11 (November 1999), pp. 2356-2364. ISSN 1529-0131

Farahat, M.N., Yanni, G., Poston, R. & Panayi, G.S. (1993) Cytokine expression in synovial membranes of patients with rheumatoid arthritis and osteoarthritis. *Annals of the Rheumatic Diseases* Vol. 52, No. 12 (December 1993), pp. 870-875. ISSN 0003-4967

Feldmann, M. & Maini, R.N. (2008) Role of cytokines in rheumatoid arthritis: an education in pathophysiology and therapeutics. *Immunological Reviews* Vol. 223 (June 2008), pp. 7-19. ISSN 1600-065X

Feldmann, M. (2009) Translating molecular insights in autoimmunity into effective therapy. Annual Review of Immunology Vol. 27 (2009), pp. 1-27. ISSN 0732-0582

Fernandes, J.C., Martel-Pelletier, J. & Pelletier, J.P. (2002) The role of cytokines in osteoarthritis pathophysiology. *Biorheology* Vol. 39, No. 1-2 (February 2002), pp. 237-246. ISSN 0006-355X

Fioravanti, A., Fabbroni, M., Cerase, A. & Galeazzi, M. (2009) Treatment of erosive osteoarthritis of the hands by intra-articular inflizimab injections: a pilot study. *Rheumatology International* Vol. 29, No. 8 (June 2009), pp. 961-965. ISSN 1437-160X

Fosang, A.J., Rogerson, F.M., East, C.J. & Stanton, H. (2008) ADAMTS-5: the story so far. *European Cells and Materials* Vol. 15 (February 2008), pp. 11-26. ISSN 1473-2262

Foxwell, B.M.J., Browne, K.A., Bondeson, J., Clarke, C.J., de Martin, R., Brennan, F.M. & Feldmann, M. (1998) Efficient adenoviral infection with IκBα reveals that macrophage TNFα production in rheumatoid arthritis is NF-κB dependent. *Proceedings of the National Academy of Sciences of the USA* Vol. 95, No. 14 (July 1998), pp. 8211-8215. ISSN 0027-8424

Gendron, C., Kashiwagi, M., Lim, N.H., Enghild, J.J., Thøgersen, I.B., Hughes, C., Caterson, B. & Nagase, H. (2007) Proteolytic activities of human ADAMTS-5. Comparative studies with ADAMTS-4. *Journal of Biological Chemistry* Vol. 282, No. 25 (June 2007), pp. 18294-18306. ISSN 0021-9258

Genovese, M.C., Cohen, S., Moreland, L., Lium, D., Robbins, S., Newmark, R. & Bekker, P. (2004) Combination therapy with etanercept and anakinra in the treatment of patients with rheumatoid arthritis who have been treated unsuccessfully with methotrexate. *Arthritis and Rheumatism* Vol. 50, No. 5 (May 2004), pp. 1412-1419. ISSN 1529-0131

Gilbert, A.M., Bikker, J.A. & O'Neil, S.V. (2011) Advances in the development of novel aggrecanase inhibitors. *Expert Opinion on Therapeutic Patents* Vol. 21, No. 1 (January 2011), pp. 1-12. ISSN 1354-3776.

Glasson, S.S., Askew, R., Sheppard, B., Carito, B.A., Blanchet, T., Ma, H.L., Flannery, C.R., Kanki, K., Wang, E., Peluso, D., Yang, Z., Majumdar, M.K. & Morris, E.A. (2004) Characterization of and osteoarthritis susceptibility in ADAMTS-4-knockout mice. *Arthritis and Rheumatism* Vol. 50, No. 8 (August 2004), pp. 2547-2558. ISSN 1529-0131

Glasson, S.S., Askew, R., Sheppard, B., Carito, B., Blanchet, T., Ma, H.L., Flannery, C.R., Peluso, D., Kanki, K., Yang, Z., Majumdar, M.K. & Morris, E.A. (2005) Deletion of active ADAMTS5 prevents cartilage degradation in a murine model of osteoarthritis. *Nature* Vol. 434, No. 7033 (March 2005), pp. 644-648. ISSN 0028-0836

Goupille, P., Mulleman, D. & Chevalier, X. (2007) Is interleukin-1 a good target for therapeutic intervention in intervertebral disc degeneration: lessons from the osteoarthritic experience. *Arthritis Research and Therapy* Vol. 9, No. 6 (2007), article no. 110. ISSN 1478-6354

Grunke, M. & Schulze-Koops, H. (2006) Successful treatment of inflammatory knee osteoarthritis with tumour necrosis factor blockade. *Annals of the Rheumatic Diseases* Vol. 65, No. 4 (April 2006), pp. 555-556. ISSN 0003-4967

Güler-Yüksel, M., Allaart, C.F., Watt, I., Goekoop-Ruiterman, Y.P., de Vries-Bouwstra, J.K., van Schaardenburg, D., van Krugten, M.V., Dijkmans, B.A., Huizinga, T,W,, Lems, W.F. & Kloppenburg, M. (2010) Treatment with the TNF-α inhibitor infliximab might reduce hand osteoarthritis in patients with rheumatoid arthritis. *Osteoarthritis and Cartilage* Vol. 18, No. 10 (October 2010), pp. 1256-1262. ISSN 1063-4584

Hashimoto, S., Takahashi, K., Amiel, D., Coutts, R.D. & Lotz, M. (1998) Chondrocyte apoptosis and nitric oxide production during experimentally induced osteoarthritis. *Arthritis and Rheumatism* Vol. 41, No. 7 (July 1998), pp. 1266-1274. ISSN 1529-0131

Hayes, A.L., Smith, C., Foxwell, B.M. & Brennan, F.M. (1999) CD45-induced tumor necrosis factor alpha production in monocytes is phosphatidylinositol 3-kinase-dependent and nuclear factor kappaB-independent. *Journal of Biological Chemistry* Vol. 274, No. 47 (November 1999), pp. 33455-33461. ISSN 0021-9258

Haywood, L., McWilliams, D.F., Pearson, C.I., Gill, S.E., Ganesan, A., Wilson, D. & Walsh, D.A. (2003) Inflammation and angiogenesis in osteoarthritis. *Arthritis and Rheumatism* Vol. 48, No. 8 (August 2003), pp. 173-177. ISSN 1529-0131

Hellio le Graverand, M.P., Vignon, E., Otterness, I.G. & Hart, D.A. (2000) Early changes in lapine menisci during osteoarthritis development Part II: Molecular alterations *Osteoarthritis and Cartilage* Vol. 9, No. 1 (January 2000), pp. 65-72. ISSN 1063-4584

Hellio Le Graverand-Gastineau, M.-P. (2010) Disease modifying osteoarthritis drugs: Facing development challenges and choosing molecular targets. *Current Drug Targets* Vol. 11, No. 5 (May 2010), pp. 528-535. ISSN 1389-4501

Hutchinson, J.W., Tierney, G.M., Parsons, S.L. & Davis, T.R. (1998) Dupuytren's disease and frozen shoulder induced by treatment with a matrix metalloproteinase inhibitor. *Journal of Bone and Joint Surgery (British volume)* Vol. 80, No. 5 (September 1998), pp. 907-908. ISSN 0301-620X

Kalliolias, G.D. & Liossis, S.N.C. (2008) The future of the IL-1 receptor antagonist anakinra: from rheumatoid arthritis to adult-onset Still's disease and systemic-onset juvenile idiopathic arthritis. *Expert Opinion on Investigational Drugs* Vol. 17, No. 3 (March 2008), pp. 349-359. ISSN 1354-3784

Kashiwagi, M., Tortorella, M., Nagase, H. & Brew, K. (2001) TIMP-3 is a potent inhibitor of aggrecanase 1 (ADAM-TS4) and aggrecanase 2 (ADAM-TS5) *Journal of Biological Chemistry* Vol. 276, No. 16 (April 2001), pp. 12501–12504. ISSN 0021-9258

Kinne, R.W., Stuhlmuller, B. & Burmester, G.-R. (2007) Cells of the synovium in rheumatoid arthritis: macrophages. *Arthritis Research and Therapy* Vol. 9, No. 6 (June 2007), article no. 224. ISSN 1478-6354

Lim, N.H., Kashiwagi, M., Visse, R., Jones, J., Enghild, J.J., Brew, K. & Nagase, H. (2010) Reactive-site mutants of N-TIMP-3 that selectively inhibit ADAMTS-4 and ADAMTS-5: biological and structural implications *Biochemical Journal* Vol. 431, No. 1 (October 2010), pp. 113–122. ISSN 0264-6021

McCulloch, D.R., Nelson, C.M., Dixon, L.J., Silver, D.L., Wylie, J.D., Lindner, V., Sasaki, T., Cooley, M.A., Argraves, W.S. & Apte, S.S. (2009) ADAMTS metalloproteases generate active versican fragments that regulate interdigital web regression. *Developmental Cell* Vol. 17, No. 5 (November 2009), pp. 687-698. ISSN 1534-5807

Magnano, M.D., Chakravarty, E.F., Broudy, C., Chung, L., Kelman, A., Hillygus, J. & Genovese, M.C. (2007) A pilot study of tumor necrosis factor inhibition in erosive/inflammatory osteoarthritis of the hands. *Journal of Rheumatology* Vol. 34, No. 6 (June 2007), pp. 1323-1327. ISSN 0315-162X

Martel-Peletier, J. & Pelletier, J.-P. (2009) Osteoarthritis: A single injection of anakinra for treating knee OA? *Nature Reviews Rheumatology* Vol. 5, No. 7 (July 2009), pp. 363-364. ISSN 1759-4790

Maini, R.N. & Feldmann, M. (2007) The pitfalls in the development of biologic therapy. *Nature Clinical Practice Rheumatology* Vol. 3 (2007), p. 1. ISSN 1745-8382

Malemud, C.J. (2004) Cytokines as therapeutic targets for osteoarthritis. *Biodrugs* Vol. 18, No. 1 (2004), pp. 23-35. ISSN 1173-8804

Moore, E.E., Bendele, A.M., Thompson, D.L., Littau, A., Waggie, K.S., Reardon, B., Ellsworth, J.L. (2005) Fibroblast growth factor-18 stimulates chondrogenesis and cartilage repair in a rat model of injury-induced osteoarthritis. *Osteoarthritis and Cartilage* Vol. 13, No. 7 (July 2005), pp. 623-631. ISSN 1063-4584

Neuhold, L.A., Killar, L., Zhao, W., Sung, M.L., Warner, L., Kulik, J., Turner, J., Wu, W., Billinghurst, C., Meijers, T., Poole, A.R., Babij, P. & DeGennaro, L.J. (2001) Postnatal expression in hyaline cartilage of constitutively active human collagenase-3 (MMP-13) induces osteoarthritis in mice. *Journal of Clinical Investigations* Vol. 107, No. 1 (January 2001), pp. 35-44. ISSN 0021-9738

Pavelka, K., Trc, T., Karpas, K., Vítek, P., Sedláčková, M., Vlasáková, V., Böhmová, J. & Rovenský, J. (2007) The efficacy and safety of diacerein in the treatment of painful osteoarthritis of the knee. *Arthritis and Rheumatism* Vol. 56, No. 12 (December 2007). pp. 4055-4064. ISSN 1529-0131

Pelletier, J.-P. & Martel-Peletier, J. (2005) New trends in the treatment of osteoarthritis. *Seminars in Arthritis and Rheumatism* Vol. 34 (2005), pp. 13-14. ISSN 0049-0172

Qvist, P., Bay-Jensen, A.-C., Christiansen, C., Dam, B.E., Pastoreau, P. & Karsdal, M.A.
(2008) The disease modifying osteoarthritis drug (DMOAD): Is it on the horizon?
Pharmacological Research Vol. 58 (2008), pp. 1-7. ISSN 1043-6618

Rudolphi, K., Gerwin, N., Verzijl, N., van der Kraan, P. & van den Berg W. (2003)
Pralnacasan, an inhibitor of interleukin-1 converting enzyme, reduces joint damage
in two murine models of osteoarthritis. *Osteoarthritis and Cartilage* Vol. 11, No. 10
(October 2003). pp. 738-746. ISSN 1063-4584

Sahebjam, S., Khokha, R. & Mort, J.S. (2007) Increased collagen and aggrecan degradation
with age in the joints of Timp3(-/-) mice. *Arthritis and Rheumatism* Vol. 56, No. 3
(March 2007), pp. 905-909. ISSN 1529-0131

Sekiya, I., Tang, T., Hayashi, M., Morito, T., Ju, Y.J., Mochizuki, T. & Muneta, T. (2009)
Periodic knee injections of BMP-7 delay cartilage degeneration induced by
excessive running in rats. *Journal of Orthopaedic Research* Vol. 27, No. 8 (August
2009), pp. 1088-1092. ISSN 0736-0266

Shahrara, S., Castro-Rueda, H.P., Haines, G.K. & Koch, A.E.. (2007) Differential expression
of the FAK family kinases in rheumatoid arthritis and osteoarthritis synovial tissue.
Arthritis Research and Therapy Vol. 9, No. 5 (2007), article no. R112. ISSN 1478-6354

Song, R.H., Tortorella, M.D., Malfait, A.M., Alston, J.T., Yang, Z., Arner, E.C. & Griggs, D.W.
(2007) Aggrecan degradation in human articular cartilage explants is mediated by
both ADAMTS-4 and ADAMTS-5. *Arthritis and Rheumatism* Vol. 56, No. 2 (February
2007), pp. 575–585. ISSN 1529-0131

Sowers, M., Jannausch, M., Stein, E., Jamadar, D., Hochberg, M. & Lachance, L. (2002) C-
reactive protein as a biomarker of emergent osteoarthritis. *Osteoarthritis and
Cartilage* vol. 10, No. 8 (August 2002), pp. 595-601. ISSN 1063-4584

Stanton, H., Rogerson, F.M., East, C.J., Golub, S.B., Lawlor, K.E., Meeker, C.T., Little, C.B.,
Last, K., Farmer, P.J., Campbell, I.K., Fourie, A.M. & Fosang, A.J. (2005) ADAMTS5
is the major aggrecanase in mouse cartilage in vivo and in vitro. *Nature* Vol. 434,
No. 7033) (March 2005), pp. 648-652. ISSN 0028-0836

Tortorella, M.D. & Malfait, A.M. (2008) Will the real aggrecanase(s) step up: evaluating the
criteria that define aggrecanase activity in osteoarthritis. *Current Pharmacological
Biotechnology* Vol. 9, No. 1 (February 2008), pp. 16-23. ISSN 1389-2010

Tortorella, M.D., Tomasselli, A.G., Mathis, K.J., Schnute, M.E., Woodard, S.S., Munie, G.,
Williams, J.M., Caspers, N., Wittwer, A.J., Malfait, A.M. & Shieh, H.S. (2009)
Structural and inhibition analysis reveals the mechanism of selectivity of a series of
aggrecanase inhibitors. *Journal of Biological Chemistry* Vol. 284, No. 36 (September
2009), pp. 24185-24191. ISSN 0021-9258

Urano, T., Narusawa, K., Shiraki, M., Usui, T., Sasaki, N., Hosoi, T., Ouchi, Y., Nakamura, T.
& Inoue, S. (2007) Association of a single nucleotide polymorphism in the WISP1
gene with spinal osteoarthritis in postmenopausal Japanese women. *Journal of Bone
and Mineral Metabolism* Vol. 25, No. 4 (2007), pp. 253-258. ISSN 0884-0431

van den Berg, W.B., van de Loo, F., Joosten, L.A. & Arntz, O.J. (1999) Animal models of
arthritis in NOS2-deficient mice. *Osteoarthritis and Cartilage* Vol. 7, No. 4 (July 1999),
pp. 413-415. ISSN 1063-4584

van der Heijden, J.W., Oerlemans, R., Dijkmans, B.A., Qi, H., van der Laken, C.J., Lems,
W.F., Jackman, A.L., Kraan, M.C., Tak, P.P., Ratnam, M. & Jansen, G. (2009) Folate
receptor γ as a potential delivery route for novel folate antagonists to macrophages

in the synovial tissue of rheumatoid arthritis patients. *Arthritis and Rheumatism* Vol. 60, No. 1 (January 2009), pp. 12-21. ISSN 1529-0131

van der Laken, C.J., Elzinga, E.H., Kropholler, M.A., Molthoff, C.F., van der Heijden, J,W,, Maruyama, K., Boellaard, R., Dijkmans, B.A., Lammertsma, A.A. & Voskuyl, A.E. (2008) Noninvasive imaging of macrophages in rheumatoid synovitis using ^{11}C-(R)-PK11195 and positron emission tomography. *Arthritis and Rheumatism* Vol. 58, No. 11 (November 2008), pp. 3350-3355. ISSN 1529-0131

Van Lent, P.L.E.M., Blom, A.B., van der Kraan, P., Holthuysen, A.E.M., Vitters, E., van Rooijen, N., Smeets, R.L., Nabbe, K.C. & van den Berg, W.B. (2004) Crucial role of synovial lining macrophages in the promotion of transforming growth factor beta-mediated osteophyte formation. *Arthritis and Rheumatism* Vol. 50, No. 1 (January 2004), pp. 103-111. ISSN 1529-0131

Wandel, S., Jüni, P., Tendal, B., Nüesch, E., Villiger, P.M., Welton, N.J., Reichenbach, S. & Trelle, S. (2010) Effects of glucosamine, chondroitin, or placebo in patients with osteoarthritis of hip or knee: network meta-analysis. *British Medical Journal* Vol. 341, (September 2010), c4675. ISSN 09598138

Wayne, G.J., Deng, S.J., Amour, A., Borman, S., Matico, R., Carter, H.L. & Murphy, G. (2007) TIMP-3 inhibition of ADAMTS-4 (Aggrecanase-1) is modulated by interactions between aggrecan and the C-terminal domain of ADAMTS-4. *Journal of Biological Chemistry* Vol. 282, No. 29 (July 2007), pp. 20991–20998. ISSN 0021-9258

Wittwer, A.J., Hills, R.L., Keith, R.H., Munie, G.E., Arner, E.C., Anglin, C.P., Malfait, A.M. & Tortorella, M.D. (2007) Substrate-dependent inhibition kinetics of an active site-directed inhibitor of ADAMTS-4 (Aggrecanase 1) *Biochemistry* Vol. 46, No. 21 (May 2007), pp. 6393–6401. ISSN 0001-527X

Permissions

The contributors of this book come from diverse backgrounds, making this book a truly international effort. This book will bring forth new frontiers with its revolutionizing research information and detailed analysis of the nascent developments around the world.

We would like to thank Dr. Bruce Rothschild, for lending his expertise to make the book truly unique. He has played a crucial role in the development of this book. Without his invaluable contribution this book wouldn't have been possible. He has made vital efforts to compile up to date information on the varied aspects of this subject to make this book a valuable addition to the collection of many professionals and students.

This book was conceptualized with the vision of imparting up-to-date information and advanced data in this field. To ensure the same, a matchless editorial board was set up. Every individual on the board went through rigorous rounds of assessment to prove their worth. After which they invested a large part of their time researching and compiling the most relevant data for our readers. Conferences and sessions were held from time to time between the editorial board and the contributing authors to present the data in the most comprehensible form. The editorial team has worked tirelessly to provide valuable and valid information to help people across the globe.

Every chapter published in this book has been scrutinized by our experts. Their significance has been extensively debated. The topics covered herein carry significant findings which will fuel the growth of the discipline. They may even be implemented as practical applications or may be referred to as a beginning point for another development. Chapters in this book were first published by InTech; hereby published with permission under the Creative Commons Attribution License or equivalent.

The editorial board has been involved in producing this book since its inception. They have spent rigorous hours researching and exploring the diverse topics which have resulted in the successful publishing of this book. They have passed on their knowledge of decades through this book. To expedite this challenging task, the publisher supported the team at every step. A small team of assistant editors was also appointed to further simplify the editing procedure and attain best results for the readers.

Our editorial team has been hand-picked from every corner of the world. Their multi-ethnicity adds dynamic inputs to the discussions which result in innovative outcomes. These outcomes are then further discussed with the researchers and contributors who give their valuable feedback and opinion regarding the same. The feedback is then collaborated with the researches and they are edited in a comprehensive manner to aid the understanding of the subject.

Apart from the editorial board, the designing team has also invested a significant amount of their time in understanding the subject and creating the most relevant covers. They scrutinized every image to scout for the most suitable representation of the subject and create an appropriate cover for the book.

The publishing team has been involved in this book since its early stages. They were actively engaged in every process, be it collecting the data, connecting with the contributors or procuring relevant information. The team has been an ardent support to the editorial, designing and production team. Their endless efforts to recruit the best for this project, has resulted in the accomplishment of this book. They are a veteran in the field of academics and their pool of knowledge is as vast as their experience in printing. Their expertise and guidance has proved useful at every step. Their uncompromising quality standards have made this book an exceptional effort. Their encouragement from time to time has been an inspiration for everyone.

The publisher and the editorial board hope that this book will prove to be a valuable piece of knowledge for researchers, students, practitioners and scholars across the globe.

List of Contributors

Judith Farley, Valeria M. Dejica and John S. Mort
Genetics Unit, Shriners Hospital for Children and Department of Surgery, McGill University, Canada

Chathuraka T. Jayasuriya and Qian Chen
Alpert Medical School of Brown University, Rhode Island Hospital, United States of America

Akihisa Kamataki, Wataru Yoshida, Mutsuko Ishida, Kenya Murakami and Takashi Sawai
Iwate Medical University, Japan

Kensuke Ochi
Kawasaki Municipal Kawasaki Hospital, Japan

Di Chen and Hee-Jeong Im
Department of Biochemistry, USA
Department of Orthopedic Surgery, USA
Department of Internal Medicine, Section of Rheumatology, Rush University Medical Center, Chicago, IL, USA

Dongyao Yan
Department of Biochemistry, USA

Michael B. Ellman
Department of Biochemistry, USA
Department of Orthopedic Surgery, USA

Qi Wu and James L. Henry
Department of Psychiatry and Behavioural Neurosciences, McMaster University, Hamilton, Canada

Elizabeth Perez-Hernandez
Hospital de Ortopedia Dr. Victorio de la Fuente Narváez –IMSS, México

Nury Perez-Hernandez
Departamento de Biomedicina Molecular, Escuela Nacional de Medicina y Homeopatía- IPN, México

Fidel de la C. Hernandez-Hernandez and Juan B. Kouri-Flores
Departamento de Infectómica y Patogénesis Molecular, CINVESTAV-IPN, México

William C. Kramer and John P. Schroeppel
Department of Orthopaedic Surgery, USA

Jinxi Wang
Department of Biochemistry and Molecular Biology, University of Kansas Medical Center, Kansas City, USA
Department of Orthopaedic Surgery, USA

Sture Forsgren
Department of Integrative Medical Biology, Anatomy Section, Umeå University, Umeå, Sweden

Kenneth W. Finnson, Yoon Chi and Anie Philip
Division of Plastic Surgery, Department of Surgery, Montreal General Hospital, McGill University, Montreal, QC, Canada

Petya Dimitrova and Nina Ivanovska
Department of Immunology, Institute of Microbiology, Bulgaria

Peter I. Milner, Robert J. Wilkins and John S. Gibson
University of Liverpool, University of Oxford & University of Cambridge, United Kingdom

Jan Bondeson
Department of Rheumatology, Cardiff University, Heath Park, Cardiff, UK

Shane Wainwright, Clare Hughes and Bruce Caterson
Connective Tissue Biology Laboratories, Cardiff School of Biosciences, Cardiff University, Museum Avenue, Cardiff, UK

Printed in the USA
CPSIA information can be obtained
at www.ICGtesting.com
JSHW011444221024
72173JS00004B/932